Multiple Personalities,
Multiple Disorders

OXFORD PSYCHIATRY SERIES

Edited by
Joseph Coyle
Michael Gelder
Samuel Guze
Robin Murray

1. Multiple Personalities, Multiple Disorders:
   Psychiatric Classification and Media Influence
   Carol S. North, Jo-Ellyn M. Ryall, Daniel A. Ricci, and
   Richard D. Wetzel   1993

Multiple Personalities, Multiple Disorders

Psychiatric Classification and Media Influence

Carol S. North, M.D.
Assistant Professor of Psychiatry
Washington University School of Medicine

Jo-Ellyn M. Ryall, M.D.
Assistant Professor of Clinical Psychiatry
Washington University School of Medicine

Daniel A. Ricci, C.M., A.C.S.W.
Psychiatric Social Work Coordinator
Grace Hill Services, Inc.

Richard D. Wetzel, Ph.D
Professor of Medical Psychology in Psychiatry
Washington University School of Medicine

New York   Oxford
OXFORD UNIVERSITY PRESS
1993

Oxford University Press

Oxford   New York   Toronto
Delhi   Bombay   Calcutta   Madras   Karachi
Kuala Lumpur   Singapore   Hong Kong   Tokyo
Nairobi   Dar es Salaam   Cape Town
Melbourne   Auckland   Madrid
and associated companies in
Berlin   Ibadan

Library of Congress Cataloging-in-Publication Data
Multiple personalities, multiple disorders :
psychiatric classification and media influence /
Carol S. North . . . [et al.].
p.   cm. — (Oxford monographs on psychiatry ; 1)
Includes bibliographical references and index.
ISBN 0-19-508095-5
1. Multiple personality.   2. Multiple personality—Public opinion.
3. Mass media—influence.   I. North, Carol S.   II. Series.
[DNLM: 1. Multiple-Personality Disorder.   WM 173.06 M961]
RC569.5.M8M85   1993   616.85'236—dc20
DNLM/DLC   for Library of Congress   92-49904

2   4   6   8   9   7   5   3   1
Printed in the United States of America
on acid-free paper

To our mentors in psychiatric nosology:
Drs. Sam Guze, Eli Robins,
Lee Robins, George Murphy,
George Winokur, Bob Cloninger,
Ted Reich, Remi Cadoret

Acknowledgments

The authors thank Dr. Sam Guze for his thoughtful insights and his help from the early stages of this project. We also wish to thank Dr. C. Robert Cloninger, Dr. Kim McCallum, and Ms. Leslie Strohm for reading and commenting on the manuscript. Mr. Jeffrey House has had a keen sense of direction and has provided superb editorial leadership, and we are grateful to him for his assistance. We are indebted to Ms. Irene Fischer, Ms. Cathy Casebolt, Ms. Shirley Mazenko, and Ms. Jenny Stout for secretarial assistance. In addition, the reference librarians at the Washington University Medical Center library have provided indispensable assistance. We are deeply indebted to Mr. William Odman for his skillful computer crisis intervention and software assistance. We thank Ms. Tobi Don, M.S.W., and Ms. Sharon Stecher, R.N., M.S.W, C.S., for providing information on reactions of beginning professional students to popular accounts of multiple personality disorder. We also wish to thank our spouses and significant others for their generous understanding, patience, and support throughout the process of putting together this work.

We are indebted to clinicians before us who have studied multiple personality disorder and reported on their findings, for without their pioneering observations we would not have such a wealth of information available as a foundation for our work. We acknowledge our intellectual debt to the tradition of research in psychiatric nosology as pioneered by Dr. Eli Robins and Dr. Sam Guze. We are grateful for the supportive academic atmosphere at Washington University that stimulated our intellectual curiosity and allowed us to germinate and develop this work. Finally, we are indebted to our patients who continue to stimulate and inspire us.

Preface

We felt we had to write this book on multiple personality disorder (MPD). The rising popularity of the disorder demands objective information about it. Currently, there exists very little balanced academic material on this disorder. The bulk of the literature is strongly biased toward proving its existence as a real psychiatric disorder, and much of the rest is devoted to claiming that it doesn't exist.

Until now MPD has been largely untouched by the Washington University model of investigation of psychiatric nosology. In this book it is our purpose to examine MPD from an empirical and agnostic viewpoint, describing the work that has been done on this disorder in order to better understand how this material fits into the framework of diagnostic validity.

It was by accident that we became very interested in MPD. At our institution, no one had ever said much about this disorder. Because of our strong diagnosis-oriented tradition in psychiatry, it simply didn't exist, and no one believed in it.

It was inevitable, however, that with rising public attention to MPD, we would in time encounter it and begin to take a serious interest in it. This happened in 1987 when one of us (C.S.N.) appeared on a television talk show with Truddi Chase, a woman with MPD who had written a book about her 92 personalities. Before appearing on the show, C.S.N. prepared by reading the book and discovered that what was most intriguing was the prominent somatoform and sociopathic symptomatology that was described but was basically ignored by both the therapist and the author.

A couple of months later, Chris Sizemore, the MPD patient described in the famous book *The Three Faces of Eve*, made a personal appearance in St. Louis, and another one of us (J.M.R.) spent a good deal of the day with her where she described many somatoform symptoms. In reading her book we were struck once again by the prominent somatoform and sociopathic symptomatology. Curious to learn more, we then proceeded to collect other published books describing personal accounts of MPD, and found that they all displayed prominent somatoform, sociopathic, or borderline personality features. There were 22 such books in all.

Perplexed by all this, we wondered what light the academic literature might shed on our clinical observations in these cases. We began collecting and reading academic publications on MPD and found a widespread tendency to focus narrowly on the fascinating components of the disorder specifically related to complaints of multiple personalities and all the problems they are purported to cause.

Although the literature contained ample evidence of high rates of somatoform disorders and sociopathy in persons with MPD, this other psychopathology was de-emphasized.

All of us in our various practices had been exposed to patients claiming multiple personalities. J.M.R. followed several MPD patients for varying periods of time and has here contributed clinical material from their histories. After a multiple presented to C.S.N. in her clinic for treatment of homeless persons, C.S.N. recruited the case manager of this program (D.A.R.) to participate in the reading and systematic assessment of the biographical books on MPD. His interest in MPD and his sensitivity to it grew as other homeless patients in the clinic reported dissociative symptoms and multiple personalities.

A request to discuss our analysis of the books on MPD at a local conference led us to recruit R.D.W. to our ranks. Considerable psychological testing material was available and we asked him to discuss it. We soon discovered that he already had an interest in MPD.

R.D.W.'s first contact with a multiple had occurred in the 1960s when he directed a suicide prevention hotline in St. Louis. A calm, concerned woman called about a severely depressed, distraught, suicidal friend who was unable to handle the death of her only son in Vietnam. The caller had a psychiatrist who was treating her for depression; the friend had no therapist and needed help. The caller indicated that she knew her friend was not home, but she would be in in about fifteen minutes, and she provided her telephone number.

He called that number fifteen minutes later and talked to a very upset woman who reported a very severe depressive syndrome of several months' duration with severe, recurrent, and intrusive suicidal ideation with some preparation for carrying out a lethal suicide plan. Hospitalization was recommended. Because she said she had no personal psychiatrist, she was accepted on the University's teaching service.

R.D.W. was amazed when two days later he was confronted by an irate psychiatrist who demanded to know why he had referred his patient to another doctor without consulting him. It turned out that the caller and her distraught friend were both different personalities of the same woman. The patient had a florid history of somatoform symptoms qualifying her for the diagnosis of Briquet's syndrome (somatization disorder). Her treating psychiatrist had recognized the somatization and the depression; he did not accept her claim of multiple personalities.

During her hospitalization, it became clear that she experienced herself as having three different personalities with some amnesia among them. Her personalities apparently predated her bereavement and had been discovered during seven years of weekly psychotherapy with another psychiatrist. Her treatment plan in the hospital focused on helping her deal with her grief and depression, along with nonreinforcement of hysterical symptoms (including multiplicity). In the end, she did not pursue discharge follow-up with members of her treatment team, and, in addition, did not return to the psychiatrist she was seeing before her admission; instead she chose to resume treatment with the psychiatrist who had first helped her discover her personalities.

Coming from a center with strong traditions in psychiatric nosology, we were inspired by our MPD patients to begin to ask specific empirical questions: What are the rates of other disorders in patients with MPD, especially somatization disorder (Briquet's syndrome), antisocial personality disorder, and borderline personality disorder? It seemed that the diagnostic overlap was extensive. Thus, we also asked: How does MPD differ from these other diagnoses? Unfortunately, there were few sources of information available to answer such questions, and we had to work hard to draw conclusions from the available literature. In fact, many key questions remain unanswered.

Ultimately, during our investigations we came to believe in MPD. We do not believe, however, that MPD has been adequately validated as a psychiatric diagnosis. We will explain here these conclusions and the sources from which we draw our arguments. Our academic investigations while preparing this manuscript have helped us further shape the ideas we developed from working with our MPD patients and from reading the published accounts of other patients. During the course of writing this book we have been in contact with additional patients with MPD. Their presentations have been consistent with our earlier clinical impressions and with our findings from our literature search.

Our investigations into MPD have sensitized us to the influence of our culture on the disorder and have led us to examine the history of MPD. We agree with Ross (1989, p. 5) who commented that "MPD must be understood in a historical and cultural context," and that "the first step in understanding MPD is to review the history, placing the disorder in a broad context" (p. 6). Social and cultural factors that must be examined in the study of the history of MPD should include media influences, which Kluft (1984b) also has recognized as significant forces in the growth and development of this disorder. Ross (1989) cautions that "the cultural and historical aspects of MPD do not make it less serious, less worthy of treatment, or a less legitimate subject of scientific study" (p. 2). No matter how the condition arrived at its current state, it deserves serious attention.

MPD has an intriguing history. Its existence and character have been debated from the time of the first case reports on MPD in the last century. The dispute has never been resolved, and MPD has become the most controversial syndrome known to mental health professionals. In the past, general understanding of MPD was guided largely by arguments in the medical literature by prominent academicians. In the middle of this century, however, the general public was widely exposed to the disorder through its presentation in the mass media, and the numbers of cases in treatment began to grow exponentially. We are now experiencing an epidemic of this disorder.

The popular literature is now bursting with personal accounts of MPD. More than half of all book-length biographical accounts were published in the last decade, and another quarter in the previous decade. These accounts are a rich source of clinical information on the subject for both professional and non-professionals. The sharp rise in the number of these publications is another indicator that MPD is an entity of increasingly widespread interest and cannot be dismissed as nonexistent or unimportant.

Because of the nature of this disorder and the individuals who are prone to develop it, it is clearly essential to examine it in light of these popular and media influences. Persons at risk for MPD have been characterized as very suggestible (Putnam et al. 1986; Fahy 1988; Coons 1980; Spiegel 1988; Bliss 1980). Therefore, information they obtain from the mass media could contribute to the occurrence and characteristics of the disorder and could conceivably have an impact on its natural history in our culture (Bowers 1991).

There is some evidence supporting this possibility. Following their widely publicized account of *The Three Faces of Eve*, for example, authors Thigpen and Cleckley (1984) received a flood of inquiries from individuals who had been diagnosed or had diagnosed themselves as multiples, often claiming psychopathology identical to Eve's. Today every patient presenting with MPD is likely to have received some media information about the disorder and therefore no one with MPD today can be considered untouched by media influence (Merskey 1992).

In response to this apparent influence on the disorder, this book provides an in-depth appreciation of how MPD has developed over the years in relation to the media. We identify the earliest origins of the MPD concept in published literature and trace the course of its development through its history in academic work and in its popular portrayal. We examine prevailing opinions about MPD through different periods of history, leading up to the current controversy over its nosology.

Bliss (1980) noted that because of the controversial nature of the MPD syndrome, ". . .most physicians and psychiatrists carefully avoid it . . . ." To the extent that this is so, this will not contribute to our understanding of the disorder. Facing the issue squarely in a detailed historical investigation of this kind will shed light on the continuing conflict over its existence and on the nature of the disorder. Our historical review and examination of the conflict over nosology is presented in the context of scientific methodology, specifically regarding accepted procedures for validating a diagnosis. Data that have been collected so far supporting the validity of this disorder as a psychiatric diagnosis are presented in the categories of clinical descriptions of the disorder, delineation from other disorders, family history studies, follow-up studies, and laboratory documentation. We further point out specific areas of research that are still needed before psychiatry can consider MPD an adequately validated diagnosis. This approach should provide direction to researchers in the pursuit of a better understanding of MPD and progress toward resolution of the controversy.

In sum, this work is a synthesis of all relevant information we could draw from the published literature about the disorder and the issue of diagnostic validity.

Contents

1. The History of MPD in Academic Literature, **3**
   Origins of MPD, 3
   MPD in the Twentieth Century, 9
   The "Epidemic", 13
   Current Trends, 19
   Conclusion, 21

2. Theory and Controversy: Validation of the Disorder, **23**
   Validation of a Diagnosis, 24
   Briquet's Syndrome: A Model for
         Diagnostic Validation, 24
   The Controversy, 26
   Proponents of MPD, 27
   Skeptics, 30
   Discussion, 39

3. Current Knowledge About MPD, **43**
   Clinical Description of MPD, 44
   Comorbidity and Delineation from
         other Psychiatric Disorders, 48
   Familial Associations, 58
   Physiologic Investigation, 59
   Natural Course, Treatment, and Outcome, 64
   Case Reports, 67
   Conclusion, 72

4. Psychological Investigations of MPD, **73**
   IQ Tests and Cognitive Testing, 73
   Objective Personality Tests, 74
   Other Scales, 100
   Tests of Dissociation, 100
   Projective Tests, 105
   Specialized Diagnostic Interviews, 107
   Experiential Time Sampling, 108
   Tests of Hypnotizability, 109
   Utility of Psychological Assessment Instruments, 109
   A Model for the Role of Psychological
         Testing in MPD, 110

5. MPD and the Popular Media in History, **115**
    Historical Review of Famous Accounts, 116
    MPD and the Media Today, 119

6. Popular Biographical Accounts of MPD:
    A Detailed Analysis of 21 Books, **125**
    Summary of Results for All the Cases, 128
    Somatization Disorder, 130
    Conversion Symptoms, 132
    Sexual Histories, 133
    Histrionic Traits, 133
    Skepticism, 134
    Antisocial Personality Disorder, 134
    Other Behavioral, Interpersonal, and
        Characterological Difficulties, 136
    Suicidality, 137
    Adult Victimization, 137
    Troubled Children, 138
    Dysfunctional Families, 138
    Mothers, 140
    Summary of Psychiatric Disorders
        in Family Histories, 141
    Assortative Mating, 141
    Psychiatric Diagnoses Applied to Cases, 142
    The Alternates, 144
    Treatments Received, 146
    Transference-Countertransference, 148
    Outcomes, 149
    Professional Knowledge and Aspirations
        in the Mental Health Field, 150
    Parapsychology and the Occult, 151
    Misinformation, 152
    Authorship, 152
    Public Attention, 153
    Afterword, 154
    Discussion of the Accounts, 155
    Conclusion, 157

7. Perspectives on MPD, **161**
    The Nosologic Status of MPD, 161
    Etiology, 177
    Nosologic Issues Affecting Treatment, 178
    Conclusion, 182

Appendix A. Synopses of Book-Length Accounts of MPD, **185**

Appendix B. Summary Tables of Book-Length Accounts of MPD, **231**

References, **251**
Author Index, **271**
Subject Index, **275**

Multiple Personalities,
Multiple Disorders

1

The history of MPD in academic literature

Our understanding of multiple personality disorder (MPD) has developed over time as the field of psychiatry has evolved. When the first reports of MPD appeared in the seventeenth century, scientific investigation in psychiatry was divided between two main approaches: "materialist" and "nonmaterialist." These embodied the original "mind–brain" clash in efforts to explain human psychological functioning. The materialist approach was anatomically and physiologically oriented, its methods based on laboratory investigation, empirical observation, and quantification. The nonmaterialist movement dealt with subjective phenomena, including spirit communication, hypnotism, altered states of consciousness, and the unconscious (Decker 1986, pp. 31–32).

When the early case reports of MPD were being published, the mind–brain problem was beginning to evolve into a slightly different form, with opposing "associationist" and "organicist" groups of scientists who similarly argued over whether the basis of psychological function was to be found in mental associations or in organic factors (Ellenberger 1970, p. 141). These "two faces of science" (Decker 1986, p. 31) have coexisted for centuries, with little agreement between them. The debate over the origins of mental functions has outlived the associationists and the organicists, and despite the contributions of modern technology in settling the dispute, it persists today.

The controversy surrounding MPD throughout its history has reflected this rift between the two factions in psychiatry. Early disagreements about the etiology and existence of MPD have changed little in character over the centuries. Much of the debate today stems from the inability of biologically oriented psychiatrists and mental health professionals of other persuasions to communicate with each other.

Origins of MPD

There is some evidence that MPD may be an ancient malady. Coons (1984) has described cases of spirit possession that "bear a remarkable resemblance" to

MPD dating as far back as ancient Egypt. The first known written reference to MPD is thought to be biblical; Miller (1989) believes Mark 5:1–3 may describe a case of the disorder. In this passage, Jesus met a man with unclean spirits who lived in the tombs in the country of Gerasenes. The man spent night and day crying out and bruising himself with stones (i.e., self-mutilation). He could not be subdued and broke all fetters and chains. Upon meeting Jesus he cried out in a loud voice, begging Jesus not to torment him. When Jesus asked him his name, he replied, "My name is Legion; for we are many." Jesus transferred the unclean spirits into a herd of swine that went rushing down a steep bank to drown in the sea.

The first clear description of a syndrome recognizable as MPD by current standards was a case reported by Paracelsus in 1646 (Völgyesi 1966, p. 16). Paracelsus himself was "considered a genius and a charlatan," claiming a doctoral degree in medicine, although no records of a degree exist (Veith 1965, p. 103). Paracelsus described a hostess of a tavern who had an alternate personality, her "second self," that stole money from her while sleepwalking. Her "original self" did not recall these activities; for some time she accused her servants, but she later found the money hidden in the roof. Another time the patient found blood on her bedclothes and pieces of broken glass and more blood on a nearby table, ostensibly left by her other personality.

Credit for the first detailed case report of MPD goes to Eberhart Gmelin, a German, who described in 1791 an "exchange [of] personalities" brought about by hypnosis (Coons 1986b; Decker 1986, p. 37; Larmore et al. 1977; Prasad 1985). More reports surfaced after the turn of the nineteenth century. In 1812 Rush described two cases of "double minds" (Rush 1812). The first American case of MPD was that of Mary Reynolds, initially reported in 1816 by Mitchell and more fully described in 1888 by Mitchell's son (Coons 1986). This patient exhibited "hysterical fits" and spells of blindness, deafness, and amnesia.

In 1822 Dyce reported a case of "divided consciousness, or double personality." This case was cited by Taylor and Martin (1944) in what was considered the most authoritative review of published cases up to that time. These reviewers dismissed the Dyce case as "too narrowly hysterical to be multiple personality." The next known recorded case of MPD appeared shortly thereafter in 1828. This was the case of Sörgel, a criminal Bavarian youth with epilepsy and double consciousness. His doubles consisted of a "decent" personality and a criminal personality. During one episode, the criminal component chopped up an old woodcutter and drank his blood (Mesulam 1981).

The first "objective" case study of MPD was published in 1840: an eleven-year-old girl who suffered "extreme pain" and who was "magnetized" by her physician, Despine. After a month in treatment she developed two personalities (Decker 1986, p. 42). Apparently Janet, who was to become an important figure in the early development of MPD, was greatly impressed and inspired by this particular case (Ellenberger 1970, p. 131). In 1845 two more cases of dual personality were reported in England. According to Taylor and Martin (1944), no reports of MPD were published for more than a quarter of a century after 1846. Something else had caught the public's attention.

A popular movement toward spiritualism was spreading over Europe in the second half of that century, a "fad [that] originated in the United States" (Decker 1986, p. 37). Associated phenomena were table tipping, spirit rapping, spirits of the dead speaking, mediumship, trances, automatic writing, divining rods, swinging pendulums, the ouija board, and spirit possession and exorcism (Carlson 1986, p. 27).

Jung (1902/1977) was very much interested in "so-called occult phenomena." He presented a number of case histories of mediums and spiritualists and dissociative phenomena. The basis for his split with Freud has been ascribed to Jung's burning interest in parapsychology and dissociation (Ross 1989, p. 27), in conflict with Freud.

The practice of exorcism was gradually replaced by a new art, mesmerism, as the popular means of curing spiritual ills and demon possession (Decker 1986, pp. 36–37). Mesmerism was born out of the controversial practice of "animal magnetism." Its originator, Mesmer, was both "hailed as a genius and denounced as an imposter" (Veith 1965, p. 221), and was apparently a colorful and charismatic character who developed a strong following. The popularity of this new practice and its associated phenomena apparently began to draw the attention formerly given to demon possession. The mesmerists observed that when people with dual personalities were magnetized (hypnotized), a third personality sometimes appeared (Abse 1982, p. 166). Veith (1965, p. 8) reported that "As cases of possession became less common, case histories of other kinds of multiple personality disorders began appearing in the mesmerist literature and other medical reports."

By the turn of the nineteenth century, however, the pursuits of both spiritualism and mesmerism had given way to new interests. These developed into the practice of "hypnosis," a term first used by Braid in 1843 (Veith 1965, p. 225). Janet, a significant figure in psychiatry of that era, devoted himself to the study of hypnosis and suggestion, eschewing any involvement with parapsychology.

The rise in respect for hypnosis was sparked largely by a paper on hypnosis that Charcot presented before the French Academy in Paris (Decker 1986, p. 44). Charcot, a widely renowned neurologist and a teacher of Janet, Freud, Babinski, and others (Veith 1965, p. 245), believed that "'major hypnotism' could only be induced in grave hysterics" (Veith 1965, p. 239). In retrospect, critics charge that Charcot's dramatic and flamboyant hypnotic demonstrations (Putnam 1989b) "unleash[ed] a psychic epidemic" in his day (Decker 1986, p. 54). His work in mesmerism and hypnosis was highly controversial. A substantial effort was made by his contemporaries to invalidate his work in hypnosis and hysteria (Veith 1965, pp. 240–241), but these concepts were already too firmly entrenched.

With the possession concept abandoned in the post-Mesmer era, the psychic phenomena it represented came to be understood as fugues, multiple personality, and personality disturbances (Decker 1986, pp. 36–37). The syndrome of demon possession is thought to have thereby evolved into MPD about 100 years ago (Coons 1986b; Ross 1989, pp. 17, 41), when the popularity of hypnosis was on the rise. Hypnosis was a fertile medium for the growth and spread of MPD. With the increasing popularity of hypnosis, the late nineteenth century saw an acute upsurge of interest in MPD, particularly in France. Two French dual personality cases were described in 1874 and 1876. In 1887 the famous French case of Félida X was reported by Azam. This patient had "many symptoms of a hysterical nature" starting at puberty, including vomiting attacks, fainting spells, and involuntary spasmodic movements (Abse 1982, pp. 165–184, 238).

Shortly thereafter, a case of "co-consciousness" from approximately 1860 was belatedly published in 1889 (Taylor & Martin 1944). A number of additional cases of MPD were described by Dana, Dessoir, Binet, Azam, Laurant, Myers, Sidis, Goodhart, and Prince (Bliss 1986, p. 117; Horevitz & Braun 1984). By the end of the nineteenth century, a total of perhaps 30 cases had been reported (Prasad 1985). One author reflected on the reporting phenomenon of that age: "The more reports appeared on multiple personality, the more cases were recognized and reported. And as this happened, the cases described became increasingly complex" (Decker 1986, p. 43).

Concerns were aired that cases of MPD could be shaped by clinicians prejudiced by the prevailing climate of psychological theory and social context (Sutcliffe & Jones 1962). Recently, Bowers (1991, p. 169) commented on this phenomenon: "The more widespread the *idea* of MPD becomes, the more such an idea can serve as an implicit suggestion to people whose natural endowments and life circumstances have honed dissociative defenses as a way of dealing with profound threat. . . . Accordingly, the more MPD gets diagnosed, the more attention is drawn to it." (This pattern, however, has been recognized in association with a variety of medical illnesses the public knows little about and is thus not unique to MPD.)

These events in the late nineteenth century took place in the context of a newly developing view of the mind as a duality of conscious and unconscious states. The idea arose that fragments of personality could split off and act autonomously. This hypothesis laid the groundwork for development of the concepts of dissociation and MPD (Decker 1986, p. 37). Although Moreau de Tours is thought to have first conceived the idea of dissociation (van der Hart & Horst 1989), Janet is credited with its discovery and it was he who provided its name (Decker 1986, pp. 47–48). Nonetheless, he did not regard MPD as an important new syndrome. A careful scientific observer, he predicted that the disorder would be of more academic than clinical interest, remarking that the phenomenon was so rare that "it is unlikely you will have to occupy yourselves with it in practice" (Janet 1907, p. 66).

At the time, many leading figures in psychiatric investigation were not aware of the importance of MPD. Now it is widely recognized that Breuer's famous patient, Anna O. (Breuer 1950, pp. 14–31), might have suffered from MPD rather than ordinary hysteria (Bliss & Jeppsen 1985; Coons 1986a); Breuer (1950, p. 101) himself, however, did note that Anna O. was split into two personalities, one apparently sane and the other insane. Anna O.'s illness reportedly began in 1880, when she was twenty years old. She had many "hysterical" features including paralysis, anesthesia, aphonia, deafness, visual hallucinations of snakes, and diplopia. She forgot how to speak her native language, split her memory and consciousness, and developed another personality that took the place of her usual one (Breuer 1950, pp. 14–31). She also threw cushions at people and tore buttons off her bedclothes (Breuer 1950, p. 76).[1]

Breuer (1950, p. 63) observed that "double conscience . . . is present to a rudimentary degree in every hysteria," a phenomenon he included with other dissociative states of consciousness under the term "hypnoid." Ross (1989, p. 6) recognizes the value of reviewing history in the study of MPD:

> By studying the past, one can learn a great deal about the range of dissociative phenomena and variations in symptomatology. One can pick up numerous clinical tips and ideas from the 19th-century specialists in dissociative disorders. One realizes by studying the history of dissociation that many recent findings were already known 100 years ago.

Ross (1989, p. 36) believes that "Correctly understood, Anna O., Breuer, and Freud have much to teach us." Breuer and Freud apparently did not differentiate dissociative phenomena and hysterical conversion. That distinction was to come later.

Janet postulated that dissociation, or splitting of mental functions, was the pathophysiologic basis of hysteria (Putnam, 1989b; van der Hart & Horst 1989; van der Hart & van der Kolk 1991), and this began a tradition that would greatly affect the course of development of MPD for some time (Velek & Balon 1986). In his series of clinical studies of hysteria, Janet's conceptualization of hysteria was broad enough to include somatization disorder, conversion disorder, psychogenic amnesia, psychogenic fugue, MPD, and other dissociative syndromes (Janet 1907). Apparently he included hypnosis in this list: "The hypnotic state has never any character which cannot be found in natural hysteric somnambulisms" (Janet 1907, p. 114). Although Janet evidently considered both dual personality and dissociation within the realm of hysteria, retrospectively it is be-

[1] Of interest, Anna O.'s real name was Bertha Pappenheim; she was one of Europe's first social workers, a feminist noted for her work toward the establishment of homes for prostitutes and unwed mothers; she was honored in a 1954 commemorative German postage stamp (Ross 1989, p. 33).

lieved that he may have discerned differences between dual personality and hysteria (van der Hart & Boon 1989).

Janet reported several cases of double personalities. These patients also exhibited florid conversion and somatoform symptoms such as forgetting everything they ever knew, "hysteric accidents," fainting spells, vomiting everything eaten, pain complaints, "diffuse insensibilities," chronic sickliness from puberty on, urinary retention, anesthesia, paralysis, deafness, and blindness. Historians have concluded that "for Janet hysteria comprised all dissociative and related disorders" (van der Hart & Horst 1989, p. 409). Given this heritage, shortly before the turn of the twentieth century the French school at Salpetriere hospital adopted a classification of dissociative symptoms together with dual personality as manifestations of "la grande hysterie" (Velek & Balon 1986). At this juncture, MPD seems to have become embedded in hysteria, with no independent identity of its own.

Binet, an important figure in neuropsychiatry in the late nineteenth century who wrote two major treatises on dissociation, apparently discovered that alternate personalities could be produced in highly hypnotizable but otherwise normal subjects. He viewed the phenomenon of doubling of consciousness as a common clinical mechanism underlying a variety of psychiatric disorders, including somatization, conversion, and dissociative disorders. He further observed that disorders of dual personality were also associated with amnesia, paralysis, auditory hallucinations, and automatic writing (Ross 1989, pp. 29–30).

Morton Prince, a giant in the field of neuropsychiatry of his era, who has been called the "father of multiple personality syndrome" (Prasad 1985), was also struck by the similarities between MPD and hysteria:

> The individual, physiological, and mental alterations observed, including the amnesias, taken by themselves are in no way uncommon as phenomena and therefore are not peculiar to this condition, but are frequently observed as elements in other symptom-complexes, particularly hysteria. (Prince 1906, p. 186)

He further remarked that "the symptom-complex observed in certain types of hysteria differs in no way from that manifested by many so-called secondary personalities without amnesia" (p. 186).

Prince thought that media influences were shaping the development of MPD in his time. He wrote, "The fact is that our conception of multiple personality has been derived entirely from those sensational cases. . . . Such cases appeal to the imagination, and, from their very bizarre character, have colored the popular conception of multiple personality" (p. 173).

The rising popularity of MPD in the late 1800s was countered by a wave of reaction against it. Skeptics pointed out cases where alternate personalities had obviously been created "conveniently" to avoid responsibility for unacceptable behavior, contending that even the highly regarded authorities Prince, Janet, Flourney, and Despine had been deceived by patients who voluntarily shaped the manifestations they were exhibiting (Ellenberger 1970, p. 141). Others suggested that multiple personalities might be an artifact of hypnosis or inadvertent suggestion by therapists (Dercum 1913, p. 254; Ellenberger 1970, p. 141; Larmore et al. 1977; Rosenbaum 1980).

Prince commented that a patient "hypnotized sufficiently often and under sufficiently varied circumstances" would develop an "extensive" second self. He implied that hypnosis could have "created the multiplicity" in Janet's patient, Madame B. (Braun 1984a; Prince 1890). According to Braun (1984a), it was Janet who first suggested that MPD could be created by hypnosis. Janet is also thought to have been the first to raise the possibility of role playing to please the therapist as a factor in the production of MPD (van der Hart & Horst 1989). Janet openly said that he believed some of his own patients were playing and acting (Decker 1986, p. 55; van der Hart & Horst 1989). He described one of his own cases as "the psychological marvel of the nineteenth century," one in which "you feel it in a kind of mystic admiration for the subject, an exaggerated seeking after surprising and supranormal phenomena, which of course inspires you with some fear as to the way in which the observation has been conducted" (Janet 1907, pp. 84–85).

Janet expressed concern about the bizarreness of the symptoms and the degree of fascination surrounding the disorder. Current postulation is that Janet, too, may have been worried that therapists of his day were reinforcing or embellishing MPD symptoms (Fahy 1989).

MPD in the Twentieth Century

In the first two decades of the twentieth century, the popularity of MPD trailed off sharply (Ellenberger 1970, p. 141). Gruenewald's (1977, p. 386) interpretation of this was that MPD "went out of fashion and perhaps took on somewhat different forms."

It appears that two major factors contributed to the diminishing popularity of MPD after the turn of the century. First, in 1909 Freud publicly discounted hypnosis, declaring it "a failure and a method of doubtful ethical value" (Ellenberger 1970, p. 802). MPD, then tightly tied to hypnosis, therefore lost standing. At the same time, Freud discarded the theory of incestuous seduction of children in favor of repression—a move thought to have been instrumental in the discrediting of MPD (because the histories of childhood abuse reported by multiples would be considered mere fantasies) (Ross 1989, p. 37). Two years later, in 1911, Bleuler brought schizophrenia into prominence with its new name and a broadly encompassing description that included many diverse forms of functional mental disorders. With the increasing popularity of the diagnosis of schizophrenia in the decades to follow, many cases that would have been previously reported as MPD may have been diagnosed as schizophrenic (Rosenbaum 1980).

Like Janet, Bleuler was not terribly impressed with MPD as an independent entity. He dismissed it as an artifactual disorder, stating that he could "produce the very same through hypnosis" (Bleuler 1924, p. 138).

In the early twentieth century, MPD came to be considered rare, if not nonexistent (Kluft 1987b), and the disorder "vanished from serious study" for many decades (Ross 1989, p. 38). Around that time, Freud had lost respect for Janet (Veith 1965, p. 253), and Janet's work with dual personalities had become suspect. According to Ross (1989, p. 47), "Janet was politically unsuccessful, which is partly why he fell into obscurity." Janet's reputation suffered—and along with it, professional enthusiasm for hypnosis and dissociation, including MPD. Hypnosis was largely forsaken for treatment of the fully awake patient on the couch.

Historically, interest in MPD has paralleled the rise of popularity of hysteria, first at the end of the nineteenth century and again after World War II (Bliss 1980; Kluft 1987b). Ross (1989, p. 44) noted that "the level [sic] of interest in hypnosis and MPD have always been intertwined and have covaried."

The early twentieth century disenchantment with MPD and lack of attention to the disorder was punctuated by the celebrated case of Christine Beauchamp reported by Prince (1906). Prince heavily invested himself in the intensive treatment of this patient over many years. He provided extensive clinical descriptions of this case to the medical community, winning professional respect and widespread publication in a prestigious psychiatric journal. One of Prince's contemporaries, McDougall (1926, p. 497), observed that "It has been suggested by many critics that, in the course of Prince's long and intimate dealing with the case, involving as it did the frequent use of hypnosis, both for exploratory and therapeutic purposes, he may have moulded the course of its development to a degree that cannot be determined. This possibility cannot be denied. Yet, even if such influence was very considerable, the fact would not seriously detract from the interest and theoretical importance of the case." Prince's handling of the Beauchamp case was later criticized by McCurdy (1941, p. 35) as a "melodrama, with facts and theater all mixed up together." McCurdy pointed out that the patient had made Prince the center of her life for a number of years, bringing up the question of potential gain for her and a strong motive to please him with her symptoms. He argued that the behavioral abnormalities Prince described reflected powerful transference effects. McCurdy and more recent critics asserted that Prince may have inadvertently caused further dissociation (Coons 1980) and may have suggested alternate personalities to patients (Sutcliffe & Jones 1962).

Another case of that period that had the potential for suggestibility in the origination of MPD was that of Bernice, discovered in 1921 and reported a few years later (Goddard 1926). Bernice was said to have been "an avid reader of newspapers and loved going to the movies" (Hacking 1991), the implication being that her symptoms constituted mimicry or theatrics.

Prince's enthusiasm for MPD did not catch on, and only a few more cases were reported until the second half of this century. By 1944, a total of 76 cases that Taylor and Martin (1944) considered to be genuine cases of MPD had been reported, although the *Index Medicus* lists many more purported cases. In the years between 1944 and 1969 only a scattering of MPD cases surfaced. One of these was the most famous case of all time, "Eve White," reported by Thigpen and Cleckley (1954). This case, described in detail in a popular book, *The Three Faces of Eve* (Thigpen & Cleckley 1957), was a woman who developed three separate personalities. Of the 14 cases reported in that 25-year period (1944–1969), 6 were reported by one clinician, Cornelia Wilbur (Aldridge-Morris 1989, p. 3).

Just three decades ago, MPD was "thought to be [nearly] extinct" (Ross 1989, p. 4). Multiple personality did not appear in official diagnostic nomenclature until 1968, when it was unobtrusively mentioned in DSM-II (American Psychiatric Association 1968, p. 40) under a section entitled "hysterical neurosis; dissociative type." Having lost its historical status as a hysterical condition established by Janet and others in the early 1900s, MPD was now considered a dissociative disorder. MPD did not actually achieve official diagnostic status, however, until 1980, when it was listed among the dissociative disorders in DSM-III (American Psychiatric Association 1980).

DSM-III also narrowed the diagnostic criteria for schizophrenia, further contributing to the recognition of MPD cases by more carefully delineating them from schizophrenia. Of note, the British were not much affected by Bleuler's broadened definition of schizophrenia and did not follow American trends toward widely inclusive definitions of this disease (Eaton 1985; Kramer 1961). Nor did the British move with American trends in the popularity of MPD, the result being a wide rift in British and American attention to the subject (Fahy et al. 1989). Only two case reports of MPD appeared in the British literature after 1960 (Cutler & Reed 1975; Fahy et al. 1989), and both doubted whether MPD could even be considered a psychiatric disorder. In 1987 Aldridge-Morris (1989, p. 15) surveyed British therapists about their experience with MPD and reported very few cases. The author stated, "the vast majority [of cases] (dare I say, 'all'?) are in the United States. Such a significant epidemiological difference cries out for explanation." One of his survey respondents wrote, "In the UK, we react to any suggestion by patients or relatives that there are two or more personalities by immediately saying that there are two or more aspects to one personality, and asserting that the individual must take responsibility for both of these aspects. It works" (p. 15).

Janet (1907) had been alerted early in the history of MPD by the fact that most cases were from America, and Taylor and Martin (1944) calculated that 57% of the world's cases were American. The geographic distribution of cases has been described as "bizarre" (Simpson 1988). Hacking (1991, p. 841) describes MPD as "strictly American with Canadian branch plants." Aldridge-

Morris (1989, p. 107) concluded, "It is . . . at least suggestive that we are dealing with a psychological disturbance which is endemic to the United States of America." He believes that compared to the United Kingdom, the United States was ripe for an epidemic of MPD due to five factors: (1) the social acceptance of role playing in the United States, (2) the greater public exposure to MPD in the United States, (3) the influence and high prestige awarded American psychiatrists and psychologists, (4) the destigmatization of psychotherapy in the United States, and (5) the American proclivity toward self-analysis and introspection (Aldridge-Morris 1989, pp. 108–109).

Skepticism related to geographical maldistribution is not unique to MPD. It has also followed the diagnosis of somatization disorder. Othmer (1988, p. 330) wrote, "In spite of the empirical validation of somatization disorder, skeptics still doubt its existence as a disorder entity." Vaillant (1984, p. 543) commented that somatization disorder is "a disorder quite as regional as kuru" and that "For unknown reasons Briquet's disease [somatization disorder] is rarely encountered outside of Missouri, Kansas, and Iowa."

MPD has not been included in major landmark studies of lifetime and current prevalence rates of major psychiatric disorders in general populations (Ross 1991), such as the Epidemiologic Catchment Area study (Robins et al. 1984). Even though such studies have covered other similarly uncommon psychiatric disorders such as obsessive-compulsive disorder, they have neglected MPD. The Diagnostic Interview Schedule (DIS) (Robins et al. 1981), used extensively in epidemiologic studies, does not inquire about the symptoms of MPD or dissociation. No systematic epidemiologic studies to determine the prevalence or clinical phenomenology of MPD in the general population have been conducted (Ross 1989, p. 90), although a preliminary population survey indicated evidence of MPD in 14 of 454 subjects, a 3% prevalence rate. (Of these 14 subjects, only 6 reported a history of childhood abuse and were "clinically diagnosed" according to their Dissociative Disorders Interview Schedule [DDIS] profiles. The other eight, with no history of childhood abuse, were "not as clinically disturbed as clinically diagnosed MPD patients" and were considered possible false-positive cases. Ross [p. 509] observed that "most of the MPD cases in the general population were radically different from clinical MPD patients.")

Fleming (1989, p. 877) and Ross (1989, p. 91) protest the invocation of the unusual nature of MPD as evidence against its veracity as a disorder, arguing that MPD has been singled out from other rare or uncommon conditions for this claim. Ross contends that the arguments of skeptics who claim that the dramatic increase in MPD indicates iatrogenesis or a false-positive diagnosis make an unfair example of MPD. He cites a systematic population survey in which rates of obsessive-compulsive disorder were found to be 40 to 60 times the prevalence estimated by Nemiah eight years earlier, but no one claimed that the apparent increase in the rate of that disorder was iatrogenic (Ross 1989, pp. 91–92). (It is quite possible that a great deal of the disparity in rates between the two reports of obsessive-compulsive disorder may be due to difficulties in comparing studies rather than to an actual increase in the reporting of cases, because the means of assessment in the two sources cited were very different.)

The "Epidemic"

The strongest surge of interest in MPD in history occurred in the United States after 1970 (Rosenbaum 1980); in that decade, the number of reported cases sky-rocketed (Boor 1982; Ross 1989, p. 44). In the following decade, Ross (1989, p. 45) described an even greater "exponential rise" in the number of reported cases.

While the average number of annual publications on MPD prior to 1970 had been fewer than 1, between 1970 and 1980 the number increased a thousand percent, to 9.1. In the next decade (1981–1990) the annual number increased to 59.8 (Goettman et al. 1991).

Interest in MPD was so widespread by 1984 that Bennett Braun convened an international conference on MPD in Chicago and an international association was founded, the International Society for the Study of Multiple Personality Disorder and Dissociation (ISSMPD&D). Ross (1989, p. 47) feels that "One cannot overemphasize the importance of the ISSMPD&D and the annual Chicago meetings in reestablishing the study of MPD." He describes a highly political process in the consolidation of the MPD movement, the mainstream of which was curiously not to include four of the early pioneers of MPD (Allison, Beahrs, Bliss, and Orne), all of whom were left behind, each with his own reasons for skepticism or deviation (Ross 1989, pp. 48–49).

The year 1984 was a landmark year for MPD, marking its transition from "a prescientific to a scientific literature" (Ross 1989, p. 47). The reawakening of interest in MPD prompted five journals (*American Journal of Clinical Hypnosis, Psychiatric Annals, Psychiatric Clinics of North America, International Journal of Clinical and Experimental Hypnosis,* and *Investigations*) to devote special issues to the topic in a period of two years (Kluft 1987b). Until the mid-1970s, many psychiatric journals had refused to publish articles about MPD because it was considered to be a rare disorder of little interest to readers (Coons 1986a). The *Cumulative Index Medicus* did not have a heading for MPD until 1979; prior to that time, the entity was listed under "dual personality." The 1980 *Cumulative Index Medicus* cited only 2 articles on MPD; a decade later, the 1990 listing contained 33 citations. The field was expanding so rapidly that the first comprehensive bibliography on MPD published in 1983, containing 350 references (Boor & Coons 1983), had to be updated only two years later with 90 additional references (Damgaard et al. 1985) and again in 1991 to include 847 references (Goettman et al. 1991). The years 1985 and 1986 were especially prolific, with "six scholarly books on MPD" published in North America (Ross 1989, p. 53).

14   *Multiple personality disorder*

By 1986, 133 full case reports had been published and more than 300 cases had been described in the literature (Bliss 1986), and it was estimated that 6000 cases had been diagnosed in North America (Coons 1986b). That year, Putnam and coworkers (1986, p. 285) wrote, "more cases of MPD have been reported within the last 5 years than in the preceding two centuries."

Figure 1-1 charts the waxing and waning growth of MPD in earlier eras and the recent exponential growth spurt in published case reports tallied by the authors. The graph shows that the peak in the late 1800s is diminutive compared to the rise in the last two decades, and particularly in the last decade, for which the bar in the figure had to be interrupted because of the large number of publications in relation to prior decades.

The published literature on dissociation and amnesia has, interestingly, recently begun to lag behind the number of publications on MPD. Apparently the more fascinating MPD has moved ahead of the other dissociative disorders of its class in the attention that has been paid to it. According to Goettman and colleagues (1991, p. iii), "MPD—with its extraordinary symptoms and clinical signs—has been the flagship of writings in the psychiatric group of dissociative disorders."

Unfortunately, the definition of MPD is still uncertain and seems to be shifting. DSM-III-R (American Psychiatric Association 1987, p. 272) lists only two basic criteria: first, that there exist at least two distinct personalities or personality states, and second, that they repeatedly take control of the person's behav-

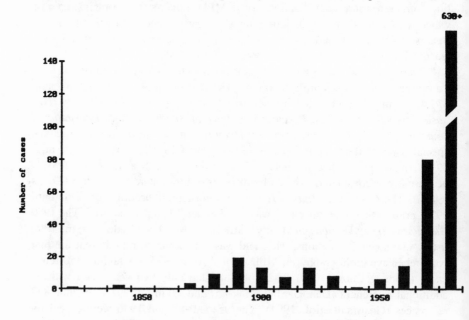

Figure 1-1. Number of cases reported by decade.

ior. There are no exclusion criteria to separate MPD from other conditions such as somatization disorder.

Aldridge-Morris (1989, p. 44) points out that there are no objective criteria of what constitutes a "personality," and he notes that the definitions given by various authors include vague terms such as " 'well developed,' 'integrated,' 'complex', [and] 'distinct'." He further cites the distinction made by Coons (1984) between "personality" and "personality fragment" as "painfully reminiscent of ancient theologians debating how many angels could sit on a pinhead." Apparently "fragments" have been included in counts of alternate personalities in some reports. Kluft (1989) has also noted the difficulties in separating "personality fragments" and "personality states" from full alternate personalities.

Not only has the prevalence of MPD apparently increased, but the usual number of personalities per case also seems to be growing (Kluft 1984a). Whereas in the last century reported cases were mostly dual personalities, almost all cases since 1944 have had three or more personalities (Boor 1982). Only one case reported prior to 1944 had more than eight alternate personalities. Modern cases average from 6 to 16 alternates apiece (Coons et al. 1988; Kluft 1984c; Ross et al. 1989e). In Kluft's 1982 series of 54 MPD patients, 44% had more than 10 personalities, and seven cases exceeded 20 (Kluft 1982). Adolescent multiples studies by Dell and Eisenhower (1990) reported a mean of 24.1 alternates. There may be a cohort effect in the number of alternates displayed, with younger cohorts having greater numbers, which would be consistent with historical trends (Dell & Eisenhower 1990). Figure 1-2 depicts recent trends in mean numbers of alternates in the studies cited by Dell and Eisenhower (1990); the increase in number in recent years is clearly evident.

In 1986 a case with 300 alternates was reported (Ross et al. 1989d), and a recent autobiographical account (Spencer 1989) claimed more than 400. The number quickly jumped to 1000 in a recent report (Mayer 1991). Putnam (1989a, pp. 39–40) and Schultz and coworkers (1989) have suggested that increased willingness and skill on the part of therapists may be helping to identify additional alternate personalities.

Clearly, there has been a population explosion in the ranks of MPD, both in numbers of cases and numbers of alternate personalities. Thigpen and Cleckley (1984) reported, however, that they found virtually no cases among patients with suspected MPD referred to them, and they thought the exponential increase in cases was spurious and overdramatized. Expressing skepticism, they bluntly remarked that MPD patients seem to have "a competition to see who can have the greatest number of alter personalities. (Unfortunately, there also appears to be a competition among some therapists to see who can have the greatest number of multiple personality cases)" (p. 64). What they were trying to describe seems to be a folie à deux. Using a similar metaphor, Aldridge-Morris (1989, p. 16) referred to the popularity of MPD as a case of "the Emperor's new clothes."

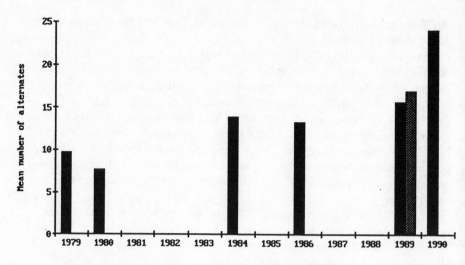

Figure 1–2. Mean number of alternate personalities by year of study.

The MPD phenomenon has clearly reached epidemic proportions (Boor 1982; Fleming 1989; Hilgard 1988; Thigpen & Cleckley 1984; Tozman & Pabis 1989). Ross (1991, p. 504) identified the movement as "an unprecedented shift in psychiatric epidemiology." The dramatic acceleration in the number of cases reported has provoked some authors to feel "quite dismayed" (Bowers 1991) and "greatly concerned" (Thigpen & Cleckley 1984). Such concern over the dramatic increase in MPD cases was the impetus for a British monograph (Aldridge-Morris 1989) written about this phenomenon (Aldridge-Morris 1989, pp. 107–108).

Recently, Bliss' group has reported the discovery of very high rates of MPD in four studies. In a series of 33 selected cases of Briquet's syndrome, 63% were alleged to be multiples or probable multiples (Bliss 1984c). Of 33 convicted male sex offenders, 21% were classified as DSM-III multiples and another 18% as probable multiples (Bliss & Larson 1985). Bliss' group found that as many as 13% of the psychiatric inpatients and 9% of the outpatients they sampled suffered from MPD (Bliss & Jeppsen 1985) and that 60% of the psychiatric inpatients with auditory hallucinations in their study were multiples (Bliss et al. 1983). Although it is recognized that these patient samples may have been selected from specialized practices and therefore may not be representative of the general patient population, the high rates in these samples are striking.

Ross (1991) reported that he and his colleagues found that 14% of a group of substance abusers, 17% of a sample of adolescent psychiatric patients, and 5% of a psychiatric inpatient sample had MPD. Other reports of the prevalence of MPD in inpatient populations range between 1% and 5% (Bliss & Jeppsen 1985; Putnam et al. 1984; Ross 1987). Among more special populations, 5% of prostitutes and 50% of exotic dancers have been reported to have MPD (Ross et al. 1990a).

Loewenstein (1989) has estimated the prevalence rate of MPD in the general population to be about 1 case per 100 people. According to Ross (1991, p. 511), "Complex dysfunctional posttraumatic MPD requiring specific psychotherapy appears to affect about 1% of the general population." Ross suspected that the florid cases of MPD may only be as prevalent as 1 in 500 in the general population. Some researchers believe the disorder is "exceedingly rare" (Thigpen & Cleckley 1984; Tozman & Pabis 1989).

Ross (1989, p. 77), on the other hand, speculated that "By the year 2000, most mental health professionals will probably have diagnosed at least one case of MPD. Not only that, people will be making a point of mentioning their MPD case, in order to let colleagues know that they are competent diagnosticians and don't miss cases. By the year 2000 the psychiatrist who has never diagnosed a case of MPD may be looked on with suspicion." Ross (1989, p. 77) also expressed the concern that "Within a span of 10 years, we may evolve from extreme underdiagnosis of MPD to a situation in which the major problem is false positive diagnoses." Observing the ubiquity of dissociation in the population, Ludwig and colleagues (1972, p. 308) facetiously wrote, "Perhaps it is not too presumptuous to presume that all individuals, no matter how well adjusted, have at least a touch of multiple personality within them."

Chodoff (1987) reported that an informal poll of his colleagues turned up very few cases of MPD; he didn't think all his colleagues lacked the clinical acumen to detect cases and wondered how they could have missed cases "being reported in the hundreds, even thousands." He suggested iatrogenesis as a likely factor operating in suggestible patients in the interest of secondary gain—for psychiatrists as well as patients.

Considerable speculation has focused on the origins of the precipitous rise in the rate of published MPD cases (Bliss 1980; Boor 1982; Boor & Coons 1983; Greaves 1980; Kluft 1986; Putnam 1989a, pp. 39–40; Rosenbaum 1980; Ross 1989, pp. 37–54; Schultz et al. 1989; Sutcliffe & Jones 1962). The possibilities considered include increased professional and public awareness of the disorder, resulting in improved recognition of more existing cases (Boor 1982), an actual increase in the prevalence of the syndrome in suggestible individuals (Thigpen & Cleckley 1984), and overdiagnosis of MPD in times of increased popularity of the diagnosis (Chodoff 1987). A less contributory factor is thought to be a decrease in misdiagnosis of actual MPD cases as schizophrenic (Kluft 1987a; Rosenbaum 1980).

In another psychiatric disorder, obsessive-compulsive disorder, the case has been clearly made that the well-documented increases in the frequency of this disorder likely reflect a "treatment-oriented diagnostic bias" (Stoll et al. 1992,

p. 638). Apparently, recent increases in publications about the disorder have influenced clinicians to consider and diagnose the condition more frequently (Stoll et al. 1992).

Another possibility is that the natural history of the biology of MPD has taken a turn (Ross 1991). Cohort and period effects have been observed in increases in other psychiatric phenomena, the most noteworthy wave being recent alarming increases in rates of teenage and young adult suicides and rates of depression (Weissman et al. 1991, p. 66; Wetzel et al. 1987). Rates of bipolar affective disorder (Weissman et al. 1991, p. 66), conduct disorder (Robins et al. 1991, pp. 266–270), and drug abuse (Anthony & Helzer 1991, pp. 133–134) have had similar rising courses.

It has been pointed out that a few clinicians may be contributing a disproportionate number of MPD cases to the literature (Ludolph 1985; Orne et al. 1984; Simpson 1988; Spanos et al. 1985, 1986) and that the literature may reflect the "personal agendas" of a few individuals, although this is vigorously disputed (Kluft 1987b). Bliss (1984b) reported that he saw more than 100 cases in four years. Kluft (1984c) saw 171 cases in 10 years of practice and a total of 250 cases in his career (Chodoff 1987). Jeppsen, Coons, Fraser, Allison, and Braun each encountered 50 or more cases (Allison 1981; Bliss & Jeppsen 1985; Braun 1984a; Coons et al. 1988; Ross et al. 1989d). These authors have been among the most prolific in the field.

In 1989 Ross (pp. 51–52) raised a concern about the MPD literature, the bulk of which is relatively recent: the most prolific authors in the MPD field are few. Thus they have unavoidably cross-referenced each other extensively, with the potential danger of forming an "in-club." This phenomenon has also been observed in different fields of psychiatric research—for example, with the Feighner criteria introduced in the most frequently cited psychiatric journal article of recent years (Feighner et al. 1972). That article was most often cited by authors affiliated or associated with Washington University in St. Louis (Blashfield & McElroy 1987).

The historical ebb and flow in the popularity of MPD lend support to those who believe that patterns of attention to MPD are faddish; it has been said that the status of MPD vacillates with the prevailing trend or "vogue" in psychiatric thinking (Gruenewald 1977; Sutcliffe & Jones 1962; Thigpen & Cleckley 1984). In this sense, the diagnosis of MPD might be considered a "designer diagnosis" (similar to the concept of "designer drugs," referring to the latest illicit synthetic substance of abuse to hit the street market).

In spite of the increasing attention to MPD, even as recently as the late 1980s "the field of psychiatry as a whole remained highly skeptical about MPD" (Ross 1989, p. 50). Some experts fear that MPD may once again fall into obscurity in the next decade or two (Ross 1989, p. 51), as it did in the past, succumbing to "disrepute again, repeating the events of the late 19th and early 20th centuries" (Ross 1989, p. 7). If MPD is to be more than "a passing fad," proponents point to the need to continue political and research efforts (Ross 1989, pp. 50–51).

Current Trends

Other countries lag behind American trends. Historically, New Zealand and Australia have not been sources of MPD reports, and in 1987 a Czechoslovakian psychiatrist stated that MPD is "unknown to the present day generation of psychiatrists" (Aldridge-Morris 1989, p. 108). According to Ross (1989, p. 5), MPD is rarely diagnosed in Great Britain and Europe today. Certain European countries have, however, started to pay attention to MPD, in particular Switzerland (Modestin 1992) and the Netherlands (van der Hart 1991). The 1992 meeting of ISSMPD&D took place in Amsterdam. According to one report, "The interest in the Netherlands in dissociation and MPD is slowly spreading to the Flemish part of Belgium, which shares a common language, and Germany" (van der Hart 1991, p. 9). Interest in MPD has also recently been reported by clinicians in "many European countries, North America, and Israel" (van der Hart 1991, p. 9) and reports of MPD have emerged from Puerto Rico, South America, and India (Putnam 1991b).

In India, the first case of MPD was reported as recently as 1956 and a second case was not reported for another 25 years (Adityanjee et al. 1989; Alexander 1956; Varma et al. 1981). The lag of MPD's appearance in India has been attributed to differences of interest in role playing in these cultures (Adityanjee et al. 1989). MPD appears to be rare in India, as well as in other South Asian and Southeast Asian countries, but reported cases are expected to increase once physicians are made aware of MPD as a diagnostic entity (Adityanjee et al. 1989).

A rise in the incidence of cases with Westernization and industrialization of culture is not unique to MPD. This phenomenon has been described in association with somatization disorder (Swartz et al. 1991, p. 255). It is also speculated that just as non-Western countries have been slow to catch on to the diagnosis of MPD, the mean number of alternate personalities per case has not yet increased in these countries; however, this is to be expected (Adityanjee et al. 1989).

Adityanjee and coworkers (1989) entertain the possibility that most MPD cases in India may be unrecognized because they are misdiagnosed as "possession syndrome," which these authors also term a "hysterical" condition. Adityanjee's group predicts that the prevalence of possession syndrome in India is likely to fall with increasing Westernization of Indian society, accompanied by a compensatory increase in cases of MPD. In an epidemic of possession syndrome in India in 1970 during a smallpox outbreak, 400 patients required psychiatric hospitalization (Varma et al. 1970). Varma and colleagues (1981, p. 114) wrote that "the question arises as to how that condition [possession syndrome] differs from multiple personality." Mulhern (1991), however, emphasizes that there are important differences between MPD and spirit possession.

Coons (1980) remarked that even today MPD may be difficult to differentiate from demon possession, mediumship, automatic writing, and hypnosis. It is interesting that women make up the vast majority of both the spirit possessed and MPD patients (Mulhern 1991). Similarities have been drawn between MPD and the occult, demon possession, satanic cults, bewitchment, mediumship, and automatic writing (Adityanjee et al. 1989; Coons 1980; Varma et al. 1981). There is a current tendency to link MPD with satanic cults (Mayer 1991; Spencer 1989, p. xviii), riding the wave of the recent rise in popularity of satanism in American culture. [The interested reader seeking more information on this latest vogue is referred to Peterson (1989), Johnston (1989), and Larson (1989).]

Kline (1984, p. 199) noted that "more developed forms" of MPD seem much like trance states of mediums and personalities of "reincarnated selves." According to DSM-III-R, symptoms may include the belief that one is possessed. Multiples occasionally report having a personality who claims to be possessed (Coons 1984). One-fourth of the 95 cases in Ross and Norton's (1989b) series reported a personality identified as a demon. Kluft (1989) has observed that demonic alternates are more common among MPD patients whose therapists have religious belief systems. Of note, informing MPD patients that their alternate personalities are demonic has apparently not proved helpful (Fraser 1991; Kluft 1989). Exposure to exorcism is thought to frighten MPD patients and cause further harm (Fraser 1991).

Paranatural and occult experiences are commonly reported by MPD patients. In one series (Ross et al., 1989c) multiples reported an average of five or six extrasensory and supernatural experiences each. Typical kinds of experiences reported include mental telepathy, telekinesis, clairvoyance, possession, contact with ghosts or poltergeists, and knowledge of past lives. All of the eight MPD patients studied by Stern (1984) believed they had experienced parapsychological phenomena. A study by Richards (1991) found that subjective "psychic" experiences, such as telepathy, clairvoyance, and out-of-body experiences, are associated with elevated scores on the Dissociative Experiences Scale. Multiples are also often said to have great facility in automatic writing (Bliss 1980).

Historical connections between hysteria and the occult, demon possession, and the supernatural have been well documented (Abse 1987, pp. 3–4; Fine 1962, p. 84; Veith 1965, pp. 40–54). In China, 49% of patients with symptoms of possession were found to have "hysteria" (diagnostic criteria not specified) (Yap 1960). The association of hysteria and the occult, and the historical connection between MPD and the occult, are consistent with Janet's incorporation of MPD into his design of hysteria.

Sybil (Schreiber 1973) was the first report to link MPD with child abuse (Coons 1986a), an association that has been increasingly underscored. Ross

(1989, p. 45) noted that in 1980 "even leading experts in the field had not yet grasped the frequency or severity of the abuse experienced by MPD patients." Adityanjee and colleagues (1989) have observed that possession syndrome in India, like MPD in America, seems to be closely associated with a history of childhood abuse. Ross (1989, p. 45) described "horrific stories" of "ritual abuse by cult members" in the childhood histories of MPD patients, one of the newer twists to MPD that has just recently started to trickle into the literature, apparently having taken hold in 1983–1984 (Ross 1989, p. 48). According to Ganaway (1989, p. 207), "Patients and therapists who validate and publicly defend the unsubstantiated veracity of these reports [of childhood satanic ritual abuse] may find themselves developing into a cult of their own, validating each others' belief systems while ignoring (and being ignored by) the scientific and psychotherapeutic community at large."

Related to the recognition of childhood abuse associated with MPD, another recent trend starting in about 1984 links MPD with posttraumatic stress disorder (Braun 1984a; Kluft 1987a, 1987b; Spiegel 1984, 1986, 1988; Loewenstein 1989; Ross 1989, p. 48; Ross 1991), and many conceptualize MPD as a posttraumatic disorder of adulthood caused by severe childhood trauma. It has been noted, however, that Janet was aware of the connection between traumatic experiences and dissociation; his work on this association has only recently come to light after a long period of obscurity in the shadow of Freud and the psychoanalytic movement (Putnam 1989b). Ross (1989, p. 44) observed that the attention to posttraumatic stress disorder generated by the Vietnam War and renewed trends to publicize the women's movement "helped to bring child abuse, and particularly incest, out of the closet" as a recognizable contributor to the resurgence of MPD.

Conclusion

This chapter has traced the development of the concept of MPD in the academic literature through history. MPD has been seen to have origins in hysteria, demon possession, and hypnosis. This chapter has provided some background to the arguments for and against the existence of MPD and its validity as a diagnosis to be presented in Chapter 2.

2

Theory and controversy: validation of the disorder

Recent proponents of MPD have met resistance at practically every turn in mainstream psychiatry. Neither of the two dominant schools of psychiatry in America fully accepts MPD as a disorder. The basic concept of MPD does not harmonize with established concepts of traditional psychoanalysis. Biological psychiatry, on the other hand, cannot assimilate MPD into its demands for rigorous scientific proof (Bliss 1988) because relevant data on MPD are not currently available and not easily obtained.

Perhaps no other psychiatric disorder has aroused as much passion within the psychiatric community as MPD. Kluft (1987b, p. 366) writes, "one can ask whether this polarized debate, however venerable, has clinical relevance." Underlying the controversy is the shortage of rigorous empirical investigation of the disorder. This leaves the field open to unsupported arguments and emotional reasoning. Kluft (1986) has pointed out the result: a "truculent clash" of "strongly worded statements of opinion" and "irrational thinking" that are the basis of many of the contentions of the skeptics, who have no "compelling hard data" to back them.

Negative reactions directed against advocates of MPD have sometimes been intense, including antagonism, open hostility, and behavior exceeding the bounds of professionalism (Bliss 1988; Dell 1988b; Hilgard 1988; Spiegel 1988; Tozman & Pabis 1989). On the surface, it is not obvious why people should be so upset about the question of the validity of MPD. Melancholia, for example, is a subclass of major depression that has never been well validated, nor has its place in diagnostic nosology been settled, yet this disorder does not elicit skepticism and ridicule. Dell (1988) surveyed clinicians to assess the reactions they had encountered as a result of their interest in MPD. Of 62 respondents who had treated patients with MPD, more than 80% said they had experienced moderate to extreme reactions from colleagues. Over half related that they and their patients had "repeatedly been subjected to malicious harassment, contemptuous ridicule, and deliberate interference in the medical care of the patient" (Dell 1988a, p. 537). Some professionals who treated MPD said attempts were made to refuse their admissions to hospitals or to force discharge of their patients, even patients they felt represented a serious suicidal risk (Dell 1988b). A few respondents said they were banned from inpatient units they staffed. Sometimes hospital staff refused to treat their patients for MPD. The clinicians also said they suffered repeated challenges in scheduled staff reviews.

On the other hand, proponents can be as impassioned about MPD as skeptics are hostile to it. There seems to be little middle ground. Dell (1988b) suggests that the emotional reactions may stem from anxiety evoked by the disorder's bizarre, unsettling clinical presentation (Dell 1988b).

To move toward resolving the question of the existence of MPD, it seems prudent to turn first to the basics of validation of the diagnosis and the steps needed to achieve it. This chapter will review that process and will then examine the various views of the validity of MPD in published works, tracing the paths that have led investigators to their strong beliefs.

Validation of a Diagnosis

In their seminal work, Robins and Guze and colleagues (Feighner et al. 1972; Robins & Guze 1970) established guidelines for determining diagnostic validity in psychiatric illness. Their methods are a contemporary extension of the work of Thomas Sydenham (1624–1689), a founding figure in clinical medicine and epidemiology (Cloninger 1989). Sydenham's approach to diagnostic validation emphasized detailed observation of the clinical features and longitudinal course of medical disorders. His methods are particularly useful in the classification of psychiatric diseases because knowledge about etiologic agents is generally lacking (Cloninger 1989). These methods should be especially useful in validating the diagnosis of MPD, given the diversity of opinion about its etiology and the controversy over its nosological status. They are empirical and atheoretical with regard to etiology, so that no assumptions are needed in their application.

There are five phases in this method of validating psychiatric disorders: (1) clinical description, (2) laboratory studies, (3) delimitation from other disorders, (4) follow-up study, and (5) family study (Robins & Guze 1970). In this way, Robins and colleagues (Feighner et al. 1972) established diagnostic criteria for 14 psychiatric disorders and provided validating evidence for most of these diagnostic categories. Cloninger (1989, p. 14) remarked, "No additional psychiatric disorders have been validated by the five-phase approach to reduce the proportion of 'undiagnosed' cases since the system was first described" 20 years ago. MPD is one of those unvalidated conditions.

Briquet's Syndrome: A Model for Diagnostic Validation

Briquet's syndrome, also called "somatization disorder" in DSM-III-R (American Psychiatric Association 1987), serves as a template for the validation methods of Robins and Guze's group. For readers with little background on this disorder, a brief summary of its history follows, beginning with the condition when it was first known as "hysteria."

Hysteria was described before Hippocrates by the Egyptians, who thought it was caused by a wandering uterus. In 1859, Paul Briquet (1859) in France provided the first systematic description of hysteria with his careful observational study of 430 patients over 10 years. Dramatic and unexplained medical complaints characterized the condition. Briquet recommended that the term "hysteria" be abandoned because of its pejorative connotations. This did not take place in his time.

Kraepelin observed that patients with this disorder exhibited social disability, hallucinations, emotional instability, and exaggeration. In later studies of hysterical women, Janet (1907) found frequent dual (multiple) personalities and considerable social disability. Savill (1909) also noted dual personalities in the hysterics he saw. In subsequent conceptualizations of hysteria, histrionic personality traits were focused upon as central to the disorder, and the association with chronic medical complaints was overshadowed (Martin 1988).

Things changed in the mid-twentieth century when Purtell, Robins, and Cohen (1951) resurrected a medical model of hysteria focusing on medical symptoms (Martin 1988). In 1962, Perley and Guze systematized the diagnostic criteria for Briquet's disorder around the characteristic complicated medical history; personality factors pertained only secondarily to the medical presentation of the complaints. According to their definition, 25 of 59 possible unexplained medical symptoms distributed in 9 of 10 categories were required for a diagnosis. In 1972 the criteria of Feighner et al. (1972) were delineated, and the condition has subsequently been well validated by their methods (Guze 1970, 1975; Guze & Perley 1963; Guze et al. 1986; Perley & Guze, 1962; Woerner & Guze 1968).

Guze (1970), harkening back to Briquet's original suggestion, proposed that the pejorative term "hysteria" should be replaced by a less evocative term. He proposed the name "Briquet's syndrome," which has been fully adopted in certain sectors of psychiatry, though not universally (Guze 1975).

Briquet's disorder is characterized as a polysymptomatic disorder that begins early in life, affects women predominantly or exclusively, and is associated with chronic and recurrent somatic complaints, often described dramatically and without medical explanation. Conversion symptoms are also very common in patients with this disorder. The disorder tends to remain constant over time and has been shown to run in families. It is a condition grossly underrecognized by the internists and surgeons who see the majority of these patients, and who experience these patients as very difficult and complicated management problems.

In DSM-III-R the condition is listed as "somatization disorder," again focusing on the medical complaints. In the description accompanying the diagnostic criteria, the associated histrionic personality features are acknowledged, though they are not required for a diagnosis. DSM-III-R criteria for somatization disorder require endorsement of 14 of 37 possible symptoms to make a diagnosis. These criteria differ from the Perley-Guze criteria in the omission of "psychoform" (as distinguished from somatoform) symptoms—that is, anxiety, de-pressive, and psychotic-like symptoms. The abbreviated list of criterion symptoms in DSM-III-R is felt to permit diagnostic assessment with less time and effort than are required by the Perley-Guze checklist for Briquet's syndrome. DSM-III-R also provides a screening index composed of seven criterion symp-toms, with two positive symptoms constituting a positive screen for somatization disorder.

Our understanding of MPD could benefit from the lines of investigation that have validated Briquet's syndrome. Such studies will yield not only clear-cut diagnostic criteria for MPD but also exclusion criteria from other disorders, and will provide necessary follow-up data and family information for validation of MPD as a psychiatric diagnosis.

The Controversy

Two basic positions dominate the controversy over the phenomenology of MPD. One is the contention that MPD represents a psychiatric disorder in its own right with a unique and stable set of core symptoms and behaviors (Coons et al. 1988; Putnam et al. 1986). These core features are felt to provide confirmation of the independence of MPD as an entity. Laboratory evidence documenting physio-logical differences between the separate personalities in MPD patients is further evidence cited in support of this position. At the other extreme are skeptical opponents who insist that MPD doesn't exist, that it has one of two major etiol-ogies: (1) it is caused by willful malingering or by misguided individuals seeking out therapists who will endorse their condition; (2) it is an iatrogenic phenome-non artifactually brought about by therapists through misdiagnosis, suggestion, and hypnosis. Heated arguments between advocates of these opposing positions have occupied volumes of printed text. The pivotal question is: "Is it real?" (Putnam 1991a).

The contention of iatrogenesis implies that the diagnosis itself reflects a lack of competence of the clinician making it. The degree of respect bestowed upon MPD by the scientific community has been compared to the response elicited by ESP (Tozman & Pabis 1989). Ross (1989, p. 109) observed, "To diagnose MPD is a bit like admitting you believe in UFOs; it calls your professional reputation into question." Therefore, if one is to openly profess a conviction about this diagnosis, one puts one's reputation on the line. On the other hand, the compe-tence of those who resist making the MPD diagnosis is challenged by claims that they are not well trained; otherwise, they would not be "missing" the diagnosis. Such high stakes—calling one's competence and reputation into question—ap-pear to be a prominent symptom of the conflict, if not an integral part of the controversy over MPD, and may help explain the degree of emotional investment in the arguments about the disorder's existence.

Proponents of MPD

Kluft (1984a, p. 22) contends that most clinicians have "low indices of suspicion and high indices of skepticism" toward the existence of MPD. MPD enthusiasts claim that the skeptics are just plain missing it, either by failing to look for it or by not recognizing it when it is present. The general professional lack of awareness of the disorder is credited for "misdiagnosis" and failure to recognize the disorder (Dell 1988b), allegedly by clinicians untrained in the sensitive techniques of detection of the syndrome (Dell 1988b). The result is the passage, on average, of four to seven years from the onset of MPD to its diagnosis (Putnam et al. 1986; Rivera 1991; Ross & Norton 1989a; Ross et al. 1989b).

Proponents of MPD argue that most patients with the disorder are quiet, unassuming, shy, reserved individuals who do not seek the limelight or public attention (Franklin 1990; Herzog 1984; Putnam et al. 1984). According to Kluft (1985), most multiples actually try to disguise their condition. They are said to be secretive and reluctant to divulge clinical information (Franklin 1990; Kluft 1987b; Putnam et al. 1984), out of fear of either meeting with skepticism and rejection or being regarded as crazy (Coons 1980, 1984; Coons & Milstein 1986; Franklin 1990; Kluft 1987a; Putnam et al. 1986). Undoubtedly, most patients diagnosed with MPD have probably encountered one or more therapists who are skeptical of the disorder and unreceptive to complaints of symptoms related to MPD (Dell 1988b; Spiegel 1988). Some, according to Wilbur (1984b, p. 27), thus "test the doctor to find out whether or not they are heard and 'believed.' They may also test to find out if he or she approves of some or any of their behavior."

Kluft (1986) found that 50% of MPD patients withheld evidence of MPD at their first assessment, and 90% said they had at some time tried to hide the manifestations of MPD. In some cases, symptoms of MPD may not be volunteered because the individuals are unaware they have the disorder (Coons 1980, 1986a; Coons et al. 1988; Loewenstein 1989). It is thought that as few as 20% of MPD patients spend the majority of their adult lives in an overt MPD state (Kluft 1991). In Kluft's (1984a) series, 40% of multiples showed only subtle hints of MPD and 40% showed no overt signs at all. In that study, the diagnosis of MPD was inversely related to the degree of clarity of the symptom presentation. Patients who sought psychiatric help as self-diagnosed multiples were the least likely to be believed, and those without clear signs of MPD were discovered only by systematic efforts to uncover the disorder.

Most multiples who enter treatment do so not because of classical symptoms of MPD but because of affective, psychotic-like, or somatoform symptoms (Loewenstein 1989). Multiple personalities are virtually never the chief complaint (Kluft 1985; Stern 1988). Kluft (1984a, p. 22) reported that "florid and straightforward presentations are the tip of the iceberg . . . quasi-physical symptoms may mask MPD." Hacking (1991, p. 860) has observed that "The multiple-movement readily grants that patients don't walk in the door with a host of alters. They are painstakingly ferreted out."

Numerous articles encourage cultivation of clinical awareness of MPD and specifically recommend vigilance for key clinical indicators such as a history of incest, headaches, amnesias, loss of time, episodes of dazes or trances, inordinately rapid shifts in symptoms, and use of the collective "we" in self-reference. Other clinical signs that should alert clinicians are recurrent nightmares, depersonalized states, substance abuse, "seizures," multiple suicide attempts, major conversion symptoms, hallucinations, accusations of lying, Schneiderian symptoms, borderline features, polysomatoform symptoms, and a history of several previous diagnoses and failed treatments (Bliss 1980, 1984a; Brandsma & Ludwig 1974; Dell & Eisenhower 1990; Fagan & McMahon 1984; Franklin 1990; Kluft 1985, 1987a; Marcum et al. 1986; Putnam et al. 1984; Ross 1989, p. 96). In particular, "psychiatric patients with excellent hypnotic skills are suspect" as potential MPD cases (Bliss 1984a, p. 201).

Because the presentation of the disorder is often subtle and covert (Bliss 1988; Kluft 1989, 1991), clinicians may have to work very hard to elicit a history compatible with MPD. Kluft (1984) has specifically mentioned that "indirect inquiries" must be made about symptoms in patients who initially deny MPD. A number of sources have elaborated specialized techniques for collecting relevant information and probing for the defining symptoms of MPD (Franklin 1990; Kluft 1984a, 1985; Loewenstein 1991). Some have suggested that clinicians should routinely and carefully watch for signs of MPD among patients at risk such as rape victims (Ament 1987).

Coons (1984) recommends obtaining additional information that might provide evidence of MPD from sources external to the patient, such as family members, friends, coworkers, and hospital personnel. Evidence of subtle signs should be sought from these witnesses, specifically personality changes, a history of imaginary playmates in childhood, school difficulties, persistent lying, use of different names, use of the third person, and handwriting changes. Others have proposed hypnosis as the surest route to ascertain the necessary information. Bliss (1984a) and Solomon (1983) have suggested a novel application of the Minnesota Multiphasic Personality Inventory (MMPI) to screen for potential MPD cases, followed by hypnosis to confirm the diagnosis.

The use of hypnosis to elicit MPD is controversial. Leading researchers agree that even if hypnosis or suggestion might account for the creation of some personalities (Herzog 1984; Kluft 1982, 1987a; Kohlenberg 1973; McCurdy 1941; Spiegel 1988) or some cases (Coons 1980; Fahy 1988; Kampman 1976; Spanos et al. 1985), hypnosis (Bliss 1988; Braun 1984a; Coons 1988b; Horevitz & Braun 1984; Kluft 1982; Ludwig et al. 1972; Putnam et al. 1986; Ross et al. 1989b,d), and iatrogenesis (Horton & Miller 1972; Ross et al. 1989b,d; Silberman et al. 1985; Spiegel 1988; Sutcliffe & Jones 1962), do not explain away MPD. An analogous situation is the recognized ability of hypnosis to produce, they say, all the symptoms of hysteria (Bliss 1984c; Bramwell 1906), yet one would hardly argue that Briquet's syndrome is simply a product of hypnotic suggestion.

Evidence supporting the argument that hypnosis does not account for all cases of MPD was found by Ross' group (1989) with the discovery that only a third of the 236 patients they studied had been hypnotized prior to receiving the diagnosis of MPD. Putnam and colleagues (1986) detected no differences in clinical presentation, symptoms, or past history between patients who had been hypnotized and those who had not. A study by Ross and coworkers (1989e) compared MPD patients of psychiatrists specializing in MPD with MPD patients of other psychiatrists and found no differences between the two groups in demographics, diagnostic criteria met, number of personalities, or length of time to diagnosis. The only difference was that patients of the MPD specialists had more often worked as prostitutes and less often reported a history of sexual abuse. The authors concluded that their data provide evidence against the contention of iatrogenesis in MPD and compelling evidence supporting MPD as a genuine disorder with a consistent set of core features.

The idea of iatrogenesis in the emergence of MPD continues to be vigorously disputed. According to Ross (1989, p. 301), "The theory of iatrogenesis has caught on without a single supporting study. There is not a single documented case of iatrogenic false positive MPD reported in the entire world literature. Yet iatrogenesis is probably the most widely accepted etiological theory in psychiatry."

Bliss (1988) and Braun (1984a) argue that the alternate personalities routinely begin in childhood, long before subjects are ever introduced to hypnosis. The mean time of first splitting is typically reported to have been between the ages of 4 and 8 (Bliss 1980, 1984b; Coons & Milstein 1986; Coons et al. 1988; Fagan & McMahon 1984; Putnam et al. 1986) and almost always before age 12 (Putnam et al. 1986). Younger patients may remember further back than do adults: in one study, 8 of 11 adolescent patients retrospectively reported alternates beginning by age 3 (mean number, 3.05 years), and two subjects reported alternates beginning as early as 1 and 1.5 years of age (Dell & Eisenhower 1990).

Proponents point to documented physiologic differences between personality states in MPD as further evidence of its diagnostic validity. These claims are supported by the argument that these physiologic manifestations cannot be fully replicated by normals or professional actors simulating different personality states (Ross 1989, p. 58). The physiologic documentation cited includes findings of distinctive patterns among the various alternate personalities in studies of positron emission tomography (PET) scans, evoked potentials (Larmore et al. 1977; Ludwig et al. 1972; Putnam et al. 1984), voice prints (Putnam 1984), visual acuity, eye muscle balance, visual field size (Miller 1989), galvanic skin response (Bahnson & Smith 1975; Brende 1984; Larmore et al. 1977; Putnam et al. 1984), electroencephalographic patterns (Coons et al. 1982; Larmore et al. 1977), electromyography (Larmore et al. 1977), and cerebral blood flow (Mathew et al. 1985). Moreover, physiologic findings specific to particular ages of the alternate personalities being tested have been reported. These various lines of neurophysiologic investigation will be further examined in Chapter 3.

In spite of a lack of consensus on whether MPD actually represents a validated psychiatric disorder, proponents of MPD have proceeded to divide MPD into subtypes. Kluft (1991) has described a typology of MPD presentations that includes the following types of MPD:

Classic MPD

Latent MPD

Posttraumatic MPD

Extremely complex or fragmented MPD

Epochal or sequential MPD

Isomorphic MPD

Coconscious MPD

Possessioniform MPD

Reincarnation/mediumistic MPD

Atypical MPD

Secret MPD

Ostensible imaginary companionship MPD

Covert MPD

Puppeteering or passive-influence dominated MPD

Phenocopy MPD

Somatoform MPD

Orphan symptom MPD

Switch-dominated MPD

Ad hoc MPD

Modular MPD

Quasi-roleplaying MPD

Pseudo-false positive MPD

Skeptics

For many, the credibility of persons claiming to have MPD may be stretched by the excessive claims made about the disorder in the media and by popular dramatic and sensational depictions of it (Prasad 1985; Simpson 1988). Even without excessive claims, the fantastic nature of the manifestations of MPD may make it difficult for patients with this disorder to convince others of the veracity of their symptoms (Cohen and Giller 1991; Jeans 1976; Kluft 1984a). Prasad (1985, p. 301) writes, "The concept that more than one person may exist within one body is so alien to common sense that it borders on the supernatural."

Because MPD patients often present as theatrical or deceptive and may appear to be avoiding responsibility, clinicians find it easy to dismiss them as "immature, hysterical, borderline, or phonies" (Bliss 1988, p. 523). Ross (1989, p. 109) remarked on the "elaborate pretending" in MPD: "The patient *pretends* that she is more than one person, in a very convincing manner. She actually believes it herself." Kline (1990, p. 538) was "struck by the play-acting quality of many of these patients. It's as if the whole presentation is a monumental put-on." Kluft (1984d) described the need for therapists to "suspend disbelief" in order to work with MPD patients. Some patients may sense it if a therapist is skeptical about MPD. As a result, some persons seeking to be diagnosed with MPD apparently "move from therapist to therapist until 'achieving' a diagnosis" (Thigpen & Cleckley 1984, p. 64).

Skeptics have dismissed MPD as an artifact of covert or overt encouragement by such therapists of their patients' dramatic fantasies (Fahy 1988; Spanos et al. 1986; Spiegel 1988). In particular, hypnosis is a main target of these criticisms. Throughout history, recurrent concerns that hypnosis may cause or worsen MPD have emerged (Congdon et al. 1961; Cutler & Reed 1975; Dercum 1913, p. 254; Fahy 1989; Gruenewald 1971, 1977; Harriman 1942, 1943; Janet 1889; Kampman 1976; Prince 1890)—that it may in effect "create an artifact which it then 'finds' " (Kluft 1982, p. 230).

Putnam (1986) outlined four lines of circumstantial evidence linking hypnosis and MPD. The first piece of evidence is the steller hypnotizability characteristic of MPD patients (Braun 1984b), an association emphasized by Fahy (1988). Putnam's group (1983) found that 73% of therapists surveyed who used hypnosis with their MPD patients ranked them as highly hypnotizable relative to their other patients. A study by Bliss (1984c) rated MPD patients near the top of the Stanford Hypnotizability Scale and much higher than a control group. Supporting evidence for the association between hypnosis and MPD includes the finding that trance-like behavior in children, an autohypnotic phenomenon, is the single best predictor of childhood MPD. Further, a childhood history of strict discipline and punishment, akin to the family backgrounds and child abuse experienced by multiples, is thought to be associated with adult hypnotizability (Putnam 1986).

Putnam's second line of evidence is that a variety of symptoms reported by multiples can be induced by hypnosis in highly hypnotizable subjects without MPD, symptoms including amnesia, anesthesia, paralysis, auditory and visual hallucinations, and other conversion symptoms (Putnam 1986). Hypnosis has been equated with both "artificial hysteria" and hysteria (Bliss 1984c; Bramwell 1906) and is also associated with major conversion syndromes (Bliss 1984c). Merskey (1979, p. 169) wrote, "Hypnosis, both separately and in association with multiple personality, is a ready means for the production of hysterical symptoms."

The third link is the association of MPD with traumatic experiences, for which hypnosis is sometimes used as a treatment (Putnam 1986). The fourth line of evidence is the demonstration of hypnotically induced MPD-like phenomena in normal subjects in a number of studies (Putnam 1986). It is conceded, however, that these latter phenomena are not true analogues of MPD because they lack a number of characteristics; nevertheless, these studies are held by some as evidence of the influential power of hypnosis.

While proponents of MPD claim that hypnosis does not adequately account for the phenomenon (Bliss 1980, 1988; Braun 1984a; Coons 1988b; Franklin 1990; Horevitz & Braun 1984; Kluft 1982, 1989; Putnam et al. 1986; Ross et al. 1989b,d), Bliss (1980, 1983, 1984c, 1986, 1988) proposes that self-hypnosis does. Bliss (1980, p. 1395) states, "It seems likely that all hypnosis is self-hypnosis, with the hypnotist being a guide who directs the subjects to use capabilities that he already possesses." According to Bliss' theory, in highly hypnotizable individuals, abuse of self-hypnosis is the central mechanism accounting for the creation of the full MPD syndrome. In agreement, Tozman and Pabis (1989, p. 708) recommend that MPD instead be called *"dissociative disorder with self hypnotic personality characteristics."* Bliss has delineated his self-hypnosis theory of MPD in great detail in several articles (1980, 1983, 1984b, 1984c, 1985, 1986 1988), and other authors (Gruenewald 1971; Loewenstein 1987; Miller 1984; Ross 1984; Velek & Balon 1986) have described similar phenomena.

Bliss (1980, 1984c) further proposes self-hypnosis as the "prime mechanism" in a variety of "severe hysterical neuroses," Briquet's syndrome, and conversion disorder. The "self delusion" process of development of MPD described by Sutcliffe and Jones (1962) is probably a version of the self-hypnosis phenomenon. Paradoxically, Braun (1980) recommends self-hypnosis in the treatment of MPD to enhance relaxation and promote access to alternative personalities.

Ludolph (1985) questions the wisdom of using hypnosis in the treatment of MPD, given the evidence that MPD-like manifestations can be hypnotically induced (Kluft 1989). While hypnosis is advocated as a valuable tool to help uncover personalities and work with them (Allison & Schwarz 1980; Bliss 1980, 1984a; Brandsma & Ludwig 1974; Braun 1984c; Kluft 1982; Putnam et al. 1986; Salama 1980), experts (Bowers et al. 1971; Herzog 1984; Howland 1975; Kluft 1989) strongly caution that only the most skilled hypnotherapists should use hypnosis in the treatment of multiples because of the potential for fostering further dissociation with inept handling. They urge the exercise of utmost care by all who use hypnosis in the treatment of MPD lest they inadvertently create new personalities. Coons (1980) advises clinicians to take care that they do not suggest alternate personalities. Kluft (1982) reported an example of this, a patient who developed 18 iatrogenic alternates and "cascades of splits" due to mishandling by an inexperienced therapist who "tried seven procedures" on his first experience with hypnosis. Previous therapy, specifically errors in interview technique, is an identified shaping influence in Kluft's (1984c) four-factor theory of the etiology of MPD, which will be discussed in detail in Chapter 7.

One important clarification is in order. Kluft (1989) maintains that although MPD-like phenomena can be induced quite readily, the actual condition of MPD with its full manifestations cannot be created iatrogenically by technical errors on the part of inexperienced therapists. Such iatrogenically induced phenomena, he explains, bear "dramatic but superficial resemblance" to MPD but are not the real McCoy. The many examples of supposed iatrogenic cases of MPD are merely transient personality fragments, personality states, or overinterpretations on the part of their creators. Given the "imprecise nature of the definition of the terms 'personality' and 'personality state' " (Kluft 1989, p. 85) and the difficulties in distinguishing personality states from multiple personalities (Ross 1985), the arguments over whether MPD can be iatrogenically created become rather muddy.

A potential pitfall in the therapy of MPD is the enticement of the "sensational appeal" of these cases and the potential for overfascination and overinvestment by therapists treating them (Coons 1986a; Gruenewald 1977), a problem that could contribute to iatrogenesis, with or without hypnosis. Thigpen and Cleckley (1954), who themselves openly claimed skepticism about MPD, also experienced the fascination, "awe," "wonderment," and "breathless excitement" (Sutcliffe & Jones 1962) associated with this then rarely recognized condition, although they were circumspect, containing their enthusiasm and maintaining their perspective and judgment. Simpson (1988, p. 565) compared clinicians' "infatuation" with new MPD cases they have discovered with the reaction of "new parents, they can never miss an opportunity to show photographs, movies, or videos of their uniquely talented offspring, or to tell you their latest cute trick." Kluft (1989) warned of this danger of overfascination but indicated that it generally seems to be a reaction of inexperienced therapists. It is well recognized that reactions of undue fascination, anger, or irritation on the part of the therapist may be a warning that he or she is being manipulated or "duped" (Stern 1988, p. 217).

Simpson (1988) suggested that therapists may sometimes have an unconscious secondary and perhaps primary gain of their own in relation to these patients. Aldridge-Morris (1989, p. 16) even suggested the possibility that gullible patients are "taken for a ride by psychiatrists seeking financial and/or personal aggrandizement." Saltman and Solomon (1982, p. 1140) warned of a potential for therapists to "voyeuristically and intrusively" elicit prurient information such as a history of incest from patients "for the sake of the therapist's own gratification." A therapist prejudiced in favor of MPD or a clinician enraptured by "incredulous fascination" with the disorder might communicate this favor or interest to the patient, with strong effects within the therapeutic atmosphere. Cases might be unconsciously shaped through subtle encouragement and unintentional selective reinforcement by the therapist in this manner (Gruenewald 1977).

Spanos (1986) and coworkers (1985, 1986) espouse a "social psychological" model of the origins of MPD, a scenario they conceptualize as a "role enactment" phenomenon along the lines of "shaping" described by Sutcliffe and Jones (1962). According to this scenario, psychotherapists play a key role in the generation and maintenance of the condition. These therapists are described as being "on the lookout" (Spanos 1986) for signs of MPD to which they are sensitized through special interest in the disorder and with specialized knowledge in identifying features or alleged subtle indicators suggesting the disorder. Their subjects tend to be unhappy and insecure individuals interested in eliciting from their therapists concern, approval, and attention. These patients, who are also highly suggestible, manage, through presentation of their symptoms, often with unwitting guidance from their therapists, to evoke interest, encouragement, and validation from their therapists, along with information on the correct representation of MPD. Kluft (1989, p. 87) has observed that "for many MPD patients their relationship to their therapist is the most powerful and/or gratifying event of their lives." These patients, eager to please their therapists, may create more alternate personalities. They may also create more personalities in the hope of prolonging therapy.

According to the social psychological model of MPD, initially the patient presents symptoms hesitantly until he or she is convinced that the therapist can be trusted to not reject or ridicule the patient as subsequent symptoms emerge. Consistent with this model, Kluft (1989) has noted that with further encouragement and guidance, symptoms are gradually disclosed and develop in complexity in the process. The alternate personalities "mature and become more complex" with time in therapy (Bliss 1980, p. 1390). In this "mutual shaping" process the symptoms are selectively reinforced by the therapist, consciously or unconsciously, and in turn are further elaborated by the patient (Simpson 1988). Given this scenario, the observation that "specialists" in MPD can manage to uncover large numbers of unsuspected cases that previous clinicians have failed to identify (Spanos 1986) is not surprising.

Others seem to agree with this depiction of the process (Horton & Miller 1972; Kohlenberg 1973). Horton and Miller (1972, p. 151) wrote, "suggestion, in a patient with a hysterical personality, can reinforce any preexisting multiple personality ideas the patient might have. If a therapist speaks to one or another of the personalities, the idea that these are separate within the self can be supported."

In some cases, therapists have to convince the patient that he or she has MPD, and may help the patient name the alternate personalities, a practice going back to Janet, who "showed the important role of name-taking or name-giving" (Ellenberger 1970, p. 139): "Once baptized, the unconscious personality is more clear and definite; it shows its psychological traits more clearly" (Janet 1889, p. 318). Janet, however, probably did not consider this a routine, recommended practice.

Simpson (1988) described MPD as a folie à deux phenomenon between doctor and patient. The same connection was made by another author in an article entitled "Sybil: Grand hysterie or folie à deux?" (Victor 1975).

Simpson (1988, p. 565) stated:

> There is no convincing evidence that MPD is a naturally occurring condition, let alone a distinct diagnosis. It is a symptom complex that may be superimposed on other psychopathologies, consequent upon the unfortunate matching of a susceptible patient with a susceptible therapist and trainer. The diagnosis is dysfunctional, focusing attention selectively in a way that will almost invariably worsen the condition. . . .

Simpson (1988, p. 565) notes that MPD arises "when a bright, suggestible patient meets a bright, suggestible physician convinced that MPD is an important diagnosis" Hacking (1991, p. 846) briefly summarized these concerns: "Skeptics worry about patients imitating and thereby faking symptoms, and about doctors training patients." In sum, he feels (p. 860), "It takes two to multiply."

Decker (1986, p. 43) remarked that cases of MPD often "started out as descriptions of short fugue states followed by amnesia; they ended up as prolonged, complicated, and mysterious cases of multiple personalities." Hacking (1991, p. 860) described alternate personalities as "roles that a patient can grow into rather than adopt." Bliss (1980, p. 1389) observed that "as the need arises more personalities may be created . . . [whose] various functions [depend] on the particular needs of the patient." It is almost the rule that increasing numbers of alternate personalities may blossom forth in therapy for MPD (Kluft 1989; Spanos 1986; Spanos et al. 1986). Sutcliffe and Jones (1962, p. 248) have commented on the tendency for "the most luxuriant growth and long life of additional personalities" to occur in protracted hypnotherapy.

Simpson (1988, p. 565) wrote:

> the extent of the patient's pathology is directly proportional to [the] amount and intensity [of therapy], and shows the most evolved and disturbed anomalies in the most intensively studied cases. It appears to be the norm that further "personalities", often more entertaining and rewarding for the audience, emerge in therapy. . . .

The course of disclosure of the personalities of the famous case of Bianchi (the notorious "Los Angeles Hillside Strangler") is an example of increasing numbers of alternate personalities with exposure to a therapist. Because one of

Bianchi's evaluators (Orne et al. 1984) suspected he was faking, he tested Bianchi by telling him that multiples usually have three or more personalities—Bianchi had only two. Almost immediately, Bianchi produced another personality. The second appearance of an alternate personality was apparently more dramatic than the first, and the next time he was evaluated, he had "changed dramatically" and "appeared as a caricature of a macho man" (Orne et al. 1984, p. 130).

A simulation study by Spanos and colleagues (1985) discovered that in 40 normal subjects receiving hypnosis to elicit multiple personalities in a manner similar to that used with Bianchi, 60% adopted a personality with a different name compared to none of 40 nonhypnotized controls. Furthermore, role-playing "multiples" presented themselves as more pathologic on posttesting than prior to the experimental manipulation (Spanos et al. 1986). The authors considered this experiment as evidence supporting the model of MPD as a role that persons learn to enact as they gain increasing exposure to information about the disorder and reinforcement of their enactment of it.

In cases where entertainment and audience factors are involved, Simpson (1988) believes that further personalities are likely to emerge. In the celebrated case of Eve there were just three personalities in the first account, *The Three Faces of Eve,* and these were said to have been successfully fused in that account, as well as in her first autobiographical account that followed. In her second autobiography (the third account overall), she reported that right before the release of her first autobiography she had developed additional personalities, and these increased to a total of 22. This case has been described as "therapy-nurtured" (Sutcliffe & Jones 1962).

Tozman and Pabis (1989, p. 709) have emphatically criticized mental health professionals, the media, and the legal system for their contributions to the genesis of MPD:

> We regard MPD as a dissociative phenomenon of exceedingly rare occurrence if it occurs at all. Unsurprisingly, it seems related to hypnotizability. The accentuation and "epidemic" of this rare, iatrogenic disorder does no justice to scientific psychiatry, generating media and literature distortions and misinformation. It distressingly often provides untenable and flamboyant legal defense maneuvers for serial killers and others of ill repute (Watkins, 1984). Psychiatry should not reinforce the mystical and bizarre.

In clinical practice, however, therapists may have to reinforce symptoms in order to uncover them. Therapists may have to "help" their MPD patients "remember" symptoms or historical events and traumas, which is often accomplished through hypnosis and typically evolves into a powerful emotional episode of abreaction. One study found that a childhood history of sexual or physical abuse is reported by hypnotized patients significantly more often than those not hypnotized—the explanation being that hypnosis facilitates access to information in heavily defended dissociated states in these patients (Ross & Norton 1989b).

Herzog (1984, p. 219) argues that some of these kinds of memories are unsubstantiated or exaggerated, "probably wishes and/or fears that became psychic reality. All of these memories, most of which are sharp and vivid, probably contain a high degree of imaginative elaboration, given the high degree of suggestibility and imagic thinking of these patients." Spanos and colleagues (1986, p. 310) assert that the retrospective recollections of MPD patients may be strongly influenced by their own "conceptions of the traumatic and childhood origins of psychopathology, and may be organized and elaborated into biographical accounts that serve to legitimate an ongoing self-presentation as a multiple personality patient."

Greaves (1980) warns about the potential for falsification of memory in retrospective interrogations of patients with numerous alternates. These patients, with recent dissociations, may experience them as historical events in the past, confusing in their memory the conditions under which the recollection arose. Ross (1989, p. 105) reported a phenomenon he termed "hypermnesia, which is an unusually complete memory." He wondered, however, "How much is accurate recall, and how much is elaboration?" Aldridge-Morris (1989, pp. 75–76) credits Gruenewald with the idea that "the separate 'life histories' apparent in multiple personalities actually represent secondary elaborations of the nuclear fantasies . . . fantasy has become reality." These concerns mirror Freud's thinking when he reformulated his ideas on early sexual molestation in hysteria, deciding that those memories were not of real experiences but constituted merely fantasies of incest (Bliss 1984c; Freud 1948a, 1954). Spiegel (1988) recommends obtaining outside corroboration whenever possible.

MPD affords several benefits to patients with the disorder. One obvious benefit is that symptoms of MPD represent a highly effective means of gaining attention, a recognized motivator of therapists as well as patients (Chodoff 1987; Simpson 1988; Thigpen & Cleckley 1984)—a process also inherent in somatization disorder.

Kohlenberg (1983) has illustrated attention-seeking factors associated with iatrogenic maintenance of the MPD symptoms in a case report. In an experiment with an MPD patient he selectively reinforced behaviors associated with one of the personalities, which resulted in a dramatic increase in the frequency of appearance of that personality. Later extinction trials brought these behaviors back to baseline in frequency. Kohlenberg (p. 139) reflected that "the glamorous and dramatic nature of multiple personality also resulted in a great deal of professional staff attention to the patient" that was in itself reinforcing.

Criminal offenders are a special patient population with a strong motivation for secondary gain, some of whom think they can escape responsibility for criminal behavior using an MPD defense. Bianchi, the Hillside Strangler, tried unsuccessfully to use MPD to avoid the consequences of his heinous crimes (Orne et al. 1984). Coons and colleagues (1988) recommended caution in making this diagnosis in forensic cases. Coons (1984, p. 63) has pointed out the special difficulties in diagnosing MPD in forensic settings where "individuals may lie and material may be unconsciously fabricated under either hypnosis or amytal." He (Coons 1988b, pp. 3, 6, 8) cited another case of "flagrant abuse of forensic hypnosis" that involved "extremely leading questions" in eliciting MPD symptoms, resulting in "grievous harm" to the patient.

MPD is also thought to be exceptionally well suited for providing all groups of patients prone to secondary gain a means of avoiding responsibility for certain behaviors (Simpson 1988; Thigpen & Cleckley 1984). Kluft (1985, 1987a) described a subset of MPD patients who "often value their MPD." On hospital wards, the other patients complain that MPD patients can evade accountability and responsibilities (Kluft 1984d), and the alternates manipulate others.

In India, where hysterical possession is considered an equivalent of MPD, Adityanjee and colleagues (1989) report that the "possessing spirit," through the patient, makes various demands on family members or significant others, who typically "humbly comply" with them. This virtually "ensures a recurrence," because this behavioral episode has gained the patient manipulative ends as well as attention from valued others.

MPD may serve as an outlet for expressing certain impulses and behaviors that would otherwise be considered unacceptable, such as sexual acting out, physical aggression, or substance abuse (Bliss 1980; Bliss & Larson 1985; Coons 1980, 1984; Putnam et al. 1986; Sutcliffe & Jones 1962; Thigpen & Cleckley 1984). An alternate personality may abuse substances or kidnap and rape women, while the core personality would never do such a thing (Bliss 1980) and thus does not "own" the behavior. This fits with descriptions of the alternate personalities as typically being irresponsible and acting out (Prince 1906; Putnam et al. 1986), with the host personality typically presenting as proper and retiring (Kluft 1985; Spiegel 1988; Velek & Balon 1986).

The alternate personalities are often created to manage unpleasant emotions that the patient does not wish to endure (Allison & Schwarz 1980; Bliss 1980; Coons 1980, 1984; Fahy et al. 1989; Kluft 1985; Larmore et al. 1977; Ludwig et al. 1972; Putnam 1984; Thigpen & Cleckley 1984; Wilbur 1984a). Specific emotions such as rage or hurt are assigned a specific personality (Bliss 1980). Some professionals (Bliss 1980; Fahy et al. 1989; Prasad 1985) have indicated that the creation of alternate personalities can be a means of ascribing to others (the alternates) strong, painful, or unattractive emotions they don't want to acknowledge—by personifying and naming them.

MPD may also provide a means of face saving to account for personal inadequacies and failings. Because many clinicians pinpoint early childhood difficulties as origins of adult psychopathology, it is thought that reports of extreme trauma in early life may dominate the histories of MPD patients as an excuse for current difficulties or anticipated failures, to explain "How I got this way" (Spanos et al. 1986).

It can be seen, therefore, how primary and secondary gain can be strong reinforcers of the condition in many ways once the syndrome is fully developed and a part of the patient's life. Simpson (1988, p. 535) writes:

> Spontaneous remission is probably the norm, unless the patient becomes engaged with a clinician already primed and interested in the condition. It seems to be one of the few conditions which almost invariably get worse in therapy. . . . Where the health care system or health insurance does not subsidize indulgence, the condition simply does not occur.

It has been suggested that MPD enthusiasts comprise a "professional subculture" of mental health professionals who share several common denominators: the practice of hypnosis, psychoanalytically oriented therapy, and intense therapy over protracted periods of time (Aldridge-Morris 1989, p. 43). While these elements may be particularly common among therapists who recognize and treat MPD, there are growing contingents of therapists working with MPD who do not share these characteristics.

Discussion

Proponents of MPD assert that MPD is real and constitutes a valid diagnosis, whereas skeptics allege that MPD is an iatrogenic or faked condition. These two sets of arguments, independently persuasive as either may seem, do not get at the essence of the validity of MPD. Evaluation of these arguments in the context of the established process of diagnostic validation will aid in determining to what extent the diagnosis of MPD is supported by research evidence.

The first step of the validation process, description of the condition, draws upon demographic and clinical information about race, sex, age at onset, precipitating factors, symptom clusters, and other descriptive items to help define the clinical picture in explicit detail. DSM-III-R lists very brief inclusion criteria for MPD: the existence within a person of two or more distinct personalities that apparently take over complete control of the self. While lacking precision, these criteria are accompanied by a more detailed textual description of the disorder.

Hacking (1991, p. 843) suggests that "it is a sensible research program to try to identify some features of these people over and above their overt behavior." Considerable information on demographics, clinical description of symptoms, and certain descriptive items is now available. Ross and colleagues (1989d) have provided some data supporting the notion that MPD is a stable disorder with a characteristic set of core symptoms that seems distinct from other disorders, although rigorous systematic studies utilizing controls are needed to confirm these indications. Current knowledge of the clinical phenomenology of MPD by itself, however, cannot be considered either proof or disproof that MPD represents a valid diagnostic entity. The clinical phenomenology and the data describing it constitute, unfortunately, only one of the five elements of the process necessary for validation of a psychiatric or any medical disorder.

In apparent agreement on the insufficiency of current data to confirm MPD as a validated diagnosis, a reviewer (Reich 1991) of a recent book on MPD (Ross 1989) has independently observed that "the field has relatively little empirical support at the present time" (p. 1085) and has optimistically stated that "The problem with this book seems to be that it was written too early. In a few years, when the empirical evidence . . . has accumulated a bit more depth, this type of book would be of more interest" (p. 1085).

Many investigators have been enticed into elaborate arguments for or against the existence of MPD by claims about whether actors can be taught to simulate MPD with documented physiologic differences between "personalities." Conclusions from experiments on normal subjects such as college students or actors, however, cannot be generalized to bona fide patients suffering from MPD (Putnam 1989b; Ross 1989, pp. 58, 66). This point is best illustrated by analogy. A study showing that college students could be taught to limp in a manner that consistently convinced physicians that they suffered from osteoarthritis would not prove that osteoarthritis is not a genuine medical disorder (Ross 1989, p. 58), and a patient who can successfully simulate a myocardial infarction does not prove that coronary artery disease does not exist (Guze 1977, 1978; Guze & Helzer 1985).

This same logical flaw was pointed out by critics (Farber 1975; Guze & Helzer 1985; Spitzer 1976) of the widely acclaimed report by Rosenhan (1973) describing how trained actors were able to fool psychiatrists into believing they were psychiatrically ill; the report claimed that diagnostic labels are therefore unreliable and worthless, if not damaging. This report has been cited as support for the notion that mental illness does not exist. Spitzer (1976) countered this report with the argument that the ability of actors to outsmart psychiatrists by their simulation of a psychiatric disorder is not relevant to whether a particular psychiatric disorder exists. Farber (1975, p. 589) concluded, "One cannot establish the unrealiability or uselessness of any diagnostic method by showing that pathological symptoms can be faked."

Experiments on actors and studies artificially producing symptoms in patients lie outside the arena of the five-phase use of the laboratory investigation of genuine MPD. Even if some symptoms can be induced by hypnosis or suggestion in normal subjects or even in some patients, this could not explain all MPD cases, such as those never exposed to hypnosis or overt suggestion (Spiegel 1988).

Discussions about the validity of MPD also need to address diagnostic issues in terms not only of inclusion criteria, but also of exclusion criteria. In medicine, similar clinical features and laboratory findings are often components of more than one or even a variety of conditions. For example, chest pain may be a symptom of a heart attack, esophageal spasm, pulmonary embolism, or a panic attack. Blood in a urine sample may result from kidney stones, a bladder tumor, a bleeding disorder, or urethral trauma. In delineating a discrete disorder for research investigation as well as for use in clinical management, it is necessary to specify exclusion criteria so that other disorders do not contaminate the disorder of interest. If patients with other disorders or borderline or doubtful cases are included in a sample that is presumed to be pure or homogeneous, further work with that population will yield muddled results (Feighner et al. 1972; Robins & Guze 1970).

Exclusion criteria have generally not been addressed in arguments over the validity of MPD or in the diagnostic criteria for MPD as specified in DSM-III-R. How is the disorder different from somatization disorder or from borderline personality disorder? Are there unique characteristics that can clearly segregate MPD from other disorders with high comorbidities to MPD? If amnesia is not present, can the diagnosis be made? Which of the coexisting disorders is primary (manifested first) or superordinate (more pertinent to the course and treatment)? These are the more pithy questions.

Most of the attention to "proving" the existence of MPD has been focused on neurophysiologic investigation in an attempt to document measurable changes in physiologic function among alternate personalities. Consistent and reliable laboratory findings are unavailable for the common psychiatric disorders, however, and are thus not considered necessary to diagnostic validation in psychiatry at this time. If such findings could be documented in MPD, this would be the first disorder to gain laboratory validation. Putnam (1986) concluded that no scientific study is likely to succeed in proving the existence of MPD by documenting physiologic differences among alternate personalities in a single patient on some measurable dimension, despite claims in popular media that this has been done. The absence of sufficient documentation, however, no more disproves MPD as a distinct entity than it does with the other common psychiatric disorders.

Although information obtained from follow-up studies is another key element in the five-phase validation process, data from follow-up studies have not occupied much space in the volumes of argument over the existence of MPD. Should patients initially identified with MPD be discovered to suffer from other disorders that could account for the original symptom picture, it would suggest that the originally identified patients constituted a heterogenous group rather than a pure sample of patients suffering from a distinct disorder; if time proved the disorder to remain unchanged, it would support the validity of the diagnosis by natural history and common prognosis. Many questions remain to be answered by follow-up studies to extend the validation process. Does MPD regularly remit or does it tend to be chronic? What problems no longer persist after the personalities integrate, and what symptoms remain? Do the comorbid disorders remit with fusion?

Finally, family studies are a valuable element in the validation of MPD. Because other psychiatric disorders have been shown to run in families, it seems

logical to look for a familial link in MPD as well. An increased prevalence of
MPD in close relatives of a distinctly defined homogeneous group of patients
with the MPD syndrome would strongly support the validity of the disorder.
Familial transmission of other polysymptomatic, polysyndromic disorders such
as Briquet's syndrome and borderline personality with MPD seems likely, but
there are as yet no systematic data with answers.

There is a great need for prospective follow-up studies in this patient population. The problem with the argument that MPD cannot be an artifact of hypnosis or therapist suggestion because MPD usually begins in childhood is that
such reports are retrospective and prone to the distortions of recollection, which
is a particular risk in studies of suggestible patients. Aldridge-Morris (1989, p.
47) speaks of a "crying need for longitudinal research which would follow up
the life careers of the dramatically increasing number of victims of child abuse."
To start with, means of identification of high-risk populations need to be developed so that they can be followed over time for prospective study.

There is much work to be done. Recent studies are now seriously struggling
with the first item of the Robins and Guze methods—outlining a consistent clinical description—and these studies are starting to provide some information that
is consistent across studies. Laboratory investigation, delineation from other disorders, follow-up studies, and family studies all have yet to yield consistent
findings.

Chapter 3 will describe in more detail the work that has been done on clinical description of the disorder, and will review available information about comorbidity, familiality, and long-term outcome. Laboratory investigation of physiologic markers will be discussed further in that chapter, followed by a review
of findings from psychological testing in Chapter 4.

The bottom line is that the impassioned and complex arguments about the
authenticity, etiology, and nosologic status of MPD cannot be resolved without
adequate information describing and delineating the disorder through systematic
investigation (Bliss 1985). Kluft (1985, p. 3) calls for "active research rather
than fruitless debate." The five-phase validation process described by Robins
and Guze and colleagues is a time-honored and well-tested model appropriate to
the task. Future studies will have many opportunities to address the challenges
these arguments pose.

3

Current knowledge about MPD

This chapter will summarize current epidemiologic knowledge about MPD. It should serve as a useful backdrop to the popular accounts of the illness that will be presented in Chapter 6.

Early publications on MPD consisted of case reports and anecdotal accounts. The first systematic study of a series of MPD patients was not published until 1980 (Bliss 1980). This was followed in the second half of that decade by a handful of similar studies. These efforts suffered from methodologic difficulties including very small numbers of subjects, unstandardized data collection, and lack of controls. Such limitations are expected in the early stages of systematic clinical research on any topic, however. Initial studies of any clinical syndrome frequently fail to meet rigorous criteria. Their greatest contribution may be clarification of the questions that further research should address and the methods it should use. In the study of MPD, the clinical descriptions provided in case reports and anecdotal descriptions have allowed more rigorous studies to proceed in a not uncharted direction.

Coons and coworkers (Coons & Milstein 1986; Coons et al. 1988) have pointed out intrinsic difficulties in the systematic study of patients with MPD. Given the uncommon nature of the disorder, a great deal of time and effort may be required for investigators to amass sufficient numbers of patients to achieve statistical power. Until recently, retrospective or anecdotal reporting has been the only realistic means of amassing data on MPD (Coons et al. 1988). In spite of the fact that other psychiatric disorders such as somatization disorder are as rare as MPD (Swartz et al. 1991, p. 227), however, adequate prospective studies with sufficient numbers of patients have been carried out for these other disorders. Theoretically, the same should be achievable with similar methodologic rigor in the investigation of MPD. Coons (1988a) has suggested that in the future, multicenter studies may provide the means for compiling enough prospective data for meaningful statistical analysis.

Several authors have presented useful information from retrospective analyses of cases (Boor 1982; Greaves 1980; Sutcliffe & Jones 1962; Taylor & Martin 1944). Others have dealt with methodologic difficulties by collecting data in novel ways, such as by sending questionnaires to colleagues inquiring about their patients, a strategy that has yielded information on large numbers of cases from many different sources (Putnam et al. 1986; Ross et al. 1989a).

A number of recent studies have collected data from consecutive series of patients with MPD, the most noteworthy example being the carefully designed and executed study by Coons and colleagues (1988a) of 50 MPD cases. Few controlled studies of MPD have been reported (Bliss 1980, 1984a; Bernstein & Putnam 1986; Coons & Milstein 1986; Kluft 1982), and these have appeared only in the last decade. Kluft, Braun, Bliss, Putnam, Coons, and Ross are among the early pioneers of the study of MPD, a subject poorly understood before their time. They have contributed a great deal to collective knowledge about MPD. These researchers and others have amassed extensive information about the clinical description and comorbidity of MPD, which will be reviewed, along with limited available family data, in this chapter.

Clinical Description of MPD

Putnam (1991b, p. 497) asserts that "Perhaps the strongest support for the construct validity of MPD as a diagnosis rests on the well-replicated clinical phenomenology of the disorder." Indeed, several recent studies have consistently reported on certain characteristic clinical features of the disorder.

A summary of selected demographic and clinical findings from recent studies is presented in Table 3-1. While these studies represent the best efforts to learn more about MPD, they contain, in addition to the methodologic limitations already mentioned, other flaws in varying combinations. Such problems include inadequate comparison with controls, selection bias, low response rates, lack of blind assessment, data collection with imprecise or unstandardized methods such as unstructured interviews, reliance on chart review, and drawing conclusions not warranted from the available data. Some of these problems have previously been pointed out by Coons and colleagues (1988) and by Putnam and coworkers (1986). Despite these limitations, however, available studies have provided a base of information that is beginning to shape the phenomenologic picture of MPD. A number of consistent findings illuminating basic aspects of the disorder have emerged from these studies.

It can be seen from Table 3-1 that MPD is a disorder diagnosed predominantly among women around the age of 30. The onset is typically in childhood, often reported retrospectively as having begun as early as 5 or 10 years of age (Bliss 1980, 1984b; Coons et al. 1988; Coons & Milstein 1986; Putnam 1991a). The mean number of alternate personalities varies from 6 to 16 in adults and is 24 in adolescents (Dell & Eisenhower 1990). Aside from a recent household survey study by Ross (1991), there have been no systematic attempts to determine the rates of this disorder in the general population (Putnam 1986; Ross 1989, p. 90), and the actual prevalence of this disorder remains unknown. The best estimates project the incidence of MPD in the general population to be around 1 in 100 (Ross 1991).

A history of childhood abuse is almost the norm for patients suffering with MPD, with as many as 96% or 98% of MPD patients reporting this (Coons et al. 1988; Putnam et al. 1986; Rivera 1991). Rates of childhood sexual abuse are higher than rates of physical abuse in all the studies reporting on both sexual and physical abuse histories in Table 3-1. A majority of patients also report having been adult victims of sexual assault or rape. A history of suicidality is quite common (Table 3-1), as it is in patients with Briquet's syndrome (American Psychiatric Association 1987, p. 262; Morrison 1989b).

Coons and colleagues (1988) reported that 84% of multiples in their series complained of sexual dysfunction, most often inhibited sexual desire and anorgasmia. Sexual promiscuity is frequent (Coons & Milstein 1986), and transvestism and transsexuality are also reported (Coons 1984). Two of the 20 subjects in the Coons and Milstein (1986) study were lesbian, and 2 of 10 subjects in Coons' (1984) series were bisexual.

Despite unusual reports of high-functioning MPD patients (Kluft 1986), individuals with this disorder have classically been severely ill and often profoundly disabled by their conditions (Dell & Eisenhower 1990; Greaves 1980; Horevitz & Braun 1984; Prasad 1985; Rivera 1991; Ross 1989, p. 6; Ross et al. 1989b; Schreiber 1973; Wilbur 1984a). Schreiber (1973) noted that the schizophrenics Wilbur had seen were not as ill as Sybil, and Ross (1989, p. 56) explains that "MPD patients are among the most disturbed individuals who seek the services of mental health professionals." Greaves (1980, p. 580) has derived confirmation of the reality of MPD by "look[ing] at the lives of persons with this condition. The pain, the chaos, and misery they experience is unsurpassed in the literature, and part of the emotional impact and drama of the condition arises out of the pathos that surrounds them."

The severity and disability that can be associated with MPD would seem to argue against iatrogenesis of the condition in the manner described by Simpson (1988), who hypothesizes the occurrence of the symptoms in the context of indulgence by medical professionals. It is difficult to imagine illness of this severity and chronicity originating in simple feigning or therapist suggestion.

In one study, 55% of MPD patients were receiving financial assistance due to their inconsistent ability to work imposed by the dissociative symptoms (Rivera 1991). Reports of expenditures of "millions of dollars" on "ineffective and counterproductive treatment and hospital care before diagnosis" (Rivera 1991, p. 81) are further testimony to the severity and chronicity that can be associated with this disorder. Recent information, however, indicates that untreated community cases may be much less disabled by the condition than these prominent patients found in medical settings, and that MPD may be more prevalent in communities than clinical information would suggest (Ross 1991).

It is likely that a wide range of disability is associated with this disorder. Many factors may underlie this variability. Examination of comorbid diagnoses with their associated disabilities may clarify additional sources of impairment in the overall social functioning of individual MPD patients.

Table 3-1 *Multiple Personality Studies*

	Putnam et al. (1986)	Ross et al. (1989a)	Rivera (1991)	Ross et al. (1990c)	Coons et al. (1988)	Coons and Milstein (1986)	Horevitz and Braun (1984)	Bliss (1980)	Bliss (1984)	Kluft (1982)
N	100	236	185	102	50	20	33	14	32	54
Methods	Questionnaires to clinicians interested in MPD (40% return)	Questionnaires to professional association members (10% response)	Questionnaires distributed at MPD conference (26% return)	Dissociative Experiences Scale, Dissociative Disorders Interview Schedule	Consecutive cases seen by author. RDC and DSM-III criteria	MMPI, interview	Chart review	Questionnaire	MMPI, questionnaire	DSM-III criteria
Controls	None	None	None		None	Nonschizophrenic inpatients	None	Hospital employees	Church members, nurses, students	None
Female	92%	88%	92%	92%	92%	85%	73%	100%	63%	73%
Mean age	31	31		29	29	29	35	30	Not reported	Range of 2 to >30

								Not reported
No. of alternates								
Mean	13.3	15.7			6.3	Not reported	Not reported	Not reported
Median	9	8			4			
Mode	3							
History of childhood abuse								
Physical	75%	75%	89%	82%	60%	60%		40% F, 32% M
Sexual	83%	79%	98%	90%	68%	65%		60% F, 27% M
Ever raped or sexually assaulted	48%	67% F 64% M			24%	30%	64%	
Attempted suicide	61% serious 71% nonlethal gestures (1% completed)	72% (2% completed)		73%		60%	91%	81% F 77% M

Comorbidity and Delineation from Other Psychiatric Disorders

Diagnostic overlap

MPD significantly overlaps with a variety of other disorders. Kluft (1987b) observed that MPD is rarely seen in the absence of other psychiatric disorders. Comorbid diagnoses reported in various studies are presented in Table 3-2. Having three or four disorders in addition to MPD is typical.

Personality disorders and somatization disorder are the most frequent comorbid disorders, and conversion disorder is very common. MPD patients also have a mix of other diagnoses, including high rates of substance abuse, posttraumatic stress disorder, affective disorder, anxiety disorders, multiple phobias, anorexia nervosa, and superobesity (Bliss 1983) (Table 3-2). There is disagreement about schizophrenia, which was a common misdiagnosis in the past. Comorbidity with schizophrenia, however, is not sustained in studies utilizing DSM-III and DSM-III-R criteria. Coons' group (1988) found that schizophrenia was definitively absent in their systematic study of 50 MPD patients.

The variety of comorbid diagnoses applied to MPD patients is understandable when the symptoms they report are examined. The literature describes high rates of a variety of symptoms of many diagnoses in widely differing categories. These patients exhibit "a plethora of symptoms referable to all major psychiatric syndromes" (Bliss 1984a, p. 146). Bliss (1984a, p. 197) compiled a list of disorders whose symptoms are common to MPD patients, including "anxiety states, hysteria, obsessional neuroses, phobic states, depression and mania, schizophrenia, alcoholism, sociopathy, and hyperactivity." Multiples also complain of a variety of autonomic symptoms (Bliss 1980). Affective complaints may include "severe" depression in 70% to 100% (Bliss 1980; Coons & Milstein 1986; Coons et al. 1988; Putnam et al. 1986), manic symptoms in 22% (Putnam et al. 1986), and "high periods" in 73% (Bliss 1980). Because of these striking associations, MPD may be best conceptualized as a polysymptomatic, polysyndromic disorder.

Putnam and colleagues (1984, p. 174) observed, "Like neurosyphilis, MPD is a chronic illness that may mimic the gamut of psychiatric syndromes, as well as many somatic conditions, especially neurologic, gastrointestinal, and cardiac disorders." Patients with Briquet's syndrome exhibit a classic pattern of reporting high rates of symptoms of practically every disorder. Descriptions of the comorbidity in Briquet's syndrome are virtually identical to the comorbidity associated with MPD: "There is scarcely one [nervous disease] which may not be simulated by this Protean malady [Briquet's syndrome]" (Gowers 1888, p. 935); "There is . . . no symptom-complex of somatic illness that may not have its hysterical 'double'" (Walshe 1963, p. 361); "hysteria" has been called the "mocking-bird of nosology" (Johnson 1849, p. v).

	Putnam et al. (1986)	Ross et al. (1989)	Rivera (1991)	Ross et al. (1990)	Coons et al. (1988)	Coons (1984)	Coons and Milstein (1986)	Horevitz and Braun (1984)	Bliss (1986)	Bliss (1980)	Kluft (1982)
Mean no. of other diagnoses	(3.6)*	(2.8)	(3)		3.8 (2.3)						
Personality disorder	(50%)	(58%)			84%						69%
Borderline			(37%)	64%	56% (10%)			70%			23%
Antisocial					45%	20%					
Substance abuse	53% (23%)	(31%)			45%						
Alcohol	27%		55%	33%	35% (24%)	10%	45%				
Drugs	31%		57%	28%†	20% (28%)	50%	55%				
Schizophrenia	(50%)	(41%)	(33%)	(46%)	0 (24%)						
Affective disorder	70%	(64%)	(46%)	91% (27%)	45% (54%)		75%				
Anxiety disorder		(44%)		(46%)							
Somatization disorder/ Briquet's syndrome	(19%)	(19%)		61%	50%	80%			76%	?100%	33%
Conversion disorder					10%	60%	40%			93%	
Eating disorder	39%	(16%)			(10%)						

*Figures in parentheses indicate diagnoses that subjects received from other physicians prior to the diagnosis of MPD, and figures without parentheses represent disorders determined by the authors of the study.

†Ten percent reported intravenous drug use.

This symptomatic heterogeneity is a challenge to the validity of Briquet's syndrome, and prompted Liskow (1988) to suggest that additional follow-up and family studies are still needed to delineate Briquet's syndrome from other disorders that frequently accompany it. Stability of Briquet's syndrome over time in the presence of the other disorders must be documented by follow-up studies that demonstrate that Briquet's syndrome does not follow the courses of its co-morbid disorders but behaves in the same way it does when it is not accompanied by these other disorders. Family studies are also needed to determine the degree to which Briquet's syndrome is transmissible in families separately from its comorbid disorders. Similar work needs to be done in the study of MPD to clarify whether the MPD or its comorbid disorders persist over time, and whether it runs in families separately from Briquet's syndrome and borderline personality.

Features specific to MPD

In spite of the broad spectrum of psychiatric and neurologic symptoms associated with MPD (Bliss et al. 1983; Kluft 1985), Ross and colleagues (1990c) maintain that MPD patients do not just report more symptoms in general but report a selective "profile" of MPD symptoms that a malingerer cannot fake unless he or she has this kind of information (which is now widely available in a variety of media sources and in extensively circulated popular biographical accounts of MPD such as *Sybil* [Schreiber 1973] and *The Three Faces of Eve* [Thigpen & Cleckley 1957]). Ross and colleagues do not explicitly list the components of this MPD profile in their article, but are apparently referring to a set of characteristic features of MPD including multiple symptoms of various disorders, a history of childhood trauma, self-destructive behaviors, extrasensory experiences, and dissociative symptoms.

In the same article, Ross and colleagues also defined a list of "secondary features" of MPD including hallucinations of voices, amnesias, depersonalization, use of the plural in self-reference, and other characteristic features. They described the secondary features of MPD as being "pathognomonic" for MPD when five or more of these symptoms occur in the presence of the MPD profile. Presumably, however, any overreporting subject could also report all these symptoms excessively. Patients with Briquet's syndrome and other subjects with a general overreporting tendency could potentially yield a profile much like that of MPD patients: large numbers of symptoms and features of virtually every diagnosis.

Psychotic features

MPD patients report very high rates of psychotic symptoms. Recent studies have reported an average of four to six Schneiderian symptoms per patient (Kluft 1987b; Ross et al. 1989e, 1990b,c), and 90% of MPD patients in one study endorsed three or more Schneiderian symptoms (Ross et al. 1990c). Specific psychotic complaints may include auditory hallucinations in 32 to 72% (Bliss 1980, 1986; Bliss et al. 1983; Coons & Milstein 1986; Putnam et al. 1986; Ross et al. 1989e), visual hallucinations in 16 to 72% (Bliss 1980; Bliss et al. 1983; Coons & Milstein 1986; Coons et al. 1988; Putnam et al. 1986), and "psychosis" in 38% (Putnam et al. 1986).

It is now well recognized that Schneiderian symptoms are not pathognomonic of schizophrenia (Pope 1983; Pope & Lipinski 1978; Silverstein & Harrow 1981) and frequently present as part of MPD. In a study of somatization disorder using Epidemiologic Catchment Area (ECA) data (Simon & VonKorff 1991), somatization disorder was found to be associated with psychotic disorders more than with any other diagnoses. The reason for this association was thought to be methodologic flaws in the ECA data whereby the DIS interview administered by lay interviewers did not provide diagnostic precision for psychotic disorders. In subjects with somatization disorder, then, psychotic diagnoses were thought to reflect high levels of nonspecific psychiatric disturbance.

MPD patients studied by Ross's group (1989c) reported significantly more Schneiderian symptoms than a comparison group of schizophrenics. The authors concluded, "Schneiderian symptoms are more characteristic of MPD than of schizophrenia" (Ross et al. 1990b, p. 111). They also advised, "The greater the number of Schneiderian symptoms reported by a patient, the more likely the diagnosis of MPD and the less likely it is schizophrenia" (Ross et al. 1990b, p. 116). Such high rates of psychotic symptoms endorsed by multiples may help explain the frequency with which these patients have been misdiagnosed as schizophrenic (Aldridge-Morris 1989, p. 107; Bliss 1980; Coons et al. 1988; Kluft 1987b). Reports of psychotic symptoms by multiples are also reflected in their MMPI profiles, in which Scale 8 (usually called a "schizophrenia scale") is more often elevated than any of the other standard clinical scales (Bliss 1984a; Coons et al. 1988).

Several groups (Coons 1986; Coons et al. 1988; Putnam et al. 1984; Ross et al. 1990b; Solomon & Solomon 1982) distinguish the auditory hallucinations reported by multiples from those of schizophrenics on the basis of observable qualitative differences. Hallucinations in MPD "are usually of a complex visual nature indicating an hysterical type of psychosis" (Coons 1986, p. 456), are often hypnogogic, and typically come from inside the person's own head, in contrast to schizophrenic voices, which are characteristically from outside (Allison 1981; Coons 1984, 1986a; Herzog 1984; Kluft 1987b; Marcum et al. 1986; Putnam et al. 1984; Ross et al. 1990b; Solomon & Solomon 1982). Kluft (1987b, p. 368) explains the voices of multiples as "the revivification of past experiences as hallucinations." The perceptual disturbances reported by multiples have been termed "pseudohallucinations" (Coons 1986a; Kluft 1985, 1986; Loewenstein 1989, 1991), and the psychotic-like symptoms they describe have been referred to as "quasipsychotic" and quasidelusional" or "pseudodelusional."

Pseudopsychotic behavior is thought to be related to somatoform behavior (Hirsch & Hollender 1969) and, like somatization, is frequently associated with conversion symptoms (Bishop & Holt 1980). At least a century ago, it was recognized that complaints of auditory hallucinations are common in patients with Briquet's syndrome, as noted by Freud (1948b), Briquet (1859), Mai and Merskey (1980), Janet, Breuer, Prince (Bliss 1983), Perley and Guze (1962), and others. As many as 88% of patients with Briquet's syndrome report auditory hallucinations (Goodwin et al. 1971), usually a voice calling the patient's name (American Psychiatric Association 1987, p. 262). In Briquet's syndrome these symptoms have historically been termed "pseudopsychotic" (Hirsch & Hollender 1969; Briquet 1859) and "pseudoschizophrenic" (Mallett & Gold 1964) and, like the pseudopsychotic symptoms of multiples, are described as being qualitatively different from schizophrenic symptoms (Bishop & Holt 1980). Pseudopsychotic features have also been noted in association with borderline personality disorder (Gunderson & Kolb 1978; Gunderson & Singer 1975).

Somatoform features

Ross and colleagues (1989a) found that multiples report more somatoform symptoms than do patients with other psychiatric disorders (not including somatization disorder, which was not considered in their study). Ross and colleagues reported a mean of 13.5 somatoform symptoms in one series of MPD patients (1989a) and 15.2 in another (1990c). This compares with a mean (calculated by the authors) of 16.1 ± 1.6 somatoform symptoms reported by nine women meeting the criteria for somatization disorder in a large population survey (Robins et al. 1984).

Coons (1980, p. 331) has observed that "hysterical conversion reactions are almost universal" in MPD and physical symptoms are "extremely common." All but one of the 14 MPD cases in Bliss' (1980) series reported multiple conversion symptoms, and one-third described limb paralysis (Bliss 1984a). Hirsch and Hollender (1969, p. 912) feel that in certain contexts "the concept of dissociation adds nothing which cannot be conveyed by the concept of conversion, and the two words can be used interchangeably."

Symptoms of amnesia or fugue are endorsed by 85 to 100% of multiples (Bliss 1980; Coons et al. 1988a; Putnam et al. 1986). Some authors require amnesia for a positive diagnosis of MPD (Aldridge-Morris 1989, p. 108; Coons 1980; Coons et al. 1988b; Osgood et al. 1976; Prasad 1985; Putnam et al. 1984; Ross et al. 1990c) even though this symptom is not required by current diagnostic criteria (American Psychiatric Association 1987). Ross and colleagues (1990c) recommend inclusion of amnesia as a mandatory symptom in the DSM-IV criteria for MPD in order to make criteria less likely to include false positives.

Headaches are an especially common symptom in MPD (Aldridge-Morris 1989, p. 55; Bliss 1980; Coons & Milstein 1986; Gruenewald 1971; Packard &

Brown 1986; Putnam et al. 1986; Ross et al. 1989e) and are often described as indicators of transitions from one personality to another (Coons et al. 1988; Prasad 1985). Bliss (1980, p. 1390) observed a proclivity for some multiples to "have many illnesses, frequent physicians' offices, invite unnecessary surgery, and take medications to excess."

Most of the 14 multiples described by Bliss (1980) met criteria for Briquet's syndrome, and he further explained (p. 1396), "all of these patients qualify for the diagnosis of hysteria as it has been denoted over the centuries." Coons (1984) reported that 8 in a series of 10 MPD patients he reviewed met Research Diagnostic Criteria for hysteria, and 6 had a history of hysterical conversion. Conversely, Bliss (1984c) reported that about half of a sample of 33 patients with Briquet's syndrome he studied were multiples.

Antisocial features

Considerable overlap in symptoms between MPD and antisocial personality disorder is well documented (Fink 1991). In most male and many female cases, antisocial personality is present, and in the rest, antisocial features are frequently apparent.

Putnam's group (1986) reported high rates of antisocial behavior problems in multiples, including assaultive or destructive behavior in 70%, homicidal behavior in 29%, and sexual promiscuity in 52%. Allison (1981) reported criminal activity in 5% of female multiples and 62% of male multiples. Rivera (1991) learned that 12% of multiples in her study had criminal records. Coons and colleagues (1988) noted a history of criminality in 32% of their 50 patients, including 3 of the 4 men in the sample. Adult crimes included assault and battery, burglary, armed robbery, prostitution, serial rape, and child abuse. The youngest male, an adolescent, had an extensive history of delinquency, including assault and battery, arson, shoplifting, burglary, and vandalism, and had been incarcerated in a boys' school twice. An essentially universal phenomenon in MPD is the use of different names when experiencing different personalities. The use of an alias or assumed name is a criterion symptom of antisocial personality disorder (American Psychiatric Association 1987, p. 345).

Compared to female multiples, male multiples report more antisocial symptoms and alcoholism, and females have more hysterical, anxiety, phobic, and obsessive-compulsive symptoms (Bliss 1984a, 1984b; Putnam et al. 1986; Ross & Norton 1989a). While women predominate in the overall population of MPDs (Boor 1982; Kluft 1984a, 1987a), men dominate the ranks of the criminal cases (Bliss & Larson 1985; Boor 1982). It is unusual for a male multiple to be seen primarily for treatment, male patients more typically coming to psychiatric attention through the criminal justice system (Allison 1981; Bliss & Larson 1985). Because of the high rate of criminality in male MPD cases, several authors (Bliss & Larson 1985; Kluft 1985a, 1987b; Ross & Norton 1989a) have speculated that the relative scarcity of male MPDs in treatment-seeking populations may be in part a product of their unavailability due to incarceration.

Bliss and Larson (1985) discovered that 13 of 33 convicted sex offenders on a forensic unit had probable or definite MPD. Cloninger and Guze (1970a) found that a substantial number of female felons they studied (80% diagnosed with sociopathy or Briquet's syndrome) spontaneously volunteered that they had a "split personality" or "multiple personality," though how many of those would actually meet the criteria for MPD is not known. In the Bliss and Larson study (1985), subjects with high hypnotizability scores had more polysymptomatic profiles. Bliss (1983) reported that criminals and sociopaths often have high rates of "hypnotic symptoms" and that patients with Briquet's syndrome, like multiples, "are good or excellent hypnotic subjects with few exceptions" (Bliss 1984c, p. 203); also, women with major conversion symptoms are "hypnotic virtuosos." Bliss and Larson (1985) have proposed self-hypnosis as a mechanism in the production of antisocial disorders and Briquet's syndrome, as well as MPD.

Features of personality disorders

Adult multiples studied by Ross' group (1990c) not only endorsed more somatoform symptoms than patients with other disorders and more Schneiderian symptoms than patients with schizophrenia, but they also reported more borderline personality symptoms than any other group of patients. A number of authors have noted strong similarities and associations between MPD and borderline personality (Benner & Joscelyne 1984; Buck 1983; Coons 1984; Harvard 1985; Horevitz & Braun 1984; Kluft 1982). In several studies a substantial portion, often the majority, of multiples had been diagnosed borderline personality (Armstrong & Loewenstein 1990; Horevitz & Braun 1984; Kluft 1982; Rivera 1991; Ross et al. 1990c). Rates of diagnosed borderline personality disorder among samples of MPD patients have been as high as 60 to 70%, although as low as 13% in one study (Fink 1991).

Clinical features of borderline personality disorder shared by MPD include impulsivity, identity disturbance, angry outbursts, marked mood changes, suicidal gestures, manipulativeness, self-mutilation, and a pattern of stormy and unstable interpersonal relationships and unhappy marriages (Coons 1980, 1984; Fink 1991; Prasad 1985). Elevated rates of reported rape by multiples (Table 3-1) are also present in the histories of borderlines (Goodwin et al. 1990). Kroll (1988, p. xiii) characterized borderlines in a manner that also seems to describe multiples, with their "dramatic symptomatology, chaotic life-style, resemblances at times to the major mental illnesses, and difficulties in treatment situations." Both borderline personality disorder and MPD are polysymptomatic, polysyndromic disorders of early onset, as is Briquet's syndrome, and all are notoriously difficult and frustrating to treat.

Ross and colleagues (1990c) reported that 91% of their sample of multiples endorsed two or more borderline personality criteria, and the mean was 5.2 borderline symptoms (therefore meeting 5 of the 8 criterion symptoms of borderline personality disorder required for a DSM-III-R diagnosis). In another study, a mean of 3.7 borderline characteristics was endorsed by a sample of MPD patients (Fink & Golinkoff 1990). Ross (1991, p. 513) stated, "If both diagnoses [MPD and borderline personality] are long-term consequences of childhood trauma, they would be expected to overlap extensively."

Self-mutilation has been reported in 34% of multiples in one series (Coons et al. 1988), and it is thought to be underreported (Kluft 1991). Several of Coons' (1984) patients had factitious dermatologic disorders and injuries due to self-mutilation during an amnestic period. Typically, an alternate personality claims credit for the act (Bliss 1980; Coons 1984). Patients often report that they feel no pain from these acts (Bliss 1980), sometimes because they were in an alternate personality state at the time of the act and sometimes due to the presence of other dissociative states or psychogenic amnesia. Ross and colleagues (1990c) learned that 40% of their MPD patients had lacerated themselves, 24% had inflicted cigarette burns or other self-injuries, 27% had used a weapon to harm themselves, 13% had attempted to hang themselves, and 57% had taken an overdose. They concluded (p. 600), "Patients with multiple personality disorder are probably the most self destructive diagnostic group among psychiatric patients."

Some suggest that MPD may actually be a subtype of borderline disorder or a special case of borderline personality (Benner & Joscelyne 1984; Buck 1983; Clary et al. 1984). Horevitz and Braun (1984) and Armstrong and Loewenstein (1990), however, argue that MPD is a separate disorder with features distinct from those of borderline personality. Because of the diverse polysymptomatic, polysyndromic picture extending beyond the usual symptom clusters exhibited by borderlines, Kluft (1985) has concluded that MPD does not lie within the domain of a borderline category. Due to the lack of supporting data, many of the arguments over the relationship between MPD and borderline personality are somewhat foggy (Greaves 1980) and have been described elsewhere as "Lewis Carrollian gobbledegook" (Aldridge-Morris 1989, p. 49).

Coons (1984) observed that MPD frequently has characteristics in common with histrionic personality disorder, including self-dramatization, irrational angry outbursts, egocentricity, demandingness, dependency, and manipulativeness. MPD has been conceptualized "usually as a mixed hysterical disorder with borderline characteristics" (Kline 1984, p. 198). This description, however, does not fully explain the disorder. MPD represents more than just borderline and histrionic personality. Others regard MPD as a narcissistic disorder (Clary et al. 1984; Gruenewald 1977). Yet others (Ross & Anderson 1988) hypothesize a phenomenologic overlap of MPD with obsessive-compulsive disorder.

Personality disorders in general appear to be ubiquitously associated with MPD. Only 14% of patients in one study series did not meet criteria for a personality disorder (Coons et al. 1988). One-fourth of the subjects in that study qualified for three or more personality disorder diagnoses. The most frequent personality disorder was borderline (56%), followed by dependent (26%) and histrionic (22%). Compulsive, avoidant, antisocial, paranoid, and passive-aggressive personality disorders were also represented. Herzog (1984, p. 211) was "impressed with the diagnostic and 'characterologic' range" of MPD patients. Coons and colleagues (1988, p. 527) reported that their MMPI profiles "generally reflected underlying character pathology."

The general study of personality disorders is currently in a state of underdevelopment and unrest. The validity and reliability of personality disorder diagnoses are still problematic, and the diagnoses overlap extensively (Pfohl et al. 1986). Leading researchers do not concur on the basic manner in which personality disorders should be conceptualized (Frances 1980; Godfried & Kent 1972; Heumann & Morey 1990; Livesley 1985a, 1985b, 1986; Livesley & Jackson 1986; Pfohl et al. 1986; Widiger et al. 1988). Available instruments of measure for personality disorders reflect these nosologic problems and may be less than adequate for systematic research (Skodol et al. 1988). These difficulties have impeded progress in the investigation of the relationship between MPD and personality disorders.

Posttraumatic stress disorder and MPD

Posttraumatic stress disorder is a common diagnosis in individuals suffering from MPD. Many believe that MPD represents a posttraumatic disorder of adulthood caused by severe childhood trauma (Braun 1984a; Coons 1986a, 1988a; Coons & Milstein 1986; Fagan & McMahon 1984; Kline 1984; Kluft 1987a, b; Loewenstein 1989; Prasad 1985; Putnam et al. 1986; Ross 1989, p. 44; Ross et al. 1989a; Spiegel 1984, 1986, 1988; Wilbur 1984). This disorder also suffers from a lack of sufficient systematic investigation, inadequate definition, and limitations in available diagnostic instruments.

Pediatric MPD

When symptoms of MPD present in younger people, the diagnostic differential includes substance abuse, dissociative-hysterical conditions, and sociopathic conditions (Fagan & McMahon 1984). Frequently a "well developed delinquent personality" is already present in childhood (Fagan & McMahon 1984). Children destined to develop MPD are described as shy, lonely, and having few friends (Bliss & Larson 1985; Dell & Eisenhower 1990). Childhood behavioral antecedents include lying, stealing, fire setting, disruptive behavior, school disciplinary problems, adolescent delinquency, physical complaints, change of temperament, hostility, precocious sexual interest, and sexual seductiveness (Bliss & Larson 1985; Dell & Eisenhower 1990; Fagan & McMahon 1984; Harvard 1985). Almost all multiples examined by Kluft (1984a) had difficulties in school as children. Given that these problems coincide with conduct disorder, research into the roots of MPD should include further investigation of childhood conduct problems.

In a study of 11 adolescent MPD cases, Dell and Eisenhower (1990) diagnosed 36% with conduct disorder and an additional 19% with oppositional defiant disorder. Two of the 11 also qualified for borderline personality disorder, and 1 had an eating disorder. In addition, almost half were diagnosed with posttraumatic stress disorder.

Attribution of symptoms

Personal bias by the clinician regarding the origins of symptoms in MPD affect how these symptoms are applied in the assessment of psychiatric diagnoses. Because some clinicians ascribe borderline features in multiples such as instability of mood and self-image, self-mutilation, and stormy interpersonal behavior to personality-specific contexts, such as in transitions between alternate personalities, these symptoms may be attributed to MPD only and may not be applied to the assessment of borderline personality in these patients (Nakdimen 1989; Putnam et al. 1984). Similarly, frequent presenting somatization symptoms such as unexplained headaches and amnesias might be discounted because they classically occur in relation to switches of personalities. The somatoform symptoms may thus be considered only for a superordinate diagnosis of MPD and not enumerated for documentation of Briquet's syndrome. Substance abuse is often confined to just one or two of the personalities (Coons 1984; Putnam et al. 1986) and may not attract attention to diagnostic consideration. Personality-specific behaviors such as suicidality, homicidality, and self-mutilation have been described (Putnam et al. 1986), and these could easily be lost in the polysymptomatic smokescreen of MPD. Diagnoses such as antisocial personality disorder or histrionic personality disorder coexisting with MPD may be overlooked because the alternate personalities, rather than the original core personality, are felt to produce the symptoms of other psychiatric disorders (Coons et al. 1988; Fink 1991; Loewenstein et al. 1987; Nakdimen 1989; Solomon & Solomon 1982). Conversely, DSM-III-R (American Psychiatric Association 1987, p. 272) cautions that the MPD diagnosis may be missed if symptoms due to alternation of the personalities are counted only toward another diagnosis.

Prasad (1985, p. 302) believes that "All the personality states can be considered to be a whole personality only when taken together." The alternate personalities are all a part of the same person (Bowers et al. 1971; Buck 1983; Coons 1984; Horevitz & Braun 1984; Prasad 1985; Spiegel 1988; Thigpen &

Cleckley 1984), even if the symptoms are experienced by different personality states. Horevitz and Braun (1984, p. 76) write, "An Axis II diagnosis for each personality, though possible, is scarcely useful." The combined symptoms of all the alternate personalities are additive and should logically contribute to the making of additional psychiatric diagnoses (Buck 1983). Horevitz and Braun (1984) speak of a "global rule" for the assignment of symptoms of the alternates to the individual.

Further study needed in diagnostic comorbidity

From the studies reviewed so far in this chapter, it is clear that patients with MPD can be readily differentiated from normal controls and from patients with certain psychiatric disorders. While some systematic studies have compared MPD with schizophrenia, anxiety disorders, eating disorders, and normal subjects, they have not included patients with the clinically most overlapping disorders—Briquet's syndrome, borderline personality, histrionic personality disorder, and antisocial personality disorder—to try to differentiate MPD from them. Rigorous systematic studies comparing multiples to patients with Briquet's syndrome, antisocial personality disorder, borderline personality disorder, and other personality disorders are imperative if we are to conclude that MPD is clearly different from any of them.

Not all patients with borderline personality and Briquet's syndrome become multiples. What accounts for the difference? Does MPD just represent the severest form of borderline or somatoform psychopathology, or is it an entirely different phenomenon? Could MPD be a special symptom complex sometimes complicating Briquet's syndrome in the way conversion symptoms do, or complicating borderline personality as dissociative symptoms do? Studies to date have scarcely addressed the possibility that MPD may be a complication of another disorder, a symptom complex common to several other disorders, or a marker of severity when it occurs in the context of other disorders such as Briquet's syndrome or borderline personality. Studies addressing these questions are possible and should be carried out.

Familial Associations

Few studies have investigated psychiatric disorders in families of multiples. There have been some family history studies (asking patients about their family psychopathology), but family studies (interviewing family members) have not been done. Family history studies, as opposed to family studies with direct interviewing of family members, are not universally considered adequate for scientific purposes.

Putnam's group (1986) reported a mean of 2.1 first-degree relatives of multiples with a psychiatric disorder, but no clear pattern of diagnoses was present. In a study of family histories of multiples, Coons and colleagues (1988) found alcoholism in 36% of fathers, 10% of mothers, and 10% of siblings of multiples. Schizophrenia, major depression, and substance abuse were each reported in about 10% of first-degree relatives. Forty percent of the multiples' children had a diagnosable psychiatric disorder, but there was no predominance of any particular disorder. Systematic family studies including somatization disorder and personality disorders in the diagnostic differential have not been done. This is an important gap in the investigation of families of multiples to date.

Although MPD is thought to be more prevalent in first-degree biologic relatives of multiples than in the general population (American Psychiatric Association 1987, p. 271; Braun 1985; Ross et al. 1989e), insufficient systematic evidence has been gathered to address this point adequately. In one study (Dell & Eisenhower 1990), 73% of adolescent multiples were found to have a parent with dissociative disorder and 36% of the mothers were thought to have MPD.

It has been observed that MPD patients frequently hail from family backgrounds that are authoritarian, excessively strict, and extremely religious (Boor 1982; Coons 1980; Saltman & Solomon 1982). Saltman and Solomon (1982) found multiples to be frequently derived from highly dysfunctional families. The extraordinarily high rate of child abuse reported by MPD patients supports this finding.

Studies of the families of multiples to date do not add much additional support to the validity of the disorder at this time. Available data are still too scant to allow us to draw firm conclusions regarding specific familial associations of MPD. It is likely, however, that families of multiples are significantly deviant from the general population.

Physiologic Investigation

Some of the most intense efforts to study and validate MPD consist of physiologic investigations. Laboratory evidence of MPD as a documentable disorder would be very desirable in validating this diagnosis by the five-stage diagnostic validation process of Robins and Guze (1970), and both physiologic and psychological lines of study have tried to provide this elusive documentation.

Isolated anecdotal reports of physiologic differences between alternate personalities in multiples by Benjamin Rush and William James (Putnam et al. 1990) date back to the eighteenth and nineteenth centuries. Since that time, numerous reports have been published describing various clinical differences between alternate personalities of individual MPD patients (Putnam 1986). These clinical findings include somatic symptoms such as headaches that are specific to certain personalities and denied by other personalities (Coons et al. 1988; Packard & Brown 1986), differential responses of personalities to the same medication (Barkin et al. 1986; Coons 1988a; Putnam 1989a; Putnam et al. 1986), and personality-specific responses to alcohol, food, and allergens (Braun 1983; Putnam et al. 1986)—all allegedly mediated through ordinary physiologic processes.

Coons (1984) reported a case of a multiple with hives that developed suddenly in one personality and abruptly disappeared after a personality switch. Other investigators have reported changes in dominant handedness among different personalities (Putnam et al. 1986; Smith & Sager 1971; Taylor & Martin 1944), changes in handwriting (Coons 1980; Taylor & Martin 1944; Thigpen & Cleckley 1954), changes in voice quality (Coons 1980; Putnam 1984; Schreiber 1973), alterations in visual acuity, color vision, and visual fields (Coons 1988a), and differences in sensitivity to pain (Wilson 1903). Changes in physiologic functions, including heart rate (Bahnson & Smith 1975), blood pressure (Larmore et al. 1977), and respiration (Bahnson & Smith 1975), have also been described.

Considerable attention has been given to autonomic nervous system function in MPD. The autonomic nervous system mediates many physiologic responses to emotional changes, such as regulation of skin temperature, blood pressure, heart rate, and gut motility. Autonomic nervous system activity is also thought to reflect dissociative cerebral activity, and it is hoped that it may provide a vehicle for objective measurement of differences between personality states. Autonomic activity can be measured through electrodermal responses, evoked potentials, electromyography, electroencephalography, and a variety of other techniques.

Morton Prince is credited as the first researcher to investigate physiologic differences among alternate personalities of individual patients (Putnam 1984). Prince and Peterson (1908) used a galvanometer and crude kymograph to measure electrical changes in skin resistance accompanying emotional responses to certain words read to the subject. This response, presently known as the "galvanic skin response (GSR)," is the basis of the polygraph or "lie detector" test still used today to help determine whether witnesses are lying or telling the truth. Methodologic limitations of Prince and Peterson's study such as failure to address habituation effects have been noted elsewhere (Putnam 1984).

Concomitant with the decline of interest in MPD in the early part of this century, no further physiologic investigations of MPD were conducted until 1950, when Thigpen and Cleckley (1954) studied electroencephalographic (EEG) changes among Eve's different personalities. Attempting to document variations in electrical brain wave activity among the different personalities, they discovered a difference in background alpha frequency of 1.5 Hz between two of the personalities. Three years later, similar EEG differences between alternate personalities in a multiple were reported by Moriselli (1953).

Thigpen and Cleckley (1954) reported differences in measurements of the degree of muscle tension among Eve's personalities, but they described this finding as "not particularly impressive" clinically in comparison with the dramatic switches of the personalities. Further study of Eve documented micro-transient strabismus, or brief divergent eye movements, across four of her personalities (Condon et al. 1969), and a parallel was drawn between these findings in MPD and the eye movement abnormalities observed in schizophrenia.

The last two decades have seen many investigations of the physiologic correlates of MPD, ranging from studies using simple GSR measurements to sophisticated studies of brain wave patterns and cerebral blood flow. Although measurable changes among personalities in MPD have been reported, the results have been inconsistent and often mixed. These studies have also suffered from many of the same methodologic limitations pointed out earlier in this chapter on the assessment of the epidemiologic studies of MPD.

In a study of one MPD patient with four personalities, Ludwig and colleagues (1972) measured differences among the alternate personalities on GSR responses to emotionally charged words and visual evoked potentials. Evoked potentials are a measurement of electrical waves generated in the brain in response to certain stimuli such as a sound or a flash of light. Measurable differences among personalities could be evidence of alterations in physiologic responses within an individual or of differences among individuals. Although the authors found some differences in GSR there were some inconsistencies, and the nature of many of the differences made them difficult to evaluate (Putnam 1984). EEG measures of brain wave activity in this patient revealed differences across personalities in visual evoked responses, muscle tension, alpha frequency, and amplitude. The authors concluded that these findings suggested "real physiologic differences" among the personalities, although they conceded that to some degree different emotional states may have contributed to the apparent differences.

A similar study of another case by Larmore's group (1977) found differences across four alternate personalities on GSR, EEG, electromyography (EMG), and visual evoked responses. Although the authors could not draw definite conclusions from the EEG and EMG studies, they concluded that the differences in the visual evoked responses were "such as would be expected if four separate individuals had been tested" (p. 39). They concluded, "Explanations of consciously faking or role playing these personalities flawlessly in such a psychologically unsophisticated subject appear quite inadequate" (p. 40). This study included no control subjects.

Bahnson and Smith (1975) found a remarkable MPD patient with "dramatic respiratory pauses of up to two minutes duration accompany transitions from one state of consciousness to another" (p. 86), as well as marked slowing of the heart rate. This patient also showed changes in GSR values with the emergence of alternate personalities. GSR differences among alternate personalities have also been reported by Brende (1984). Ludwig and colleagues (1972) documented differences in EEG measures and visual evoked responses among the personalities of one MPD patient. Mathew and coworkers (1985) observed marked variations among personalities in regional cerebral blood flow, with hyperperfusion of the right temporal lobe.

This last report is consistent with predominantly right-sided EEG changes across personalities reported by Coons and colleagues (1982). They compared two MPD patients with a normal control (Coons himself) simulating multiples. This report is credited as the first controlled study of neurophysiologic changes in MPD, the earlier studies having been uncontrolled and largely anecdotal (Putnam 1984). Coons and his colleagues actually found few differences among the various personalities in either patient, and the control showed more marked differences across simulated personalities than did the MPD patients. The authors wrote (p. 825):

> We conclude that the most likely explanation for the differences found in the frequency analysis involves changes in intensity of concentration, mood, and degree of muscle relaxation, and duration of recording involved in such studies. It is not as if each personality is a different individual with a different brain. Instead, to put it simply, the EEG changes reflect changes in emotional state.
>   Thus, until otherwise demonstrated, it is better to attribute the EEG differences found in our patients and our control to the same underlying mechanism.

Herzog (1984) concurs. He believes that differences in GSR, visual evoked response, and alpha waves on the EEG among personalities in MPD "can probably all be explained by differences in emotional, rather than physiological states" (p. 214).

Putnam and colleagues (1990) tested skin conductance differences between the right and left sides of the body in nine subjects with MPD against five controls simulating alternate personalities through hypnosis or deep relaxation. The investigators found no consistent between-personality differences in electrodermal laterality in the MPD group as a whole or within any individual patient, and they reasoned that such phenomena may be rare. Some of the control subjects were able to produce "alternates" with a degree of differentiation equivalent to the most differentiated MPD patients. This pattern was attributed to differences in general physiologic arousal accompanying the various simulated states of the controls. The investigators felt that this effect was not produced by the same mechanisms as the personality changes in the MPD subjects. They concluded (p. 259):

> alter personality states of MPD are physiologically distinct states of consciousness. Equivalent differences can be generated by some control subjects using hypnosis or simulations based on experiential material. Muscle tension and level of arousal appear to play an important mechanistic role. . . .

Other controlled studies have reported more definite differences between MPD patients and controls on physiologic measures of change. Miller's (1989) study comparing MPD patients with control subjects role-playing MPD found significantly more variability across alternate personalities in the MPD patients than in the controls on measures of visual acuity (with and without correction), visual fields, manifest refraction, and eye muscle imbalance. Putnam (1984) described a study he carried out with colleagues comparing visual evoked potentials and habituation of an MPD patient with a normal control subject simulating alternate personalities. They found greater statistical variation across personalities in the MPD patient than in the control. Putnam concluded that "normal control subjects are not able to simply 'fake' this condition" (p. 35) but conceded that good professional actors might be able to produce these differences.

We conclude that even if actors were consistently able to reproduce the physiologic responses accompanying the switches documented among personalities in MPD, this would not prove that MPD is not real. In Chapter 2, the reader may recall, it was explained that just because a condition can be successfully faked does not mean that it does not exist.

MPD is not the only disorder known to produce psychophysiologic changes within patients. Coons (1988a) points out that many of the psychophysiologic alterations associated with distinct personalities in MPD have also been observed in patients with conversion disorder—including "phenomena such as anaesthesia, paralysis, pain, seizure-like activity, and alterations in vision, hearing and voice" (p. 51). The demonstrated physiologic differences among alternate personalities in uncontrolled studies of MPD could theoretically be explained by differences associated with the well known fluctuations in extreme mood states of individuals with certain psychiatric disorders (Thigpen & Cleckley 1984). Extreme moods are certainly characteristic of patients with MPD, as well as those prone to conversion disorders and the other disorders known to be highly associated with MPD within individuals (Briquet's syndrome, borderline personality).

Greden and colleagues (1986) stated that ordinary depressive and nondepressive states can be reliably discriminated by levels of muscle tension. Zahn (1986) found that retarded habituation such as reported by Putnam's group may represent a characteristic of ordinary anxiety states. Studies comparing MPD and other disorders such as conversion disorder, Briquet's syndrome, major depression, and borderline personality disorder on physiologic measures of their various states must be done to address the issue of uniqueness of MPD in this respect.

In summary, no laboratory measurement has been developed that can differentiate MPD from other disorders (Coons 1984; Putnam 1984). Even if laboratory evidence such as EEG markers of MPD becomes available, Aldridge-Morris (1989, p. 51) points out problems that will remain, because "Evidence which relies on physiological correlates such as altered electroencephalograms is dogged by the problem of . . . chicken and egg." We are brought back to the basic question: are these physiologic phenomena the essence of the mechanisms producing distinct personalities in MPD, or are they a by-product—through ordinary physiologic responses—of the extreme emotional displays of severe mood instabilities seen in patients tested for MPD?

Natural Course, Treatment, and Outcome

Descriptions of the treatment of MPD from the point of view of therapists are colorful. Patients' transferences include dependence, hostility, seduction, and manipulativeness; countertransference responses are overfascination, overinvestment, intellectualization, withdrawal and abandonment, disbelief, bewilderment, feeling overwhelmed, frustration, exasperation, anger, and exhaustion (Bliss 1980; Coons 1986a; Harvard 1985; Horevitz & Braun 1984; Saltman & Solomon 1982). Coons (1986c) found the most common countertransferences reported by therapists of multiples to be exasperation (reported by 75%), anger (in 58%), and emotional exhaustion (in 33%). One in three reported a "desire to rescue" and 17% reported vicarious enjoyment.

One therapist described his first observation of a patient's alternate personalities as a "hair-raising" experience (Davis & Osherson 1977). Wilbur (1984b) reported that "rather unusual transferences" may occur in the form of switches to a diverse and dramatic variety of alternates. Horevitz and Braun (1984) warned of "an ever-present danger of intense involvement with these patients" that "can lead to the development of a countertransference that threatens the therapist as well as the therapy." Saltman and Solomon (1982) warned the therapist to "monitor his own voyeurism to avoid becoming absorbed in fascination or entertainment with the patient's exotic pathology."

It is recognized that MPD patients "may act seductively toward the therapist and unconsciously evoke seductive feelings in the therapist" (Saltman & Solomon 1982, p. 1140). Cornelia Wilbur reported that Sybil behaved in ways that "were specifically displeasing and which provoked negative feelings" (Greaves 1980, p. 580). Herzog (1984, p. 218) described countertransference feelings ranging from "lustful passion to murderous rage—sometimes all within the same session" in dealing with MPD patients. Difficulties in treating MPD patients have been described as "similar to those described in the literature regarding borderline patients" (Horevitz & Braun 1984, p. 72).

Multiples are said to be very difficult hospital inpatients and to have conflicts with rules and limitations (Harvard 1985; Kluft 1984d). They "question procedures, protest regulations, and make complaints" (Kluft 1984d, p. 54). They polarize staff members, engender antagonism, and are seen as manipulative and divisive, precipitating "chaotic" situations. To protect the staff, other patients, and the MPD patient from conflict and chaos, Kluft (1984d) recommends that MPD patients be given private rooms.

Multiples can be difficult outpatients as well, being abusive to therapists (Kluft 1984d) and calling at all hours with intolerable emotional demands (Harvard 1985). Kluft (1984d) learned that many psychiatrists find these patients "extraordinarily demanding." Their patients consumed substantial amounts of their professional time, intruded into their personal and family lives, and led to difficulties with colleagues. Psychiatrists consulting him reported difficulty in setting reasonable and nonpunitive limits. They found they had to monitor themselves very carefully lest the patient sense withdrawal by them and feel abandoned and betrayed.

Treatment of multiples has been described as "difficult," "grueling," "arduous," "enervating," and an "emotional drain" (Bliss 1980; Horevitz & Braun 1984; Kluft 1984d), these patients being "among the most draining and manipulative of patients" (Kluft 1984d). The therapist's patience may be "sorely tested" (Kluft 1984d). Kluft (1984d) reported that patients often sabotage therapy. One complicating problem is the propensity for patients "to dodge into hypnotic states" during the process or to become addicted to drugs as a "convenient escape" or to block hypnotic intervention (Kluft 1984d).

Bliss (1980, p. 1393) summarized the treatment of MPD patients as "difficult and frustrating, with successes counterbalanced by distressing failures." Bliss uses hypnosis aimed at fusion of the personalities and encourages patients to assume responsibility for their actions; this can be a "stressful exercise" that "can also result in turmoil." Horevitz and Braun (1984, p. 71) reported "serious difficulties in treatment" of MPD patients, including "frequent crises, episodes of acting-out, affect swings, as well as real or threatened outbursts [that] make therapy tempestuous." Therapists consulting Kluft (1984d) reported that their treatment "often exacerbated their patients' distress." Bliss (1980, p. 1393) noted a pattern of "threats of suicide, grand hysterical episodes, and the emergence of personalities" for a period as treatment proceeds. Bliss said he "searched for ways to reduce the pyrotechnics" (p. 1393).

At the same time, Saltman and Solomon (1982) underscore the need for the therapist to treat the MPD patient with respect, empathy, and concern, developing rapport and allegiance. This will require a "high degree of resilience, patience, and tolerance" on the part of the therapist, who must also remember to do what is best for the patient, which is to focus on integration rather than pursuing unnecessary investigation of the symptoms out of curiosity. Spiegel (1988, p. 535) describes the ideal approach as "a fine blend of credulity and criticism, of caring for the patient and rational assessment of him or her."

Bowers' group (1971) recommends that "Once a multiple personality is suspected, *no hypnosis should be done*" unless the therapist is highly experienced and trained in hypnosis, because "undisciplined intervention can further separate the subpersonalities, increase fugue states, and evoke new subpersonalities, with a concomitant decrease in integration of the total individual" (p. 62). They furthermore "suggest not dramatizing an acute amnesia" (p. 62). They also recommend "hospitalizing [the patient] in humane but ungratifying surroundings. In this way he is not encouraged to develop a new personality" (p. 63). Although there is still no systematic research support for these behavioral methods, Black (1987) has recommended a similar strategy for the management of conversion symptoms in patients with Briquet's syndrome.

Kluft (1984c, p. 11) reported encountering "the reappearance of personalities alleged to have fused. . . . I wondered whether this pointed toward the condition's untreatability or the instability of gains." Ross and colleagues (1989e) noted a median of two alternate personalities at presentation for treatment, a figure that over the course of therapy eventually increased to eight. They wrote, "It is the rule to uncover personalities during treatment" (p. 417). An analysis of case report data (n = 33) reported by Kluft (1984c) yielded a significant correlation (r = .48, p = .005) between the length of treatment until fusion and the number of alternate personalities revealed.

MPD symptoms often remit with therapy directed at reintegration (Boor 1982; Dell & Eisenhower 1990; Franklin 1990; Herzog 1984; Kluft 1985, 1987b; Putnam et al. 1984; Rivera 1991; Ross 1989, p. 3; Wilbur 1984a), although one out of four multiples who successfully integrate may relapse (Kluft 1984c). Even with adequate intervention and fusion, problems remain. Bliss (1980, pp. 1393–1394) called integration of the personalities "a minor miracle, [but] it is hardly the end. Patients do regress, the problems of life do not vanish. The patient should be followed up and helped to cope with the realities, which may still be oppressive." Bliss (1986, p. 219) reported that five or six years of intensive therapy are required to achieve symptom relief and stability. Bliss (1986, p. 219) observed that in his patients "fusion was a way station; prolonged follow-up and reassessment were shown to be essential . . . therapy that terminated at the point of apparent fusion was rarely complete or stable." Kluft (1982, p. 233) agrees: "Fusion, however dramatic, is only one aspect of a patient's treatment needs. When feasible, therapy should be continued 1–2 years after fusion."

These observations are compatible with the possibility that the prevalent comorbidity of other serious disorders with MPD leaves the patient with other disorders remaining after the multiples are fused. The patient may continue to suffer from Briquet's syndrome, antisocial personality, or borderline personality, preexisting conditions unlikely to have been ameliorated by the fusion of the personalities. Furthermore, these other conditions are notoriously chronic and recalcitrant to all psychiatric interventions, and are severe and disabling in their own right (Aronson 1989; Briquet 1859; Katon et al. 1991; Nestadt et al. 1990; Robins et al. 1991, p. 290; Silver 1985; Slater 1965; Widiger & Rogers 1989; Zoccolillo & Cloninger 1986b). No follow-up studies provide specific data about remaining comorbidity. Ross and colleagues (1989a), however, have reported that in their clinical experience, comorbid somatization and personality disorders improve or remit with integration.

Bliss (1986, p. 219) reflected on the magnitude of problems typical of MPD patients:

> Other problems posed by these patients are not restricted to multiples, since they are commonly encountered in many persons being treated by psychotherapy. How

does one more rapidly change erroneous convictions, faulty attitudes, and inappropriate emotional responses engendered during childhood? How does one more rapidly alter maladaptive behaviors that were learned early in life? Both these problems are major obstacles to change in multiples, and both at present are unanswered questions.

The alternate personalities may be the relatively smaller portion of the pathology in patients with MPD.

Kluft (1983, 1984c) has hinted that poor treatment outcomes seem to occur in patients with other disorders historically associated with a poorer prognosis such as substance abuse, sociopathy, and narcissistic, borderline, and masochistic character problems. The possibility remains that the overall outcome for MPD patients may depend more on the course of the comorbid disorders.

Case Reports

The following illustrative case reports describe patients in the authors' practices, delineating the clinical course and comorbidity of representative cases.

Mrs. A

Mrs. A first came to psychiatric attention at the age of 20 at her university clinic. There she was diagnosed as having "hysteria" and was referred for psychotherapy, which continued for about a year. During that period she had the first of several hospitalizations for depressive symptoms and some psychotic-like symptoms. During her many hospitalizations, she was treated with multiple antipsychotic and antidepressant agents and once with lithium, with poor results. A subsequent auto accident, after which she claimed considerable pain and disability, led to abuse of pain medications and an alcohol problem.

In general, her psychotherapy did not go well. Her therapist felt she lacked motivation to work on her problems, was defensive, and had distorted perceptions of the therapist. Her diagnosis at that time was developmental character disorder. Discouraged, she changed therapists. Her new therapist discovered that she had multiple personality disorder. Therapy with this therapist was oriented to helping her integrate her alternate personalities, which grew to a total of 39. These personalities included six alternates under the age of 5, most of whom talked baby talk or sucked their thumbs, a lesbian and two gay men, a set of twins, two self-abusive personalities, a psychotic alternate, and a dyslexic alternate.

On referral to her current psychiatrist, Mrs. A produced a document listing her various personalities and a description of each. During an inpatient stay for suicidal behavior, she demonstrated several different personalities to the hospital staff. In the presence of her psychiatrist she switched into her 9-year-old character, Jimmie. The patient seemed to be genuinely experiencing herself as having changed into a different person. The psychiatrist told Mrs. A that she did not treat children and asked the patient to turn back into an adult. Mrs. A rapidly transformed back into her 39-year-old self.

While in the hospital, Mrs. A was not given support to appear in her various personalities, and ideas of integration were discussed. She was consistently encouraged to "own" the feelings her different personalities represented. By the time of discharge she had, by her own efforts, reduced the number of her personalities to three.

During her hospital stay the patient completed a Millon Clinical Multiaxial Inventory. Her test was considered invalid because of excessively elevated scores on all of the scales. When asked about this, the patient stated that "Arnold," a 13-year-old personality, and "The Mutterer" had taken the test for her.

A subsequent careful review of systems revealed 42 unexplained medical symptoms in 10 categories on the Perley-Guze checklist for Briquet's syndrome, and the patient acknowledged a history of sickliness throughout her adult life. She reported a number of conversion symptoms, including blindness, paralysis, anesthesia, aphonia, pseudoseizures, amnesia, visual hallucinations, and unexplained urinary retention.

Mrs. A also had a history of self-mutilation involving cutting, especially around the genital area. She now began to feel strong urges to cut off her legs. Instead, she took a chain saw to a bush in her yard.

This case illustrates several points addressed in this chapter. First, the patient clearly met the criteria for Briquet's syndrome, and she exhibited prominent features of borderline personality disorder as well. Due to the attention to her multiple personalities, these other problems were not recognized until well into her therapy, although the diagnosis of hysteria in college hinted at Briquet's syndrome. Her multiple personalities were not discovered until she entered therapy with a "specialist" in MPD. This temporal sequence might tempt some to conclude that her previous therapists may have missed the diagnosis, or that the specialist may have "created" the syndrome in this suggestible patient. Present knowledge, however, does not permit us to draw any firm conclusions about the origins of the alternate personalities in this case, and we will withhold judgment on this issue.

Regardless of the origin of the alternate personalities in this patient, she exhibited remarkable control over them. When her psychiatrist asked her to change back to her original personality, she was able to do so voluntarily, immediately, and completely. Some might say that this is evidence that her multiple personalities were not real multiples, but others might conclude that this is evidence of voluntary control over the personalities in MPD. It is not possible to resolve these differences without more precise criteria for MPD or more complete knowledge of the disorder.

The patient's long-term course was chronic and seemed to be consistent with both Briquet's syndrome and borderline personality disorder, even after the reduction in the number of alternate personalities with discouragement of their presentation. This case also illustrates principles of treatment, in particular related to a comorbid diagnosis of Briquet's syndrome in this case. The "benign neglect" of her personalities, together with support of healthier aspects of her personality taking control of her life, apparently served to diminish the dissociation and enhance her level of function.

Mrs. B

Mrs. B was a 41-year-old divorced woman with a long, complicated history of psychiatric problems including a "force" that made her hurt herself. She dissociated at the times she cut herself. During the course of her therapy, she attended a center specializing in the treatment of victims of sexual trauma and began working with a psychologist who treated multiple personalities. After they began working together, the patient began explaining the force that made her hurt herself as a separate personality that wanted to destroy her. The psychologist engaged the patient in drawing pictures of her personalities, and she named seven of them. These personalities included herself, a male personality her brother's age, a little girl approximately 6 years old, a 17-year-old girl who was unkempt and wore pants and a belt for protection, a caretaker, a Good One, and a Bad One who cut her. Upon divulging the secret of her alternate personalities to the therapist, she went home and cut her arms, legs, and breasts more severely than before and was readmitted to the sexual trauma unit.

Mrs. B's psychiatrist never witnessed any of the reported changes in personality but did observe times when the patient allowed herself to express strong reactions such as crying, which was thought to represent a tentative or incomplete version of what the patient said she experienced as different personalities.

The psychiatrist frequently received calls in the middle of the night from emergency rooms where the patient had gone for suturing of her self-inflicted lacerations. Following a surgical operation, the patient opened one of her incisions, for which she claimed no pain; this resulted in a serious wound infection.

Mrs. B also described her previous involvement in a satanic cult. A careful review of systems revealed 37 medically unexplained symptoms in 10 categories on the Perley-Guze checklist for Briquet's syndrome. Some of these symptoms were dramatically described, including absent bowel movements for 3 weeks, severe dysmenorrhea, and irregular and excessive menstrual bleeding with passage of large clots. Conversion symptoms included paralysis, anesthesia, aphonia, amnesia, visual and olfactory hallucinations, unexplained urinary retention, and inability to comprehend what was said. The patient reported sexual indifference, frigidity, constant dyspareunia, and burning pains about the vagina and rectum. Her somatoform symptoms had begun at an early age, and as a child she had been repeatedly sent home from school for recurrent nausea and vomiting.

Mrs. B, like Mrs. A, met criteria for Briquet's syndrome and, in addition, had features of borderline personality. Both had seen therapists who had a special interest in MPD.

Mrs. C

Mrs. C was a 38-year-old white, separated, unemployed, bisexual, homeless woman. Her chief complaints were insomnia and depression. Mrs. C had a long history of psychiatric symptoms going back to at least age 5 when she felt depressed. At age 10 she considered suicide. She recalled intermittent brief "manic" symptoms such as hyperactivity and staying up all night since age 11 or 12. She recalled being a destructive child, tearing up her dolls and doll clothes, and cutting up a living room chair with scissors. She admitted to persistent lying in childhood. She ran away from home many times, beginning when she was a small child.

Mrs. C had a history of polysubstance abuse and dependence beginning at age 14, including cannabis, hallucinogens, intravenous heroin, amphetamines, crack cocaine, PCP, and a variety of other illicit substances. She had also abused alcohol in a binge pattern since age 16. She supported her drug habit by prostituting. She had intermittently stayed sober for a few weeks at most. She also admitted that she abused the amitriptyline prescribed her for depression.

Mrs. C reported a history of burning herself with cigarettes and cutting her hands and arms with razors since the age of 12. She said that she did not feel pain when she injured herself in these ways.

Other adult behavior problems reported by the patient included sexual promiscuity for more than 10 years, lying, dealing drugs, writing several thousand dollars' worth of bad checks with serious legal consequences, and periodic homelessness.

Review of systems was positive for multiple physical complaints, and she reported 31 medically unexplained somatic symptoms in nine categories on the Perley-Guze checklist for Briquet's syndrome. Her conversion symptoms included anesthesia, aphonia, amnesia, deafness, hallucinations, and loss of the ability to read and talk.

Mrs. C did not do well in therapy. She did not comply with homework assignments and continued to complain of amnesia and somatoform symptoms. She failed to keep follow-up appointments and, despite intensive case management, was lost to follow-up.

Mrs. C had Briquet's syndrome with borderline personality features, but in addition she met criteria for antisocial personality and polysubstance abuse. She too had first discovered her alternate personalities with the help of a therapist who was interested in MPD. Aside from her MPD, she has three very disabling comorbid disorders.

Mrs. D

Mrs. D was a 47-year-old divorced woman referred for hospitalization by her therapist because she was expressing suicidal ideas.

The patient said she felt she had been leading a double life since the age of 2 years. Her background was that of a very religious woman who held an advanced degree in religion. She had managed to compartmentalize all of her psychological difficulties and maintain her functions as a wife, mother, and professional. She was self-employed as a teacher, and she also ran adult religious self-help groups. She had been a virgin at the time of her only marriage, which she described as excellent up to the time her husband left her. She described her parents as alcoholic codependent.

The patient stated that a few years previously, when she was going through complicated personal problems, she began remembering that she had been involved in a satanic cult and that her entire family was involved (which the family did not validate).

She was referred to a psychologist who worked with victims of satanic cults, and during therapy sessions she recounted memories of torture, murder, and burial of bodies. Mrs. D reported that living inside her were a pair of Jekyll-Hyde-like personalities, one good (the working professional, religious, responsible wife and mother) and one bad (the one who engaged in the sadistic and evil activities of the cult). Her psychiatrist could not determine whether these represented full-blown alternate personalities or a fanciful way of explaining to herself and others how a good Christian model citizen could do all the horrible things she claimed to have done. She had no history of somatic complaints or self-mutilative behaviors.

After leaving the hospital, Mrs. D found a counselor with religious training who agreed to hypnotize her to help her regain more memories. She also resumed psychotherapy with a therapist with religious training who had previously counseled her. The patient remained adamant in her belief about the cult. In spite of these ideas and her complaints of alternate personalities, she managed to maintain occupational function and stay out of the hospital. In subsequent months, while in treatment undergoing hypnosis, Mrs. D's bad personality split into several distinct personalities which she named for her emotions, such as "Angry D" and "Mean D."

Mrs. D had no obviously apparent psychopathology aside from her multiple personalities. She did not meet criteria for Briquet's syndrome, borderline personality disorder, or antisocial personality disorder. Of the four cases presented, hers had the best therapeutic outcome and occupational function and would be considered an equivalent of one of Kluft's "high-functioning" MPD cases (Kluft 1986). The lack of diagnosable conditions in addition to her MPD may explain her more favorable outcome.

Conclusion

In summary, much remains to be done before we can better understand this disorder and place it in its proper nosology. It is a polysymptomatic, polysyndromic disorder with onset early in life. The polysyndromic nature makes it difficult to delineate exclusion criteria needed to help differentiate it from other disorders. In accordance with the validation model of Robins and Guze, knowledge about MPD is limited, not only about the exclusion factors for its separation from other disorders, but also about family transmission and prognosis, because family studies and systematic, prospective follow-up studies are lacking. Although rigorous laboratory studies have not been done, the next chapter will cover the progress to date in psychological lines of investigation of MPD.

4

Psychological investigations of MPD

In this chapter, we will review studies of patients with MPD, borderline personality disorder, and Briquet's syndrome (or somatization disorder) by means of psychological tests. Comparisons of psychological test results in these disorders are quite interesting: first, because combinations of two or three of these disorders often occur in the same patient and second, because these comparisons may help one understand what the tests are measuring in patients with MPD.

Many clinicians are not very familiar with the details of psychological tests. We will therefore provide a brief introduction to each test.

IQ Tests and Cognitive Testing

IQ tests were designed to predict which children could succeed in regular schools and which would need special educational settings in order to do grade school work. The original tests developed an "intelligence quotient (IQ)" by dividing the "mental age" (the age at which the student's performance would be average) by the student's actual age and then multiplying it by 100. Since knowledge does not expand in all areas beyond the early teenage years, it became clear that there were limits to this method and "deviation IQs" were substituted. With a deviation IQ, the test taker is compared to his or her age cohort. The average person, in theory, is given an IQ of 100. The standard deviation is set at 15 or 16, depending on the test. Some IQ tests were not normed on adequate population samples, and eventually it was realized that the "real mean" was not 100. Revisions of the IQ test usually correct these problems for a number of years.

IQ tests and other tests of cognitive ability have been given to patients with MPD. MPD patients are normal in many ways. Coons (1980) noted that one patient performed normally on a cognitive reasoning test—the proverbs test. Putnam's group (1984, p. 174) observed that "neuropsychological functioning generally remains normal in MPD, despite apparently severe memory defects." Coons and coworkers (1988) reported that neurologic examination, EEG, and the WAIS (Wechsler Adult Intelligence Scale—an individual IQ test) make no contribution to neuropsychiatric investigation in MPD.

Coons and Sterne (1986) reported a mean verbal IQ of 101.1 in MPD patients, with a range of 76 to 123, in 18 patients (16 women, 2 men). The patient with the lowest IQ appeared to have a borderline IQ in all of her alternate personalities. Coons and Milstein (1986) reported a mean IQ (on WAIS or the Shipley Hartford Intelligence Test) of 101.5, with a range of 77 to 123, in 17 women and 3 men with MPD. Coons' group (1988) found that in a series of 50 patients, 21 had received the WAIS (mean full-scale IQ, 101.8), 11 had received the Shipley-Hartford Test (mean verbal IQ, 111), and 1 had received the Wechsler Intelligence Scale for Children (WISC) (IQ, 95). The IQ range in the 33 patients tested was still 77 to 123.

Amstrong and Loewenstein (1990) tested 14 MPD patients using a battery that included intelligence testing. IQ scores ranged from 92 to 129 with no common pattern of scores, similar to the results of Coons' group. A few abnormalities were detected, however. The intrascale variability was marked. The authors also reported that cognitive styles became concrete when "traumatic associations" were evoked and, "In addition, these patients showed partial or alternating responses indicative of different cognitive levels operating side by side" (p. 451). Apparently, on some material relevant to the patients' past, internal debates affected both answers and response times. The authors stated, "without attention to dissociation, switching, state changes, and traumatic responses, many of these [MPD] patients would have received a borderline [IQ range 70–80, i.e., from about the third to the tenth percentile of the population] diagnosis on testing" (pp. 452–453). The inference from their qualitative report is that a nonstandard examination may be needed to obtain the best estimates of the patient's true abilities.

As a group, patients with MPD do not appear to have significant cognitive or neuropsychological deficits on the tests described to this point. More sophisticated batteries may be more informative.

Objective Personality Tests

Probably more studies have been done of psychiatric patients in the United States with the Minnesota Multiphasic Personality Inventory (MMPI) than with any other psychological test. This is also true for patients with MPD. The MMPI was developed by selecting items from standard psychiatric interviews in use before World War II. The items are presented to the patient in a True-False format. The items are combined into a number of scales. These scales frequently have overlapping content; in other words, the items sometimes appear on several scales. Because few people would ever memorize the means and standard deviations of up to 100 scales, these scores are traditionally converted to standard scores called "T-scores." "Z-scores" (normal deviations with a mean of 0 and a standard deviation of 1) are computed and then transformed into T-scores with a mean of 50; therefore, half of normal persons will score below 50 and half above, with a standard deviation of 10 (Table 4-1). Most scoring programs or

Table 4-1 Frequency of T-scores in Normal Subjects

T-score	Percent of normal (subjects equaling or exceeding the) T-score
100	0.00003
90	0.003
80	0.135
70	2.275
60	15.865
50	50.000
40	84.135
30	97.725

procedures produce T-scores by using lookup tables rather than actually computing them each time.

One can indicate what percentage of normal persons will obtain a specific T-score by consulting the appropriate tables in statistics books. Table 4-1 shows some figures; they assume that the scores on a scale are normally distributed; most MMPI scales can be reasonably approximated in this way. A few scales cannot (L and F, for example). A new revision of the MMPI, the MMPI-2, standardizes the scales in a slightly different way (uniform T-scores). The difference between T-scores and uniform T-scores in understanding test results is negligible.

Psychiatric patients are not normal, and their mean T-scores on many MMPI scales are usually quite different from normal subjects' mean of 50.

Validity scales

The MMPI has an excellent set of validity scales that give the clinician considerable information about the patient's approach to the testing situation. These scores can be used in a wide variety of ways—to detect problems with reading or understanding the items; to identify scoring problems; to detect malingering, defensiveness, or carelessness; to assess the patient's approach to seeking help, level of distress, ability to cope; and in some degree to understand personality or psychopathology. These scales can be used to evaluate the test at hand, but they also tap somewhat more enduring patient characteristics that seem to affect the patient-therapist relationship over time.

The Q scale is a simple count of the number of questions that are not answered either True or False or that are unscorable (both answers marked). Unanswered items are not counted on any other scale. A significant number of omissions can mask psychopathology.

The L scale is a lie scale. It consists of 15 items that are improbable, such as marking False on the item "At times I feel like swearing." A False answer to this statement may imply perfection. A high score on this scale probably represents a naive denial of faults in oneself. A high score on this scale might also occur because of splitting when the test is taken by an alternate personality unable to admit to or unaware of personal defects.

The K scale is a correction scale for more subtle kinds of defensiveness. To some extent, it measures one's ability to cope with the stresses and demands of daily life. A high score indicates defensiveness, and a low score indicates a denial of psychological assets and feelings of inadequacy. The K scale is correlated with education and socioeconomic level. A T-score of 65 would be expected in a physician and would be average; a T-score of 50 might represent defensiveness in a schizophrenic.

The F (infrequency) scale is used to detect the faking of a psychiatric disorder. Less than 10% of normal persons, on average, endorse (respond in the scored direction) any one item, and they have an average raw score of 3 (out of 64 items). The scale was validated, in part, with the help of prisoners and schizophrenics. The prisoners were asked to feign psychosis. Prisoners under these instructions endorsed many more F scale items than did the real psychotic patients. At higher levels, the F scale measures malingering, random answering without regard to content, and deviant response sets about test taking. At lower levels, the F scale functions something like a psychological thermometer, with increasing scores implying increasing severity of a psychiatric disorder. A cutoff score of 23 items endorsed is frequently used to detect an invalid MMPI. Occasionally, schizophrenics in acute psychosis score at or above this level, leading to an inappropriate rejection of their profiles.

Orne and colleagues (1984) note in an interesting footnote that Grant Dahlstrom (one of the leading experts in the United States on the MMPI) indicated that no research on the effect of role playing on MMPI profiles had been done; Dahlstrom speculated that role playing could avoid detection by the usual validity indicators. The implication seems to be that it would be difficult to predict how validly the validity scales would operate in detecting persons faking MPD or how well they would work with real patients with MPD.

The ratio between the raw scores on the F and K scales is frequently used to assess the patient's approach to the testing situation. The raw score for K is subtracted from the raw score for F to obtain the ratio. In psychiatric patients, even in-patients, this number is usually negative (less than 0). It is generally accepted that if the difference between F and K equals or exceeds, 12 the MMPI profile should be discarded as invalid and not used clinically. A very high difference between F and K scores can indicate malingering, inability to read, a desperate plea for help, or interference from hallucinations or other conditions that prevent an appropriate response to the testing situation. Some authors also advocate the use of − 12 as a cutoff for extreme defensiveness. For a more detailed discussion of these issues, one can consult Dahlstrom and colleagues (1972) or Greene (1988).

The F-K ratio represents to some degree the patient's attitude toward revealing his or her psychological strengths and weaknesses. This attitude can be highly influenced by the situation (such as applying for a job or for parole), but usually it represents a somewhat stable (over weeks or months) attitude toward self-disclosure. The patient's approach to the test is crucial to the results obtained.

Five scales (depression, hysteria, psychopathic deviant, paranoia, and mania) have had their items classified as either obvious (obviously related to what the scale measures even to a layperson) or subtle (not obvious to laypersons) by Wiener and Harmon (Dahlstrom et al. 1972). This yields five obvious scales and five subtle scales. The difference between the sum of the T-scores for the five obvious scales and the sum of the T-scores for the five subtle scales is used as a validity index to indicate defensiveness, exaggeration, or malingering. If the sum of the obvious scales exceeds the sum of the subtle scales by too large a margin, the test is considered invalid (Greene 1988).

A variety of lists of items have been selected as "critical items"—those of interest to the clinician independent of scale score. Two items[1] usually on critical item lists are:

True 156.   I have had periods in which I carried on activities without knowing later what I had been doing.

True 251.   I have had blank spells in which my activities were interrupted and I did not know what was going on around me.

According to some authors, these items may reflect dissociation.

Lachar and Wrobel (1979) developed a list of 111 such items organized into 11 areas of psychological dysfunction or discomfort. The Lachar-Wrobel items assess multiple somatic symptoms, as well as a multitude of psychological and interpersonal problems. The number of items endorsed on their list has been used as a validity indicator: if the number is too high, the MMPI is considered invalid (Greene 1988).

The usual validity scales (L, F, and K, F-K, difference between subtle and obvious scales, and the Lachar-Wrobel critical items) all basically operate on the assumption that individuals faking or exaggerating psychopathology will report too many symptoms of too many kinds. Conversely, it is assumed that those faking normality will present themselves as too able to cope or as unbelievably perfect.

---

[1]These two items are exact quotes from the MMPI. The MMPI is copyrighted by the University of Minnesota.

There is a different class of validity scales that evaluate consistency of responses to the same or similar questions. The TR (test-retest) scale looks at 16 items that are repeated on the MMPI. Disagreements are counted. Disagreeing with oneself five or more times is generally considered sufficient to call the validity of the MMPI into question. The CLS (carelessness) scale examines 12 pairs of items, 6 opposite and 6 quite similar. Inconsistency on many items is rare in both normal and psychiatric populations. TR and CLS scores are said to be independent of the degree of psychopathology (Greene 1988). Normal scores on these scales indicate that the problem with an apparently invalid test by the L, F, or K scale is not due to reading problems, scoring misadventure, random responses, carelessness, or varying motivation. The patient meant to respond in the way he or she did. These interesting validity scales are seldom reported in the MPD literature. The recently published MMPI-2 has a more extensive set of these kinds of validity scales; because we know of no studies of patients with MPD using the MMPI-2, we will not discuss them.

Validity Scale Results

Solomon (1983) attempted to give MMPIs to the primary personality of 18 MPD patients. Three or four refused (the text and abstract differ on the number). Five (according to the text, six according to the abstract) profiles were "invalid" because of high F scales. Solomon noted that dissociative responses on the two MMPI dissociation items are also scored (increase the total score) on the schizophrenia scale.

Bliss (1984a) reported on the MMPI profiles he obtained from 15 women with multiple personality. The means for the profiles showed a huge inverted V on scales L, F, and K. This indicates a marked lack of defensiveness and a willingness to report, and even to emphasize, psychopathology. The mean T-scores on the L and K scales were 46 and 45, respectively, equivalent to scores at approximately the 38th and 31st percentiles of the population. The mean T-score on scale F was 85, a score attained by fewer than 1 in 1000 normal subjects. The F-K ratio would be about 18.5–9.5 or 9.0; this would usually indicate a valid MMPI profile from a patient giving a "strong plea for help." Given the standard errors of the mean reported by Bliss, one would expect that a few of these profiles would be at least three items higher on the F-K statistic and hence could be called invalid by the F-K ≥ 12 criterion. With the small standard deviations on these three scales, one would not expect any of them to be 21 points below the mean and therefore disqualified by the F-K ≤ − 12 criterion; in other words, none of the subjects was attempting to minimize or hide his or her psychopathology.

Coons (1984) reported on the MMPIs obtained from 10 of his patients with MPD. He also reported a huge inverted V on the validity scales—L: mean of 47, F: mean of 84, and K: mean of 50. This pattern is extremely similar to that shown by Bliss and would again seem to indicate no hiding of psychopathology.

Coons and Sterne (1986) reported on 18 MPD patients (16 women, 2 men) given MMPIs. These patients had an inverted V on the L, F, and K scales. The mean F scale score was 82. Five patients had raw scores on F > 22 (technically invalid scores). Mean scores on the L and K scales were below a T-score of 50. The inverted V was still present in the final MMPI of nine MPD patients who did not achieve fusion and also in the three who did appear to fuse (mean L = 47, F = 78, and K = 44). This again agrees with the findings of Bliss and suggests that the pattern is stable. The authors also reported on the two critical items suggestive of dissociation. The critical items were examined in 14 of the 18 patients. Item 156 was endorsed by 12 (of 14) and Item 251 by 9 (of 14). The mean difference between the sum of T-scores of the five obvious scales (depression, hysteria, psychopathic deviant, paranoia, and mania) minus the sum of T-scores of the five subtle scales was 24, with a range of 1 to 64. Greene (1988) cites data showing that the mean difference between combined obvious and combined subtle scale scores for psychiatric patients is 51 for males and 56 for females. This suggests that by this measure this group of patients described by Coons and Sterne with MPD did not exaggerate their pathology.

Coons and colleagues (1988) reported on a still larger series of 50 patients with MPD seen by Coons. The mean profile showed mean T-scores on the L, F, and K scales of 49, 84, and 49, respectively. Scores on the F scale were quite variable, ranging from 46 (slightly below average) to 120 (seven standard deviations above the mean). The other two scores also showed some variability, indicating that a minority of the patients had a different response set than the majority.

Griffin (1989) gave the MMPI to 30 male Veterans Administration patients with a diagnosis of MPD. They had the typical inverted V on the validity scales (L = 49, F = 93, K = 44). This is the highest mean F scale score reported in any study of MPD. The equivalent raw scores would be 28 for F and 6 for K, yielding an F-K ratio of 22 on average. Griffin suggested using a cutoff of F ≥ T-score 90 to identify MPD.

1. Borderline personality patients. Pitts and coworkers (1985) used the Lachar-Wrobel critical item list to differentiate patients with borderline personality disorder from patients with other personality disorders. Eighty-eight of the 111 items were endorsed in the pathologic direction more often by borderline patients than by other patients. Eleven of the 88 items were different enough to be statistically significant. Borderline patients reported significantly more substance abuse (one of the 11 areas) than other patients.

Gartner and colleagues (1989) identified 13 articles on MMPI scores in patients with borderline personality disorder. They went so far as to state that the validity scales may be more sensitive to borderline personality disorder than are the clinical scales (p. 434). The F scale is typically elevated above T-score 70, and the L and K scales are usually below T-score 50. On this basis, one would expect many MMPI profiles obtained from patients with borderline personality disorder to have F scale scores above the usual validity cutoffs. The authors offer three interpretations of these data, all of which they seem to find acceptable:

a. Extreme scores on F represent a general pathology factor in polysymptomatic borderline patients.

b. Extreme scores on F represent the presence of thought disorder.

c. The pattern of L, F, and K suggests that borderline patients present their difficulties in an exaggerated and dramatic manner.

We tend to believe that only the first and third explanations may be valid; the thinking of borderline patients is unusual but does not represent a consistent, true form of psychotic thought disorder. Gartner and coworkers further noted that the available studies have not agreed on any subset of the 10 clinical scales that have discriminated borderline patients from others as well as these three validity scales have done.

2. *Patients with Briquet's syndrome.* Liskow and colleagues (1977) compared MMPIs obtained from 21 patients with Briquet's syndrome and 29 patients with hysteria diagnosed on the basis of psychological functioning rather than the presence of multiple somatic complaints. Both groups showed virtually identical inverted V's on the L, F and K scales, indicating a help-seeking or dramatizing tendency. Extrapolating from the rather large standard deviations of the F scale, both groups should have had patients with F scores above the usual validity cutoffs.

Liskow's group (1986) noted that 16 patients with Briquet's syndrome had a typical inverted V on the L, F, and K scales. They noted that all 16 patients had F scale T-scores > 70. The mean for L was 52 and that for K was 47.

Wetzel (1992, unpublished data) selected MMPIs from 33 patients clinically diagnosed with Briquet's syndrome. The group showed an inverted V with T-scores of 52, 74, and 49 on the L, F, and K scores, respectively. Using the cutoffs suggested by Greene (1988) for detecting deception, two were too defensive by both the F-K ≤ − 12 and the sum of the Obvious-Subtle scale totals; three were too defensive by the F-K ≤ − 12 rule and suspect by the Obvious-Subtle scale rule; and three more were suspect by the Obvious-Subtle scale rule. Thus, five were invalid (15%) and three suspect (9%). Four patients produced invalid (exaggerating) profiles by the F-K ≥ 12 rule and the Obvious-Subtle rule; three were rejected by F-K and suspect on the Obvious-Subtle rule; and six more were suspect by the Obvious-Subtle rule. A total of 13 (40%) were suspected at least of exaggerating their symptoms by these usual criteria. Only 12 profiles (36%) were normal by these rules.

Comment

Patients with MPD, borderline personality, and Briquet's syndrome typically appear to emphasize psychopathology on these validity scales. This to some extent represents a significant degree of distress, a willingness to dramatize that distress, and an eagerness to obtain help. It also represents to some degree accurate reporting of a polysyndromic, polysymptomatic disorder. A small minority, however, do not present in this way. Some may be defensive and reluctant to admit psychiatric problems. Coons and colleagues (1988) show that some MPD patients present in a defensive manner, and reliance on high "invalid" validity scale scores would lead to a failure to detect a small minority of these patients.

Most experienced MMPI clinicians would also expect the MMPI profile to be affected by the situation in which it is obtained. The profiles of patients with Briquet's syndrome on a surgical service are not usually as florid as their typical profiles on a psychiatric service (Wetzel 1992, unpublished data). In addition, their MMPI profiles vary from test to test with the degree of depression, stress, and other factors. Similarly, one would expect MPD patients desiring to remain hidden to perform differently on an MMPI than those patients who are in longer-term treatment with MPD experts fully aware of their condition. These differences in trust and openness would frequently be picked up in the configuration of the validity scales. Future MMPI studies of MPD patients would be easier to evaluate if more of the available validity scales were reported. Undoubtedly, the truly invalid MMPIs from MPD patients "blowing off the test" because of anger or distrust by an alternate personality could be picked up by the TR and CLS scales without resort to the use of the F or F-K cutoffs.

These validity scale patterns present a clear problem in forensic settings. Because many patients with MPD, borderline personality disorder, and/or Briquet's syndrome present invalid test results, one cannot confidently attribute the production of invalid profiles to malingering alone. In clinical settings, invalid profiles should cause one to suspect that the patient has one of these disorders. In forensics, one must simply conclude that one's test data are equivocal to some extent and that the scientific conclusions that can be drawn from them are quite limited.

Clinical Scales

Ten clinical scales are routinely scored on the MMPI. MMPI experts now tend to refer to these scales by number (1 to 9 and 0), but this is confusing to most clinicians; therefore, we will use the original names. Scales do not necessarily measure what their names imply, either now or at the time they were originally developed. We shall also discuss these scales in terms of the Harris and Lingoes description of subscales based on face validity inspection of their items. (In parentheses, we will offer an opinion about what we think a scale really measures—this is inherently subjective.) Later in this chapter, we argue that MPD patients, borderline personality patients, and Briquet's syndrome patients share many kinds of psychopathology; these problems each affect a number of MMPI clinical scales. To understand the argument, the reader should appreciate the heterogeneity of the 10 MMPI clinical scales.

Scale 1 (Hs) is a *h*ypochondria*s*is scale; its items inquire about many different symptoms in various organ systems. Hs without the K correction is highly correlated ($r = 0.92$) (Wetzel 1992, unpublished data) with the number of symptoms on a Perley-Guze review (Perley & Guze 1962) of symptoms for Briquet's syndrome. Most studies report hypochondriasis scale scores with the K correction for defensiveness; this correction lowers the correlation with the total number of symptoms on the Perley-Guze review. This scale is heterogeneous only in the sense that the physical symptoms refer to many different organ systems.

Scale 2 (D) is a *d*epression scale. (The criterion group for the scale had severe endogenous depression.) The Harris-Lingoes subscales are subjective depression, psychomotor retardation, physical malfunctioning (somatic symptoms characteristic of depression), mental dullness (perceived intellectual inefficiency), and brooding. A number of items on somatic complaints characteristic of hysteria were added and scored, so that denial of these symptoms increased the depression scale score. The Subtle items on this scale reflect solidity and stability and are due in part to the "antihysteria" correction factor.

Scale 3 (Hy) is a *h*ysteria scale. It shares many items with the hypochondriasis scale. It measures, in addition, aspects of histrionic behavior. The Harris-Lingoes subscales are denial of social anxiety, need for affection, lassitude-malaise, somatic complaints (more characteristic of hysteria than of depression), and inhibition of aggression. Strong use of denial would raise one's score on this scale even if somatic complaints were average in number.

Scale 4 (Pd) is an antisocial personality (*p*sychopathic *d*eviant) scale. Its subscales, according to Harris and Lingoes, are familial discord, authority problems, social imperturbability (ability to resist social pressure easily), social alienation, and self-alienation. A history of family dysfunction could raise one's score on this scale even if one were not a psychopathic deviant/antisocial personality/ sociopath. (While sensitive to antisocial personality disorder, it is not specific to it. Any patient with a cluster B personality disorder in DSM-III-R may have an elevated score on this scale.)

Scale 5 (Mf) is a *m*asculinity-*f*emininity scale. It seems to measure stereotypical gender interest patterns. Its subscales have been described by Pepper and Strong (1958) as personal and emotional sensitivity, sexual identification, altruism, feminine occupational identification, and denial of masculine occupations.

Scale 6 (Pa) is a *p*a*r*anoia scale. Its Harris-Lingoes subscales are persecutory ideas, poignancy, and naivete. (At the high end of the normal range or the low end of the pathologic range, it may reflect problems with trust and intimacy.)

Scale 7 (Pt) is a *p*sychas*t*henia (obsessive/compulsive/anxiety/phobic) scale. It has not been given subscales.

Scale 8 (Sc) is a *sc*hizophrenia scale. Its Harris-Lingoes subscales are social alienation, emotional alienation, lack of ego mastery—cognitive, lack of ego mastery—conative, lack of ego mastery—defective inhibition, and bizarre sensory experiences. (The item content of this scale is quite diverse, and one can easily obtain a very high score without having schizophrenia.)

To illustrate this point further, we cite a study by Ben-Porath and colleagues (1991) who gave MMPIs to inpatients at three psychiatric institutions. Diagnoses were made clinically by the usual psychiatric evaluation teams (psychiatry, psychology, social work and nursing) without access to MMPI data. Patients were selected if they fit one of two selection criteria:

1. Schizophrenia without any affective disorder diagnosis.

2. Major depression without any schizophrenic spectrum diagnosis.

Eighty-seven men and 73 women met these criteria; the sex by diagnosis breakdown was not reported. Only one clinical scale significantly discriminated between the two diagnoses in both sexes: the D (depression) scale was significantly higher in patients with major depression. The Sc (schizophrenia) scale did

Sex	Dxx	D	Sc
Male	Scz	68 ± 13	82 ± 20
Female	Scz	62 ± 15	71 ± 16
Male	Dep	78 ± 16	78 ± 22
Female	Dep	72 ± 16	73 ± 18

not discriminate between the patients with depression and schizophrenia. The probability values for the D scale were 0.002 in men and 0.009 in women; for the Sc scale they were 0.52 and 0.69. One may reasonably infer that the schizophrenia scale is a measure of general distress that suggests schizophrenia when depression, anxiety, agitation, and mania are not present. Subscales like Sc3 (Sc6 on the MMPI-2) that indicate hallucinations or BIZ (bizarre mentation on the MMPI-2) help to indicate that the score on the schizophrenia scale is elevated by a disease process that may include psychosis.

Scale 9 (Ma) is a hypo*ma*nia scale. Acutely manic patients are seldom able to finish a 566-item test before dashing off. Harris and Lingoes called its subscales amorality, psychomotor acceleration, imperturbability, and grandiosity.

Scale 0 (Si) is a pure *s*ocial *i*ntroversion-extroversion scale. High scorers are introverted; low ones are extroverted.

In order to illustrate the heterogeneity of the MMPI clinical scales, we took a sample of 5334 MMPI profiles from the records of the Psychological Assessment Laboratory at the Washington University Medical Center. The file contained MMPIs obtained from patients evaluated in the psychiatry department between 1981 and 1991. The sample contained 3013 (56.5%) females and 2321 (43.5%) males. The average age was 37.9. Invalid MMPI profiles were screened out by computer. Profiles from extremely defensive patients were eliminated by excluding profiles with a T-score for the K scale higher than 70 (222 profiles). Profiles from patients exaggerating their pathology were eliminated by excluding profiles where the difference between the raw score on the F (infrequency) scale minus the K scale $\geq$ 12 (475 profiles). These two rules together eliminated 655 cases (42 met both rules). The final sample included 4679 MMPI profiles. The correlation matrix showed that the correlation ($+0.88$) of scale 7 (psychasthenia, not K corrected) with scale 8 (schizophrenia, not K corrected) was higher than the correlation between scale 8 and any of its subscales.

An oblique factor analysis was used to illustrate the composition of the MMPI clinical scales. Oblique analyses, unlike orthogonal analyses, allow the data to control the degree of correlation between factors or clusters of variables. Essentially, one is asking a computer to construct the fewest number of hypothetical or speculative variables that could account for a pattern of correlations between variables. If the clinical scales are homogeneous, then subscales from the same scale should load on the same cluster; if they are not, then subscales should be scattered from cluster to cluster.

Proc varclus of Statistical Analysis System (SAS) (version 6.04) was used to perform the oblique factor analysis on the set of MMPI scale scores. When Harris-Lingoes subscales existed for standard scales (depression—5, hysteria—5, psychopathic deviant—5, paranoia—3, schizophrenia—6, and mania—4), the subscale scores were used. Because no Harris-Lingoes subscales exist for hypochondriasis and psychasthenia, those scale scores were entered. Overall, 2 scales and 28 subscales were entered into the analysis.

The analysis produced six factors that accounted for 68% of the variance in the 30 scales and subscales. Table 4-2 shows the factor or cluster structure derived. It can readily be seen that the subscales of each clinical scale are heterogeneous; in other words, subscales have their highest correlations on different clusters. No clinical scale has all of its subscales load on only one cluster; depression comes closest, with four of its five subscales having their highest loading or correlation on cluster 1. Cluster 1 has subscales of five scales (depression, psychopathic deviant, paranoia, psychasthenia, and schizophrenia) having their highest correlation with it. It seems to be a depression–anxiety–low self-esteem cluster. Cluster 2 seems to measure interpersonal alienation and problems; three scales have subscales correlating highly with it.

Cluster 3 gathers together scales sensitive to somatic complaints; it includes the hypochondriasis scale and subscales from the depression, hysteria, and schizophrenia scales. Cluster 4 picks up the subscales that reflect coolness under pressure or imperturbability; these subscales come from three different scales.

Cluster 5 has high positive correlations with a somewhat naive need for approval and a negative correlation with pathologic ego inflation. It has its high-

Table 4-2 *Cluster Structure of Clinical Subscales of the MMPI*

Cluster 1	*correlation*
Subjective depression (D1)	.94
Mental dullness (D4)	.93
Psychasthenia (PT)	.93
Lack of conative mastery (SC2B)	.93
Brooding (D5)	.91
Self-alienation (PD4B)	.86
Lack of cognitive mastery (SC2A)	.85
Emotional alienation (SC1B)	.84
Poignancy (PA2)	.72
Psychomotor retardation (D2)	.56
Cluster 2	*correlation*
Social alienation (SC1A)	.92
Social alienation (PD4A)	.88
Persecutory ideas (PA1)	.84
Lack of inhibition (SC2C)	.73
Family discord (PD1)	.69
Cluster 3	*correlation*
Hypochondriasis (HS)	.96
Somatic complaints (HY4)	.90
Lassitude-malaise (HY3)	.85
Physical malfunctioning (D3)	.80
Bizarre sensory experience (SC3)	.79
Cluster 4	*correlation*
Denial of social anxiety (HY1)	.92
Social imperturbability (PD3)	.92
Imperturbability (MA3)	.85
Cluster 5	*correlation*
Naivete (PA3)	.97
Need for affection (HY2)	.89
Grandiosity (MA4)	$-.69$
Cluster 6	*correlation*
Amorality (MA1)	.71
Psychomotor acceleration (MA2)	.67
Inhibition of aggression (HY5)	$-.60$
Authority problems (PD2)	.57

est loadings from single subscales from three scales. Cluster 6 picks up some antisocial features on four subscales from three scales; it has positive correlations with amorality and high energy from the mania scale, authority problems from the psychopathic deviant scale, and a strong negative correlation with inhibition or denial of aggression on the hysteria scale.

Table 4-3 shows the intercluster correlations (oblique factors can be correlated). It shows that all of these clusters are significantly correlated with each
other (except for clusters 4 and 6). This indicates in general that patients reporting more difficulty on one cluster are more likely to report more difficulty on
the others. The exceptions are cluster 4, which reflects the report that one is
relatively unaffected by criticism or pressure, and cluster 5, which seems to
reflect a more naive denial of problems. Higher scores on these two clusters are
associated with lower scores on the other four clusters.

Again, the point of this excursion into factor analysis was to document the
heterogeneity of the standard scales and to indicate, first, that specific problems
can raise the scores on multiple scales and, second, that multiple problems can
raise the scores on one scale.

Interpretation of MMPIs is somewhat complicated. To oversimplify it to an
extent, standard interpretation depends on the pattern of relationships between
the 10 clinical scales considered in the light of the pattern of the validity scales.
Generally, if two of the 10 clinical scale scores are higher than T-score 70, the
patient is likely to be a psychiatric patient. If almost all of the 10 clinical personality scales are elevated above T-score 70, the profile is sometimes called a
"floating profile." (Some authorities would reserve this term for profiles with
all 10 scales at T-score 70 or higher.) Floating profiles are associated with deviant response sets (pleading for help), acute distress, or specific syndromes
(borderline personality, Briquet's syndrome).

MMPI enthusiasts frequently talk about "high point codes." This refers to
the two or three highest clinical scale scores. A 2-7 profile, for example, is one
in which scales 2 (depression) and 7 (psychasthenia) are higher than all other
clinical scales. When only a few scales are elevated above 70, it is frequently
very informative to know which scales are elevated. Establishing that a subset
of two or three scales was elevated in a particular disorder and that other scales
were less regularly elevated would give one some insight into the essence of the
clinical presentation. In our opinion, depression and anxiety can affect the
depression (2), psychasthenia (7), and schizophrenia (8) scales. Personality disorder can affect the psychopathic deviant (4), paranoia (6), schizophrenia (8),
and mania (9) scales. Psychosis can affect the paranoia (6), schizophrenia (8),
and mania (9) scales. Hysteria (somatization disorder/Briquet's syndrome) can

Table 4-3 *Intercluster Correlations*

Cluster	1	2	3	4	5	6
1	—	0.72	0.66	−0.53	−0.28	0.18
2		—	0.48	−0.41	−0.53	0.41
3			—	−0.26	−0.19	0.15
4				—	0.25	−0.03
5					—	−0.43

affect the hypochondriasis (1), hysteria (3), and schizophrenia (8) scales. Note that we believe that each of these problems can elevate scores on the schizophrenia scale. The factor analysis reported above supports our opinion.

When multiple scales are elevated, this may suggest that either multiple problems are present or a superordinate diagnosis with subordinate diagnoses might be present. The presence of many elevated scales (suggesting many psychiatric symptoms) may be more important than which scale is the highest.

Clinical Scale Research Results

1. Multiple personality disorder. Solomon (1983) gave MMPIs to 18 patients with MPD. He found that 16 of them had elevated schizophrenia scale scores as one of the two highest scale scores. Noting multiple high point codes in his group, he suggested that a modification of the schizophrenia scale might be useful in detecting dissociation.

Bliss (1984a) showed that in his 15 female MPD patients, 8 of the 10 standard clinical scales were elevated into the pathologic region. These included all the scales except Mf and Ma. The Mf scale mean was 38, indicating that this group of 15 female MPD patients had stereotypical passive, feminine interest patterns. The Ma (hypomania) scale mean was 69, just under the usual cutoff of T-score 70. The highest scale score was on Sc (schizophrenia mean = 100), indicating marked complaints of social and emotional alienation; perceived loss of control of thoughts, feelings, and behavior; and bizarre sensory experiences. The next group of elevated scales included D (depression), Pd (psychopathic deviant), Pa (paranoia), and Pt (psychasthenia).

This suggests that these women could be characterized as depressed (D), alienated from self and others, having a history of family discord, rebellious, and perhaps resistant to social pressure to conform (Pd), anxious, worrying, and obsessed (Pt), and suspicious and showing major problems with intimacy (Pa). Finally, problems with hypochondriasis (Hs), histrionic personality features (Hy), and social introversion (Si) are indicated. One could describe this mean profile as an assertion that psychologically almost everything is wrong. Bliss (1984a) also recounted the number of symptoms reported in multiple problem areas on interview. Some of these patients admitted relatively few symptoms. It is noteworthy that the MMPI did not seem to reflect the same minimizing of pathology in a small subset of MPD patients.

Coons (1984) reported the mean MMPI scale scores from 10 patients with MPD. The means of 5 of the 10 scales were above T-score 70, and the means of 2 scales were above 80. Sc (schizophrenia) was the highest, indicating, as Bliss (1984a) observed, marked alienation; perceived loss of control of thoughts, feelings, and behavior; and possible hallucinations. This was followed by Pd (psychopathic deviant), suggesting further alienation from self and others, a history of family discord, rebelliousness, and perhaps resistance to social pressure to conform. The MMPI means also indicated considerable depression (D), anxiety and worry (Pt), and suspiciousness and problems with intimacy (Pa). The three scales primed (over T-score 70) in Bliss's report were slightly lower in

Coons' sample—hypochondriasis (T = 64), hysteria (T = 68), and introversion-extroversion (T = 69). Masculinity-femininity was again the lowest scale score.

Coons and Sterne (1986) reported on 18 (16 female, 2 male) patients with MPD. Initial MMPIs showed seven scales elevated to T-score 69.5 or higher. The mean mania and social introversion scale scores were in the 60s, while the mean Mf scale was below T-score 50. The highest scale was schizophrenia (mean = 91). Follow-up MMPIs on nine patients who did not achieve fusion were essentially similar, except that the mean hypochondriasis score fell from T-score 69.9 to 64 and the hysteria scale score fell from 71 to 67.

Three patients did achieve fusion, and their mean profiles were basically unchanged; five scales remained primed (depression, psychopathic deviant, paranoia, psychasthenia, and schizophrenia). It may be noteworthy that fusion was associated with a reduction only on the two scales most sensitive to conversion symptoms (hypochondriasis and hysteria). Because the number of fused cases was only three, confirmation of these findings awaits future studies.

High point codes in the valid MMPI profiles were very variable; one was described as K+ profile: a defensive profile with all clinical scale scores below T-score 70. By definition, this is a profile in which all psychopathology is hidden to a great extent.

Coons' group (1988) reported on 50 patients with MPD. Seven of the 10 scales were primed (over 70): depression, hysteria, psychopathic deviant, paranoia, psychasthenia, schizophrenia, and social introversion-extroversion. The hypochondriasis and mania scales both had T-scores > 65 (approximately the 90th percentile). Only masculinity-femininity was below average (T-score < 50). Reported ranges showed that at least some subjects must have presented normal profiles. Four scales appeared to have variances that were larger than expected in a normal population: depression, psychasthenia, schizophrenia, and paranoia. The first three are sensitive to depression, which would lead one to expect that a subgroup may have presented without depression at the time of testing.

Griffin (1989) compared the MMPI profiles of 30 MPD male patients with those of 60 other psychiatric patients. The MPD patients were higher than the others on 8 of the 10 clinical scales (Hs, D, Hy, Pd, Pa, Pt, Sc, and Si). The two groups had quite similar scores on masculinity-femininity (mean of 67.2 compared to 66.6), and the MPD patients were slightly higher on the mania scale (mean of 73.6 compared to 68.7, p <0.10). The schizophrenia scale had by far the highest mean T-score (109.2).

Figure 4-1 shows the average MMPI profiles of the four independent studies of patients with MPD (Bliss 1984a; Coons & Sterne 1986; Coons et al. 1988; Griffin 1989). Note the amazing similarity in shape among the four profiles. Scores on the validity scales—L, F, and K—are virtually identical in the three mean profiles obtained from women, and the men's mean scores are similar but slightly higher. All of the women's profiles are dominated by the so-called "characterologic V" on scales Pd, Mf, and Pa. The Mf scale in men is inverted,

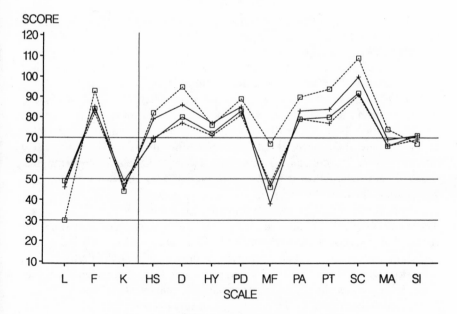

Figure 4–1. MMPI profiles of patients with MPD.

which explains the difference between the other three profiles and this one on Mf. It is interesting to note that male MPD patients show either more psychopathology or more exaggeration of psychopathology than women with MPD do.

Coons and Fine (1990) used a checklist of identifying characteristics to distinguish between the MMPI profiles of 25 patients with MPD, 11 borderline patients, 11 depressed patients, 5 schizophrenic patients, and 6 with other disorders. The features evaluated included:

a. High F and Sc scale scores

b. Technically invalid (F or F-K)

c. Numerous critical items

d. Critical items 156 and 251 positive

e. Polysymptomatic profile simulating borderline profiles

f. Obvious scores generally much higher than subtle scores

g. Lack of blatant psychosis except internal auditory hallucinations

h. Relatively low Hs scale scores

They also suggested that some other features—low Es (ego strength—Barron), high Pd1 subscale (family problems—Harris and Lingoes) score, high Wiggin's Fam (family problems) scale score, and critical items with a sexual content—be examined.

Using these criteria in a qualitative manner, Coons and Fine correctly identified 17 of 25 (68%) multiples and 28 of 38 (73%) non-MPD patients. They concluded that the MMPI has some diagnostic utility in detecting MPD.

2. *Borderline personality disorder.* Several studies have reported MMPI test results of patients diagnosed with borderline personality disorder. Snyder's group (1982) reported the mean MMPI profiles of 26 Veterans Administration inpatients with at least six DSM-III criteria for borderline disorder. Seven of the first nine clinical scales were above T-score 70. (Hysteria and masculinity-femininity were 68, and social introversion-extroversion was 65.) The two highest scales were psychasthenia and schizophrenia.

Resnick and colleagues (1983) examined the MMPIs of 19 schizotypal personality disorder patients divided into 10 patients who also had borderline personality disorder and 9 who did not. Five of the 10 clinical scales were primed (> 70) in the borderline patients compared to only 1 in the nonborderline group. Elevations were noted on the depression, psychopathic deviant, paranoia, psychasthenia, and schizophrenia scales. They suggested that the MMPI could be used as a coarse initial screen for borderline personality disorder.

Evans and coworkers (1984) reported the mean MMPI scale scores of 45 inpatients with borderline personality disorder. Six of the 10 scales were over T-score 70: depression, hysteria, psychopathic deviant, paranoia, psychasthenia, and schizophrenia. It is worth noting that borderline patients had higher mean scores on the schizophrenia and mania scales than did control groups of chronic schizophrenics and acute psychotics; the differences were not significant on these two scales, but this finding supports our opinion that one can achieve high scores on these scales without being schizophrenic or psychotic. The borderline patients were significantly higher than the two control groups on the depression, hysteria, psychopathic deviant, and psychasthenia scales.

Evans' group (1986) investigated the stability of MMPI profiles of 14 inpatients with borderline personality disorder, reporting mean scores and later mean scores at readmission for 11 of these patients. At both times of testing, the mean F scale T-score and 7 (Hs, D, Hy, Pd, Pa, Pt, and Sc) of the 10 clinical scale scores were at or above T-score 70.

Resnick and colleagues (1983, 1988) stated that the MMPI has utility as a screening tool for borderline personality disorder. They recommended the use of elevations on the F, depression, psychopathic deviant, paranoia, psychasthenia, and schizophrenia scales.

Widiger and colleagues (1986) obtained MMPIs from 44 state hospital inpatients who had borderline personality disorder. Patients with major depression, schizophrenia, and chronic organic mental disorder were excluded. The authors diagnosed all 11 Axis II personality disorders. Their data showed that the mean MMPI profile obtained was a function to some extent of the concomitant Axis II diagnoses. Borderline patients were divided into groups on the basis of the presence or absence of other common Axis II diagnoses—those with/without schizotypal personality, those with/without histrionic personality, and those with/without antisocial personality. The MMPI correlates were then examined. The presence or absence of schizotypal personality disorder was associated with significant changes in the depression, paranoia, psychasthenia, schizophrenia, and masculinity-femininity scales (6 of the 13 scales). The presence or absence of histrionic personality disorder led to significant differences on the F, hypochondriasis, depression, paranoia, psychasthenia, schizophrenia, and social introversion scales (7 of the 13 scales). The presence or absence of the diagnosis of antisocial personality led to a change on only one scale—the psychopathic deviant scale. The authors noted that the MMPI profile for borderline personality disorder differs in degree but not in shape from the MMPI profile associated with other disorders. The borderline profile is more elevated "because the BPD [Borderline Personality Disorder] group differs from the comparison group in having an additional diagnosis that may be primarily an indication of severity of disturbance" (Widiger et al. 1986, p. 549).

Gartner and colleagues (1989), in their review of MMPI studies of patients with borderline personality disorder, noted that 13 MMPI studies of borderline patients have shown that the mean score on Sc is higher than T-score 70. They indicate that they believe that this elevation occurs because the Sc scale measures thought disorder in part. (Note that, as indicated earlier, we believe it measures many other things—alienation from others, emotional alienation, and loss of control of emotions and of behavior, in addition to perceived inability to control thoughts. Because almost all patients with major depression have high scores on this schizophrenia subscale, one can say that formal thought disorder is not required to obtain a high scale score.) Eleven studies reported elevations on Pd; this is said to reflect impulsivity and low frustration tolerance.

The authors further, and importantly, note that elevation on Pd is the best discriminator between patients with borderline personality disorder and psychosis. In the comparison groups studied (no MPD or antisocial groups were included), no group had a mean score on Pd as high as that of patients with borderline personality disorder. They noted that scales D (depression) and Pt (psychasthenia) are frequently elevated in borderline patients, indicating the frequent presence of dysphoria, depression, anxiety, and worry in these patients. Typical elevations on the Pa (paranoia) scale are noted in MMPI studies of patients with borderline personality disorder; Gartner's group links this finding to problems with intense, inappropriate anger and lack of control of anger. We would add that it probably also relates to problems with intimacy and developing trust in others.

Gartner and colleagues noted that borderline personality disorder patients do not have just a few high point codes.

Figure 4-2 shows the mean MMPI profiles of 10 different studies of patients with borderline personality disorder (Edell 1987; Evans 1984, 1986; Gustin et al. 1983; Kroll et al. 1981; Resnick et al. 1983, 1988; Snyder et al. 1982; Trull

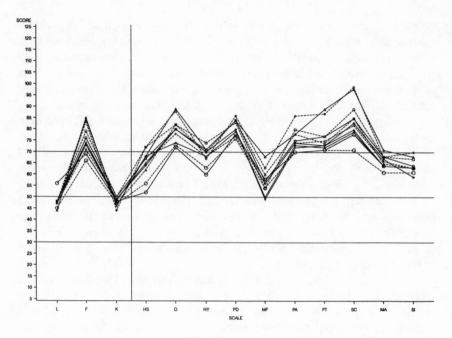

Figure 4–2. MMPI profiles of borderline patients.

1991; Widiger et al. 1986). Some variation in the profiles can be seen. Note that every borderline profile shows marked problems on the depression, psychopathic deviant, paranoid, psychasthenia, and schizophrenia scales. On the hypochondriasis, hysteria, and masculinity-femininity scales, however, there is considerable variation. One could infer that "borderline" means different things in different locales. While some borderline profiles could easily include many patients with Briquet's syndrome, others would not appear to be able to do so.

Our interpretation of the MMPI results in borderline patients includes the following observations:

a. Borderline personalities are somewhat heterogeneous; it matters what other personality disorders are present. Borderline patient groups with high concentrations of histrionic, antisocial, passive-aggressive, or explosive personality disorders resemble patients with MPD more than borderline patient groups with avoidant, schizoid, or dependent personality disorders without the above group B disorders. (DSM-III-R classifies personalities into three groups designated A, B, and C. Group B includes antisocial, histrionic, explosive, borderline, and antisocial personality disorders.)

b. High point codes are not very useful when many scales are elevated; the presence of many primed scales is more important than which primed scale is the highest. The schizophrenia scale will be highly elevated, although it will be the highest in less than half of patients.

3. Briquet's syndrome. Liskow's group (1977) showed that the 21 patients with Briquet's syndrome in their study had on average seven MMPI scales with means of T-score 70 or higher. The primed scales were hypochondriasis, depression, hysteria, psychopathic deviant, paranoia, psychasthenia, and schizophrenia. The mean scores for the 29 patients with hysteria were very similar, except for a 1.1 standard deviation difference on the hypochondriasis scale. This difference is probably a function of the criteria rather than of severity. Criteria for Briquet's syndrome explicitly require somatic symptomatology, while those for hysteria do not. This study does make it clear that the pathology in patients with Briquet's syndrome is not limited to multiple medical complaints; it also includes multiple psychological and interpersonal complaints.

Liskow and coworkers (1986) reported the MMPI results of another group of 16 female inpatients with Briquet's syndrome. The focus of this report was the frequent presence of comorbidity in patient's with Briquet's syndrome. Eight of the 10 standard MMPI scales were elevated above 70. The pattern, very similar to that of the earlier study, was almost indistinguishable from that seen in MPD and in borderline personality disorder. Sc was the highest scale score, with a mean of 88. Hypochondriasis, depression, hysteria, psychopathic deviant, paranoia, psychasthenia, and mania were all above T-score 70. Only the score on masculinity-femininity was normal (below T-score 50). The authors comment that "female psychiatric patients with Briquet's syndrome invariably have several . . . additional psychiatric syndromes." They "may simply report a great number of all types of psychiatric symptoms, just as they report a great number of all types of medical symptoms" (Liskow et al. 1986, p. 466).

Figure 4-3 shows the mean profiles for patients with Briquet's syndrome in the four studies described above (Liskow et al. 1977, 1986; Slavney & McHugh 1976; Wetzel 1992 unpublished). The marked characterologic V is present on scales Pd, Mf, and Pa. All of the "neurotic" scales (Hs, D, Hy) are elevated, and most of the "psychotic" scales (Pa, Pt, Sc, and Ma) as well.

Liskow and colleagues (1986) concede that Briquet's syndrome may occur in the course of another psychiatric disease, and that the illness of patients with both that disease and Briquet's syndrome might then follow the course of that superordinate disease. Their list of possibly superordinate diseases includes schizophrenia and MPD. They quite rightly, we think, emphasize that only careful follow-up studies of patients with a combination of syndromes can provide the information crucial to this point.

The research studies indicate that patients with MPD, borderline personality disorder, and Briquet's syndrome frequently have MMPI profiles that can be characterized as markedly elevated, with many scales primed (or types of problems reported). Typically, these patients approach the test by reporting as many symptoms as possible, and that approach affects the validity scales in a way that

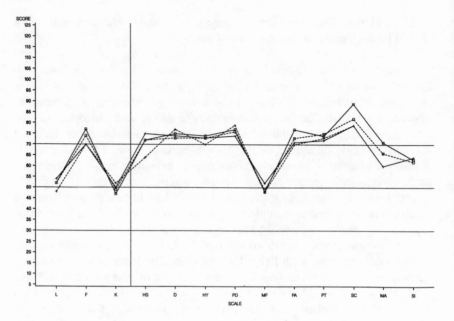

Figure 4–3. MMPI profiles of patients with Briquet's syndrome or hysterical personality disorder.

may lead the clinician to discount the message given by the test—"I am in great distress and have too many problems with which to cope." At the present time, we cannot confidently label this approach as accurate, or histrionic, or malingering. We do need, however, to recognize the pattern.

Having said this, we should also note that the clinical detection of patients with MPD on the basis of their MMPI profiles does not seem as easy as the above clinical research studies might make it seem. There is a clear mean performance in these groups that tells us what we will usually see, but individuals vary considerably from time to time. The problem is aggravated by the varying response sets of the patients to self-disclosure.

In 1991, one of us was asked to evaluate a young man with apparent MPD. He reported at least two personalities, with amnesia between them. Both had control from time to time, and each had his own circle of friends and preferred activities. Alternate A was described as a shy, introverted, passive avoidant person constantly vigilant for threats from the external world. Alternate B was "British," had a notable bad accent, was very outgoing, and loved to party by his own report. The MMPI was taken by alternate B, who produced a typical 4-9 profile (psychopathic deviant and mania above T-score 70), which is characteristic of antisocial personality. The clinical interview did not support the diagnosis of antisocial personality in this patient or this alternate. It was clear that both personalities saw this personality in this light and wanted personality B to be this way, as a way of obtaining some relief from the stultifying and depressing existence of alternate A. Since this was a one-time referral for psychometric evaluation, we do not have further information on the development of this interesting case. Bliss's comments about self-hypnosis or self-direction seem relevant. Patients with MPD (and, of course, many others) can control to a considerable extent how they present themselves to clinicians and to themselves. This control affects or determines the paucity or richness of the clues available to the diagnostician from which to formulate a differential diagnosis and an eventual diagnostic formulation.

N	L	F	K	Hs	D	Hy	Pd	Mf	Pa	Pt	Sc	Ma	Si
5	59	52	64	65	59	70	63	46	58	57	57	65	41
21	51	69	48	71	71	73	75	48	69	75	79	62	62
7	47	102	43	82	87	76	89	55	98	90	112	79	75

The major impact of response set on profile configuration is clearly illustrated by the following division of the patients with Briquet's syndrome reported in Table 4-4 and repeated above.

These data show the crucial effects of response set on the MMPI profile. The 33 patients with a clinical diagnosis of Briquet's syndrome were assigned to one of three groups on the basis of the F-K (raw scores) result. The first group of five patients had an F-K of − 12 or less; that is, they were very defensive in their general approach to the test. This group had only one primed (T-score ≥ 70) scale—hysteria. While the mean scores suggest neurosis, one would be uncertain that this was a case, let alone what type of case it is. The second group included all patients whose F-K was ≥ − 12 and ≤ 12 (a normal approach to the test). This group included 21 (63%) of the patients. The mean scale scores included six primed clinical scale scores, with schizophrenia ranking highest and an F scale T-score of 69. The third group of seven patients all had F-K ≥ 12. Nine of the 10 clinical scales were primed; only masculinity-femininity was close to average. The F scale T-score was 102, five standard deviations above average.

The reasonable interpretation of these data seems to be that patients, even those with polysymptomatic, polysyndromic disorders, can control how they present themselves to clinicians at any given time. This is independent, we believe, of the use of dissociation.

The following profiles were produced by a young white male patient who received an eventual diagnosis of MPD. He had the typical history of repeated childhood abuse (physical and sexual), a long history of psychiatric treatment with multiple diagnoses, including schizophrenia, and reported multiple personalities with amnesia between personalities (see MMPI data, p. 98).

Table 4-4 Mean MMPI Scores

Group	Author	Year	N	L	F	K	HS	D	HY	PD	MF	PA	PT	SC	MA	SI
MPD	Bliss	1984	15	46	85	45	79	86	77	85	38	83	84	100	69	71
MPD	Coons	1984	10	47	84	50	64	76	68	85	47	74	79	87	62	69
MPD	Coons	1986[M1]	18	48	82	47	70	77	71	81	48	79	77	91	66	69
MPD	Coons	1986[M2]	9	46	82	47	64	76	67	84	47	76	74	86	67	67
MPD	Coons	1986[M3]	3	47	78	44	62	78	60	77	53	82	82	94	68	69
MPD	Coons	1988	42	49	84	49	69	80	72	83	46	79	80	92	66	71
MPD	Griffin	1989	30	49	93	44	82	95	76	89	67	90	94	109	74	67
BDL[2]	Edell	1987	51	48	74	49	65	80	70	80	49	72	73	80	64	63
BDL[1]	Edell	1987	17	47	71	49	65	78	68	77	56	74	75	82	66	63
BDL	Evans	1984	45	48	76	50	67	80	71	84	57	75	77	85	68	64
BDL	Evans	1986[B1]	14	48	79	50	72	82	74	83	54	80	77	89	68	67
BDL	Evans	1986[B2]	11	50	78	50	71	80	75	84	56	79	81	90	64	67
BDL	Gustin	1983	29	44	85	46	68	89	71	84	68	78	89	98	71	68
BDL	Kroll	1981	21	48	84	47	62	82	70	84	60	78	74	85	65	63
BDL[1]	Resnick	1983	10	56	69	48	52	72	60	78	58	70	71	78	64	63
BDL[5]	Resnick	1988	37	45	66	47	56	73	63	76	54	70	71	71	61	61
BDL	Snyder	1982	26	46	86	45	75	86	68	85	68	79	88	98	72	65
BDL	Trull	1991	61	48	73	49	64	80	70	80	50	73	72	79	64	63
BDL	Widiger	1986[1]	22	47	83	44	72	88	67	86	63	86	87	99	68	70
BDL	Widiger	1986[2]	22	47	73	48	68	74	68	79	56	74	73	83	67	59
BDL	Widiger	1986[3]	25	48	83	44	73	87	67	85	59	84	86	98	70	68
BDL	Widiger	1986[4]	19	47	72	48	65	73	67	79	59	74	73	83	65	60
BDL	Widiger	1986[5]	21	48	78	46	71	80	68	87	63	81	80	91	66	64
BDL	Widiger	1986[6]	23	47	78	45	68	82	66	78	57	79	80	91	66	64

BDL	Widiger	1986[7]	10	52	70	45	70	70	68	78	59	74	72	76	62	60
BDL	Widiger	1986[8]	13	48	79	45	74	85	68	81	60	82	82	99	66	71
BRQ	Liskow	1977	21	54	70	50	75	74	73	74	52	71	72	79	60	64
HYS	Liskow	1986[Q1]	29	48	70	52	64	77	70	79	48	70	73	79	67	62
BRQ	Liskow	1986	16	52	77	47	72	75	74	77	48	77	74	89	71	63
BRQ	Wetzel	Unpb	31	52	74	49	72	73	73	76	49	73	75	82	66	62
BRQ	Wetzel	Unpb[Q2]	5	59	52	64	65	59	70	63	46	58	57	57	65	41
BRQ	Wetzel	Unpb[Q3]	21	51	69	48	71	71	73	75	48	69	75	79	62	62
BRQ	Wetzel	Unpb[Q4]	7	47	102	43	82	87	76	89	55	98	90	112	79	75

MI MPD—pretreatment profile.

M2 MPD—posttreatment profile: unfused patients.

M3 MPD—posttreatment profile: fused patients.

1 Borderline patients with schizotypal disorder.

2 Borderline personality without schizotypal disorder.

3 Borderline patients with histrionic personality.

4 Borderline patients without histrionic personality.

5 Borderline patients with antisocial personality.

6 Borderline patients without antisocial personality.

7 Borderline patients with only five criteria.

8 Borderline patients with seven or eight criteria.

B1 1986 study—initial MMPI.

B2 1986 study—second MMPI.

Q1 Hysterical patients reported by McHugh and Slavney.

Q2 Patients with Briquet's syndrome—$F-K \leq -12$.

Q3 Patients with Briquet's syndrome—$F-K > -12$ and <12.

Q4 Patients with Briquet's syndrome—$F-K \geq 12$.

Date	L	F	K	Hs	D	Hy	Pd	Mf	Pa	Pt	Sc	Ma	Si
09/03/87	60	66	53	75	77	71	69	65	64	69	86	78	54
10/14/87	70	70	74	85	92	78	69	69	65	71	86	65	60
12/14/88	60	50	74	59	70	69	62	67	53	64	61	40	58
12/21/88	56	62	59	54	63	62	60	71	59	56	65	73	50

The MMPI profiles obtained do not reflect the usual mean patterns produced by patients with this disorder. The first profile, obtained in 1987, reflects a modest attempt to disguise psychopathology, seen with the L scale score of 60 and the modestly elevated F scale score of 66. The validity scales suggest a mildly neurotic young man. The clinical scales show the highest scores on the schizophrenia and mania scales, which would usually indicate either an atypical depression, an atypical mania, or a schizoaffective disorder in this medical center. Elsewhere in the United States, it would be likely to be interpreted as indicating schizophrenia.

The second profile is noteworthy for the extreme defensiveness indicated by the validity scales. Scales L and K were both > 70, indicating a strong intent to appear unrealistically well-functioning. Almost all authorities would regard this profile as invalid. The profile is remarkably florid for a patient this defensive. The profile, if accepted as valid, indicates severe depression in a neurotic young patient. This may have been the patient's desired picture of himself.

The third profile is equally invalid. The K scale score is still 74, high enough to disqualify the profile. The clinical scales still show a remarkable amount of pathology for so defensive a patient. The profile of clinical scales suggests a depression in a neurotic patient; disregarding the validity scales, this could be a typical outpatient profile.

The fourth profile was produced by the patient about one week later. He was told to be as "open as possible." The validity scales are now acceptable. The patient appears mildly hypomanic or at least as having enormous energy. Note the three standard deviation increase on the mania scale.

If the checklist approach of Coons and Fine (1990) had been applied, none of these MMPI profiles would have been identified as likely to have been produced by a patient with MPD.

Comment

The MMPI appears to be sensitive to the presence of polysymptomatic, polysyndromic disorders. Figure 4-4 shows the weighted (by sample size) mean of the MMPI for each of the three diagnostic groups (MPD, borderline, Briquet's syndrome) in studies described earlier in this chapter. The similarity is quite striking. All three show similar panpsychopathology across the entire MMPI profile. Patients with any of these disorders are likely to share a significant amount of

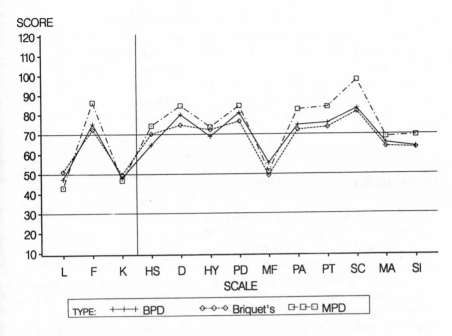

Figure 4–4. Average MMPI profiles.

similar pathology. When one of these types of patients presents openly, the MMPI profile will have many elevated scales.

Profiles with seven to nine scales elevated to T-score 70 or higher are likely to come from a patient who has MPD, borderline personality disorder, or Briquet's syndrome. If only one of these conditions is present, its identity will be difficult, if not impossible, to determine on the basis of the MMPI. The MPD patient will probably have this elevated profile because of the subordinate or coordinate diagnoses present, not because of the superordinate diagnosis of MPD. We can say this because the MMPI has only two items clearly tapping dissociative symptoms. Two items out of 566 or 567 will not shape the profile. Other tests will need to supplement the MMPI in order to obtain a full picture of the psychopathology. Because MPD presents frequently with multiple psychiatric problems, however, the more problems suggested by the MMPI profile, the higher the index of suspicion for MPD should be.

Scale 8 of the MMPI (commonly considered a schizophrenia scale) can be understood as a reasonable first pass at an MPD scale. It has subscales assessing alienation from self and others (sc1a sc1b in the MMPI; sc1 sc2 in the MMPI-2), a common correlate of childhood abuse. It has subscales measuring loss of control over one's thinking, emotions, and behavior (sc2a, sc2b, sc2c in the MMPI; sc3, sc4, sc5 in the MMPI-2), clearly a central experience in the inner life of patients with MPD. Its last subscale, sc3 (sc6 on the MMPI-2), has items on internal voices and on one of the two dissociative items. We note that every study we have located on patients with MPD shows that this scale (scale 8, the MPD scale) has the highest mean of any of the standard clinical scales. We remind our readers again that Ben-Porath and colleagues (1991) showed no significant difference between schizophrenics and depressives on scale 8, which is exactly what one would expect of an MPD scale, but not of a schizophrenia scale.

Other Scales

Horevitz and Braun (1984) used the Global Assessment Scale (GAS), a visual analogue scale ranging from 0 to 100 with anchors describing different levels of social and psychological functioning, to describe the lowest and highest levels of functioning in 33 patients with MPD. Twenty-three of the 33 also met criteria for borderline personality disorder. The GAS ratings for borderline and nonborderline patients were significantly different. Borderline MPD patients showed much greater variability in functioning and had periods of much lower-level functioning than nonborderline MPD patients. The authors noted that the percentage of MPD patients with a concomitant diagnosis of borderline disorder varied greatly among samples and may reflect the referral bases of the authors rather than true disease effects. The GAS scores do not seem diagnostic of MPD or of any other particular psychiatric entity. Patients with more psychiatric problems have lower GAS scores than those with fewer problems. Low scores suggest MPD patients with multiple syndromes; the lowest scores, however, are seen in the most dysfunctional psychotic patients. Thus, as a diagnostic tool, the GAS is not likely to be as useful as the MMPI.

This study by Horevitz and Braun makes a very interesting point: how well patients with MPD do is a function of their comorbid diagnoses. Obviously, if this finding is replicated, it means that treatment studies of patients with MPD must include all relevant diagnoses and must break down the results in terms of these diagnoses. This study could be interpreted as challenging the concept that MPD is always a superordinate diagnosis. When the diagnosis is known, it can be useful in describing the course of therapy.

Tests of Dissociation

Dissociation involves "at least momentary unbridgeable compartmentalization of experiences. . . . The concept does not require that the (compartmentalized) processes be completely independent of each other" (Spiegel & Cardena 1991, p. 367). In their review, Spiegel and Cardena assert that three instruments—the

Dissociative Experiences Scale (DES), the Dissociative Disorders Interview Schedule (DDIS), and the Structured Clinical Interview for DSM-III-R-Dissociative Disorders (SCID-D)—"exhibit particular promise, are widely known, have sound psychometric properties or are being used in programmatic research on the dissociative disorders" (Spiegel & Cardena 1991, p. 368).

Putnam and his associates (Bernstein & Putnam 1986) developed the DES, a 28-item test with a possible score between 0 and 100 on each item. DES scores reported here represent either the mean or the median score for the 28 items. The test was initially validated on eight different populations (see Table 4-5).

Test-retest reliability was acceptable (+0.84) in a normal control group with a time interval of four to eight weeks. Psychological tests with good test-retest reliability in normal subjects may be considerably more variable in psychiatric populations. Bernstein and Putnam (1986) asserted that the DES is a useful screening instrument for MPD but was not intended to be a diagnostic instrument.

Riley (1988) developed a 26-item True-False test from statements in the literature about dissociative experiences (the Questionnaire of Experiences of

Table 4-5   *Median DES Scores in Various Study Groups*

Source	*Population*	*N*	*Median DES Score*
Bernstein & Putnam (1986)	Normal adults	34	4.38
Bernstein & Putnam (1986)	Alcoholics	14	4.72
Ross et al. (1989a)	Neurologic patients	28	5.20
Bernstein & Putnam (1986)	Phobics	24	6.04
Ross et al. (1989a)	Partial complex seizures	20	6.70
Bernstein & Putnam (1986)	Agoraphobics	29	7.41
McCallum et al. (1992)	Eating disorders	38	11.60
Bernstein & Putnam (1986)	Adolescents	31	14.11
Ross et al. (1991b)	Schizophrenics	37	14.40
Bernstein & Putnam (1986)	Schizophrenics	20	20.63
Reagor et al. (1991)	Dissociative-NOS	57	21.70
Pribor et al. (1992)	Abused psychiatric patients	30	22.49
Pribor et al. (1992)	Briquet's syndrome	51	23.39
Armstrong (1990)	Dissociative-NOS	6	24.10
Bernstein & Putnam (1986)	PTSD patients	10	31.25
Ross et al. (1989a)	MPD patients	20	38.30
Reagor et al. (1991)	MPD patients	166	39.70
Armstrong (1990)	MPD patients	7	44.20
Loewenstein (1991)	Male MPD patients	15	48.75
Loewenstein (1991)	Female MPDs	36	56.25
Bernstein & Putnam (1986)	MPD patients	20	57.06

Abbreviations: NOS = not otherwise specified; PTSD = posttraumatic stress disorder.

Dissociation [QED]). Cronbach's alpha for internal reliability was 0.77, an acceptable level. Riley found significant differences between normal subjects (mean = -9.92), Briquet hysterics (somatization disorder) ($N = 21$, mean = 13.9), and multiples (mean = 24.6). The patient groups were very small, however.

Ross and colleagues (1989a) gave the DES to 20 patients with MPD, 20 with partial complex seizures, and 28 neurology patient controls. The median DES scores were significantly higher in patients with MPD than in the two neurologic control groups.

Steinberg and coworkers (1991) used the Structured Clinical Interview for DSM-III-R (SCID-III-R) to assess 45 subjects, 36 psychiatric patients, and 9 normal subjects. The psychiatric patients had all been in active therapy for at least six months. The therapists' diagnoses included eight patients with schizophrenia or schizoaffective disorder, eight with major depression, and five with posttraumatic stress disorder (PTSD) and generalized anxiety disorder. Fifteen patients were known to have dissociative spectrum disorders—one depersonalization disorder, six multiple personality disorder, and eight dissociative disorder—not otherwise specified (NOS). Patients with dissociative disorders had a significantly higher mean DES score (37.2 ± 18.2) than other psychiatric patients (9.4 ± 17.0) and normal subjects (2.33 ± 2.67). The mean score for the six patients with MPD was 40.6. All but 1 of the 15 previously identified dissociative patients had DES scores ≥ 15. Six newly diagnosed patients had scores > 15 as well, suggesting that the DES can be used to screen for dissociative disorders in previously undiagnosed populations.

Carlson's group (1991) presented a report of a factor analytic study of the DES at the eighth annual meeting of the ISSMPD&D in Chicago. The sample included patients from seven centers in North America; these patients had 11 different bases for ascertainment. Three factors were identified by a principal components analysis; these factors were named amnesia, absorption, and personalization/derealization. They were highly correlated despite the statistical methodology. At the same session, Schwarz and colleagues reported a confirmatory factor analysis on two different populations. A normal population yielded a single factor primarily reflecting absorption. The data from clinical populations yielded a three-factor solution quite similar to that of Carlson's group. Again, the three factors were highly correlated. These data indicate that the results obtained depend on the method of analysis used and the population sampled. One could extract a single higher-order factor with three subfactors or force the data into three orthogonal (but highly correlated) factors. It is not clear what difference this would make. Very limited clinical exposure to the DES suggests that the depersonalization factor score may be a better screen for that disorder than the other factors are for dissociative disorders in general.

A study by Antens and his colleagues (1991) at the Rush North Shore Dissociative Disorders program examined the susceptibility of the DES to malingering. They gave the DES to 102 patients with dissociative disorders (45 with MPD, 57 with dissociative disorder-NOS), to 22 staff members familiar with dissociative disorders who were asked to fake MPD on one occasion and dissociative disorder-NOS on another, to 58 persons unfamiliar with dissociative disorders who were asked to fake MPD, and to two groups of students (group A: $N = 259$; group B: $N = 287$).

Group	No.	DES Score	Amnesia	Depersonalization	Absorption
MPD	45	50.4 ± 19.0	39.4 ± 26.9	53.6 ± 23.7	54.3 ± 20.5
Staff members	22	70.1 ± 10.7	75.2 ± 13.5	61.7 ± 19.9	71.4 ± 10.5
Naive simulator	58	65.9 ± 19.0	68.8 ± 23.3	62.5 ± 23.5	64.7 ± 19.3
Dissociative-NOS	57	40.8 ± 19.7	27.7 ± 22.3	39.7 ± 22.8	47.5 ± 10.5
Staff members	22	47.3 ± 16.7	39.4 ± 24.6	41.3 ± 19.6	63.4 ± 15.2
Students A	259	23.8 ± 14.1	14.0 ± 13.3	13.4 ± 14.9	39.0 ± 22.1
Students B	287	21.8 ± 13.3	12.2 ± 11.9	10.7 ± 12.8	36.6 ± 21.1

Even the staff personnel most experienced with these two disorders overestimated the frequency with which dissociative disorder and MPD patients would report dissociative experiences. They suggested cutoffs to maximize the discrimination of faked from real tests. However, the mean difference between real and faked tests was less than one standard deviation. This means that one cannot confidently assign tests to one category or another. At the best cutoff, they obtained about a 70% correct classification; on replication, one would expect the results to be somewhat worse.

Gilbertson and colleagues (1991), in a paper presented at the same conference, reported their study of the susceptibility to malingering of three measures of dissociation (DES, Perceptual Alterations Scale-2, and QED). A total of 320 nursing students (253 female) were assigned to one of four groups. The "normal" group was asked to answer honestly, the "fake good" group was asked to appear symptom free, the "fake bad" group was asked to appear emotionally unstable, and the "MPD" group was read the DSM-III-R description of MPD and asked to reflect that disorder. The students were given the three scales and selected items from the MMPI F scale.

High correlations were achieved under all conditions among the three dissociative scales; in other words, they measure the same thing. The mean scores of the "normal" and "fake good" groups on the four scales were virtually identical, as were those of "fake bad" and "MPD" groups. The similarity of the "fake bad" and MPD test conditions suggests that college students do not require specialized knowledge about MPD in order to fake it. It was also reported that their abbreviated F scale correlated with the DES, the Perceptual Alterations

Scale, and the QED equally highly ($+0.69$ to $+0.85$). In the normal instruction group, the shared variance between the F scale, the Perceptual Alterations Scale, and the DES ranged from 25 to 30%.

The authors concluded appropriately that all of these scales are very transparent to individuals taking the test and thus are easily faked in either direction.

Westergard's group (1991) from the Rush Hospital group reported on a study of 217 college students, correlating DES scores with scores from two measures of hypnotizability (the Harvard group scale of hypnotizability and a self-rating scale). Although the two measures of susceptibility to hypnosis correlated significantly with each other, the measures of hypnosis and dissociation shared at most 2% of their variance. In the population studied, the DES scores may have represented primarily the absorption factor (see Schwarz et al. 1991). A replication of this finding in a clinical population of dissociative patients would represent an interesting challenge to current theory or to the validity of the instruments used.

The same Rush Hospital group reported on the correlation between the DES and Tellegen's Absorption Scale and Sanders' Perceptual Alteration Scale in the same student group. The DES correlated $+0.34$ with the Absorption Scale and $+0.60$ with the Perceptual Alteration Scale.

McCallum and colleagues (1992) administered the DES to 38 patients with eating disorders (anorexia, bulimia, or both). The median DES score was 11.60. They divided their patients into three groups: 11 without dissociative disorder and no history of physical or sexual abuse (mean DES $= 11.6 \pm 8.6$), 16 with a history of abuse and no dissociative disorder (mean DES $= 11.9 \pm 7.9$), and 11 with a diagnosis of dissociative disorder (4 with MPD; mean DES $= 24.3 \pm 20.1$). Patients with dissociative disorders had significantly higher DES scores than the other patients ($p < 0.05$). Using the cutoff of a DES score of ≥ 15, one nondissociative/nonabused, seven nondissociative/abused, and six dissociative disorder patients would have been selected. It is noteworthy that five dissociative disorder patients were not detected by this cutoff.

Pribor, Dean, and Yutzy (personal communication) administered the DES to 100 female patients with hysteria, suspected hysteria, or psychiatric or medical illnesses sometimes mimicking hysteria (multiple sclerosis, chronic fatigue syndrome, somatization only with depression) as part of the DSM-IV field trial for somatization disorder in St. Louis. Using the Perley-Guze criteria for Briquet's syndrome (Perley & Guze 1962), they identified 51 patients with definite or probable hysteria. They found that patients who met the rigorous criteria for Briquet's syndrome had a mean DES score of 23.4. Patients who did not meet the criteria had a mean DES score of 18.0. This difference was not statistically significant. Pribor's group also inquired about histories of sexual, physical, and emotional abuse. Patients who had been abused had significantly higher mean scores on the total DES and on each factor ($p < 0.05$). Patients with Briquet's syndrome were more likely to report abuse (92.2% vs. 62.5%, $p < 0.05$). Because so few patients with Briquet's syndrome denied abuse, they were analyzed

	Briquet's Syndrome (N = 51)	Other, Abused (N = 30)	Non-Abused (N = 18)
Total DES	23.39	22.49	10.54
Amnesia	17.63	18.58	8.87
Absorption	28.49	25.38	12.35
Depersonalization	17.37	17.05	4.46

as a single group. All differences are statistically significant ($p < 0.05$). This study demonstrates that patients with Briquet's syndrome report both frequent sexual, physical, and emotional abuse and significant use of dissociation.

The DES is very promising as a screening tool for MPD. It may eventually function for MPD just as the Beck Depression Inventory does for major depression—in other words, to measure a central and core component of a syndrome. Like the Beck Depression Inventory for depression, the DES is not diagnostic; it is sensitive to, but not specific for, MPD. One could easily conceive of it as an 11th scale on the MMPI, measuring dissociation. A polysmptomatic, polysyndromic patient with marked use of dissociation would be a most plausible candidate for the diagnosis of MPD.

Projective Tests

The literature on projective tests in MPD lacks systematic information on large groups of patients. Coons (1980) cited a study by Leavitt in which it was noted that hypnotically induced personalities in an analogue study of a single non-MPD patient produced "markedly different responses" to the Rorschach and Thematic Apperception tests when the patient was hypnotized.

Coons noted that psychological testing was performed on a patient named Gretchen. An angry personality, "Billie," produced an angry-looking male on the Draw-A-Person test. Two other personalities, "Gretchen"—described as soft-spoken and introverted—and "Veronica—described as seductive and flirtatious—took the MMPI. Both personalities, despite their clinical differences, produced MMPIs characterizing an "impulsive, rebellious, antisocial individual with a curious tendency to over-control her impulses" (1980, p. 334). Coons observed that this testing was not helpful because all three personalities participated. One is tempted to conclude that the same personality took all three tests from the description of the results.

In case 4, Coons (1980) noted that psychological testing (tests and results unspecified) showed that the patient had a hysterical personality, which was consistent with his diagnostic impression based on the absence of amnesia. Apparently in this case, testing was helpful in confirming that multiple personalities did not exist and that the patient was consciously playing different roles.

Griffin (1989) obtained Rorschach examinations from 30 male Veterans Administration patients with clinical diagnoses of MPD. He hypothesized that patients with MPD would differ from other psychiatric patients on 10 variables. They did differ significantly on four of the hypothesized variables—one or more percepts with a dissociative content (67% MPD patients vs. 20% controls), high human movement (more than four responses) or more than 40% of all responses involving movement (80% vs. 41%), more than three fabulized combinations (e.g., "two chickens throwing basketballs" [Griffin 1989, p. 70]) or incongruent combinations (e.g., "a dog with his hands out" [p. 70]) (46% vs. 10%), and for fictional or mythical human content (53% vs. 18%). These results suggest that these patients had a strong fantasy life, with fantasy relatively less bounded by reality than is true for many patients. One might say that for these patients, fantasy is an escape from an intolerable reality rather than a coping mechanism.

Armstrong and Loewenstein (1990) reported the results of Rorschach examinations of 14 patients: 8 with MPD and 6 with dissociative disorders. Twelve of the patients also met criteria for PTSD. According to the authors, the results were "best described as variable." Reality testing was mixed, with almost all records showing some signs of distortion and inaccurate perception and, at the same time, no developmental arrest. The patients' reality testing was described as "unusual, not severely distorted." They showed good capacity for self-observation, awareness of ambiguity, and complexity of processing. Strong indications of depression and absorption in traumatic experiences were noted.

Surprisingly, the authors found the group to be constricted, internalizing, and intellectualizing as opposed to borderline or histrionic. They emphasized the importance of paying attention to the processes of dissociation, switching, state changes, and traumatic responses during testing; doing so clarifies the cognitive processes and prevents misdiagnosis (overdiagnosis) as borderline personality. This emphasizes a truism about psychological testing (and clinical interviewing): the more the examiner knows about the patient, his or her clinical state, and his or her history, the more accurately the examiner can understand what is seen and interpret it for others. From the account of these authors, one can infer that the Rorschach is unlikely to be a good screening instrument for detecting currently undiagnosed cases of MPD. Pride of place, in their eyes, goes to the DES.

Gartner and colleagues (1989) commented extensively on the use of projective test results using the Rorschach with borderline patients. They pointed out that it has long been known that a subset of patients who show indications of thought disorder on the Rorschach do not demonstrate it on other psychological tests (e.g., the IQ test) and who rarely demonstrate it clinically when stressed. The unusual responses by borderline patients "are more likely to be idiosyncratic rather than grossly distorted. Thus, once again, BPDs appear to be discriminable from neurotic and psychotic records by their preponderance of moderate disturbances of thinking" (Gartner et al. 1989, pp. 427–428).

These authors also cited a number of studies suggesting that borderline patients show "a number of poor form responses which received a high developmental score on the Blatt (Developmental Object Relations) scale" (p. 430). Two studies they cited failed to show that borderline patients had poorer scores on this developmental scale than patients with other personality disorders. A controlled study with both blind ratings of Rorschach protocols from patients with MPD, borderline personality disorder, and Briquet's syndrome, as well as careful delineation of the diagnosis and subordinate diagnoses of each patient, might be valuable in clarifying the role of projective tests in the diagnosis of these disorders.

Specialized Diagnostic Interviews

Ross' group (1989a) developed the Dissociative Disorders Interview Schedule (DDIS), a 131-item structured interview. They administered the DDIS to 20 patients with MPD, 20 patients with partial complex seizures and documented electroencephalographic (EEG) abnormalities, and 28 neurology patient controls. The DDIS allows four dissociative disorder diagnoses (psychogenic amnesia, psychogenic fugue, depersonalization disorder, MPD) and three others (borderline personality disorder, somatization disorder, and major depressive episode).

The DDIS interviews correctly diagnosed 19 of the 20 MPD patients with MPD and all of the others as not having MPD. Five of the 20 patients with partial complex seizures and 4 of the 28 patients with other neurologic diagnoses, however, received the diagnosis of psychogenic amnesia. The patients with MPD were significantly more likely than both control groups to have somatization disorder (35% in MPD), depression (85% in MPD), and borderline personality (60% in MPD).

Steinberg and coworkers (1990) developed a 200-item structured interview, the Structured Clinical Interview for DSM-III-R Dissociative Disorders (SCID-D), to assess five dissociative disorder symptom areas: amnesia, depersonalization, derealization, identity confusion, and identity alteration. The interview was administered to 48 patients. Videotaping or audiotaping was used to allow a second blind rater to score the interviews. Interrater reliability was excellent; kappas ranged from 0.65 to 0.95.

The patient pool included (based on treating therapists' diagnoses) 18 patients with dissociative disorders (8 with MPD), 23 with other psychiatric disorders, and 7 normal subjects. The two raters diagnosed 25 patients each as having a dissociative disorder (a 38% increased rate of diagnosis above the treating therapists) and 23 as not having a dissociative disorder. They apparently disagreed on the presence or absence of dissociative disorder in only 2 of the 48 cases. Of the seven "new" cases of dissociative disorder, four were subsequently confirmed clinically. The raters reported 93% agreement on the presence of MPD. One rater diagnosed eight cases and the other seven cases of MPD with 93% agreement. This suggests that the raters agreed, on the basis of the same interview, that six subjects had MPD. They apparently disagreed on three cases where only one rater made the diagnosis of MPD. Two of these three must have been given another dissociative spectrum diagnosis by the other rater, and conceivably this could have been true of all three. (The article does not make this clear.) No comment was made about the agreement between therapists' and raters' diagnoses of MPD.

Boon and Drajier (1991) adapted the SCID-D for use in the Netherlands. They used this instrument on 42 women and 2 men, "most of whom had been referred for evaluation of dissociative disorders" (p. 459). One author diagnosed a dissociative disorder in 22 cases and the other in 23 of the 44; the authors disagreed on only 1 case. Both agreed that the same 12 patients had MPD. They reported mean ratings in five symptom areas in each of four patient diagnosis groups. Patients with neither dissociative disorders nor other personality disorders ($N = 10$) had the fewest dissociative symptoms, while patients with MPD ($N = 12$) had the most. Patients with dissociative disorder-NOS ($N = 11$) had more dissociative symptoms than patients without dissociative disorder but with personality disorder ($N = 11$) in four of five symptom groups. The agreement reported here was better than in the original article by the developers of the instrument.

Steinberg and colleagues (1991) gave the SCID-D to a population of 36 psychiatric patients and 9 normal subjects. Fifteen (six multiples, one depersonalization disorder, and eight dissociative disorder-NOS) patients had previously been identified as having dissociative disorders. The SCID-D identified 21 persons as having a dissociative spectrum disorder. No information was reported on the association between interview diagnosis and therapist diagnosis.

Experiential Time Sampling

Dissociation, when it occurs to the degree seen in MPD, makes the patient by definition a poor reporter of his or her history. According to dynamic theory, the goal of the defense is to avoid experiencing the intolerable or to seal it off from the rest of the personality (or in some cases to manipulate). Hence, amnesia for events is very frequent or even mandatory. In theory, then, one would expect patients with MPD, even those in appropriate psychotherapy, to be poor historians.

Loewenstein's group (1987) developed a procedure requiring a patient with MPD to record at randomly selected times (1) time of day, (2) alternate in charge, (3) whether a switch in control or amnesia for time was present since the last recording, (4) situational information, (5) a description of ongoing activity and the reasons for it, (6) a mood checklist, (7) physical symptoms, and (8) the main feeling state. Six days in two sets of three consecutive days were sampled. The results showed, as one would expect, that there was significant agreement between what therapists believed about the patient based on therapy accounts given by the patient on some variables and significant disagreement on others.

The authors noted (citing Kluft) that the internal experience of a patient with MPD may be far more complex than the patient's explanations of his or her behavior, especially early in treatment. That patients (or therapists) have difficulty describing the variations and complexities of a psychiatric disorder without systematic, recorded observations over time is hardly unique to MPD. The techniques of systematic behavioral analysis seem to have much to offer in the future study of patients with MPD.

Tests of Hypnotizability

Bliss (1984a) reported scores on the Stanford Hypnotic Susceptibility Scale (Form C) in five groups of subjects. The possible range of scores on this test is from 0 to 12, with higher scores associated with greater hypnotizability. A group of 18 multiples, by DSM-III criteria, had a mean score of 10.0 ± 0.44 (presumably the standard error of measurement, not the standard deviation). A second "probable" multiples group of 10 had a mean score of 10.3 ± 0.65. This indicated that at least half of all patients with MPD would have scores ≥ 10 on this test. A control group of 49 smokers had scores with a mean of 6.6 ± 0.37. Assuming that these scores are approximately normally distributed, less than 10% of normal subjects would have scores ≥ 10. In the differential diagnosis of two disorders with equal base rates in the population, this kind of mean difference would be quite useful. Bliss and Jeppsen (1985) reported that the mean Stanford Hypnotic Susceptibility Scale score for six inpatients with multiple personality was 10.2.

Bliss and Larson (1985) studied 33 convicted male sex offenders; 29 were given the Stanford Hypnotic Susceptibility Scale. Thirteen were diagnosed as having or probably having MPD. The mean scale score was 9.2 ± 0.34 (SEM).

Utility of Psychological Assessment Instruments

Coons (1980, pp. 335–336) concluded that, in general, psychological testing has "*not proved helpful in diagnosing multiple personality* but has been helpful in investigating other personalities" (italics added). In a later paper (1984), he noted that psychological testing is useful in providing relevant information once the diagnosis of MPD has been made. Rarely has the psychological tester been the first to diagnose MPD, according to Coons.

Benner and Joscelyne (1984) assert that psychological tests have not been particularly useful because they typically have been administered to the main personality (rather than to the main personality and most of the significant alternates). A further complication, they indicate, is that any given personality may resemble any known Axis I or Axis II disorder. They add that this has also been true of diagnostic interviews administered only to the main personality. Buck (1983) points out that the true clinical picture in a case of multiple personality can only be appreciated by looking at all the personalities together as a whole; it is not helpful, he states, to regard "dissociated personalities as being in fact separate individuals" (p. 65).

We tend to agree with most of these sentiments. Only adequate information about at least a number of the personalities and a careful clinical history will allow competent diagnosis of MPD and of the patient's subordinate or comorbid diseases. Very highly functioning MPD patients with few manifest problems will be difficult to detect by any means. Once the diagnosis has been made or is suspected, psychological testing can make its proper contribution by providing systematic assessment and quantification of patient characteristics.

A Model for the Role of Psychological Testing in MPD

Psychological testing is not a clinical test in the same sense that an x-ray or a hematocrit is. The latter laboratory tests provide clinicians with information different from that available when obtaining a clinical history or conducting a mental status examination. Psychological testing simply takes the data from the clinical history or the mental status exam and processes them in a more intensive fashion—assigning numbers and comparing them to norms so that finer distinctions become possible. IQ tests clearly do that in a useful way for evaluation of a fund of information. Scales for dissociation do that for the assessment of dissociative phenomena. As they develop and are refined, these measures will become quite useful in assessing the time course of dissociative experiences in MPD, the response to treatment, and the like, just as depression scales have proved highly useful in depression research. However, like depression scales, dissociation scales will not be diagnostic in themselves. They will contribute to the data base of the clinician but will not control his or her analysis of it.

Dissociation is apparently central to MPD and the other dissociative disorders, but other phenomena are also relevant. Kluft (1987b, p. 367) states, "Multiple personality disorder rarely presents as a free-standing condition. Almost invariably its manifestations are embedded in a polysymptomatic presentation suggestive of one or more commonplace conditions." The results of studies with psychological tests clearly confirm his opinion. The MMPI and the other tests pick up elements of the total picture of psychopathology seen in patients with MPD. No one element is so confined to MPD that it becomes diagnostic or almost diagnostic of MPD. Psychological testing that demonstrates the presence of multiple forms of psychopathology (anxiety, somatoform, depression, borderline, and histrionic characteristics; frequent use of dissociation; pseudohallucinations in the absence of formal thought disorder) will raise the index of suspicion of MPD and thereby increase the probability of an accurate diagnosis. No test has been developed that determines the existence of alternates or the presence of periods of amnesia.

The literature often states that one does not always find MPD patients with a florid polysmptomatic presentation. Certainly, in our clinical experience, patients with MPD have not always presented in a way that made the diagnosis obvious. The MMPI literature makes it seem that the diagnosis should be obvious in the sense that these patients have many disorders, not just one. This finding could be an artifact in that people collecting MMPIs for research papers give them to patients long diagnosed and no longer hidden. It would be interesting to ascertain whether the defensiveness (compartmentalization) seen in clinical interviews is found to be breached in test taking. Greater openness in testing than in interviews does happen in patients with other disorders or in forensic settings.

The four-factor theory of etiology (Kluft 1984a) proposes that MPD depends on

1. The potential for dissociation/hypnotizability

2. Overwhelming traumatic life experience unable to be handled by nondissociative defenses

3. Shaping influences that determine the form taken by the dissociative defenses

4. Lack of countervailing support and experiences provided by significant others

Tests for dissociation and hypnotizability can quantify these variables and indicate the ranges for them in which MPD can occur. Methods to assess the other three factors proposed by Kluft await development or adaptation for research in MPD. Moos and Moos (1986) and Robins (Holmes and Robins 1988; Robins et al. 1985) developed procedures for reliable assessment of the childhood family environment; how these instruments would work in patients with extensive childhood amnesia and how they would need to be modified remain to be worked out. Such procedures might be of diagnostic utility (by documenting amnesia), as well as of quantitative use for assessing environments.

Anecdotal reports of children at high risk for schizophrenia have indicated that some children compensate by forming attachments to supportive and nurturing neighbors, teachers, and others. This research, when published, might be useful in directing the development of instruments to assess countervailing influences in the environment that allow children to cope without becoming multiple. As knowledge accumulates about patients with MPD, better instrumentation will follow to measure relevant pieces of clinical history and mental status—a typical sequence for psychological testing.

Currently available tests can assess and quantify some aspects of the ways in which patients with MPD and patients with other psychiatric disorders (Briquet's syndrome, borderline personality disorder) are similar. Considerable research, however, is needed to determine the ways in which these disorders are dissimilar when they do not overlap within the same patient. Further, when the disorders do overlap in the same patient, we need to know which aspects of the clinical presentation are likely to be due to each disorder. Careful clinical and family studies using these newly developed instruments or batteries of instruments will clarify the relationship of MPD to other psychiatric syndromes as a superordinate, coordinate, or subordinate diagnostic entity.

Early attempts to diagnose a disorder may look naive to later observers. The psychometric literature on patients with dissociative disorders can be easily criticized. We think the following variables need to be examined for successful psychometric research:

1. Patient characteristics
   a. Who took the tests (which alternate, the alternate's role/character, whether switching occurred, whether there was "internal discussion", etc.).
   b. The test taker's attitude toward test taking and self-disclosure (defensive, considered, impulsive, careless, embellishing).
   c. Stage of treatment (prior to detection of MPD, unfused in active treatment, fused but still needing active treatment, and fused with therapy consensually terminated).
   d. The comorbid diagnoses (while this is controversial, we don't think that MPD patients with borderline personality should have the same test results as MPD patients without it).
   e. Current stress level and mood states (depressed vs. nondepressed, etc.).
2. Situational Characteristics
   a. Purpose of the evaluation (diagnostic, treatment outcome, forensic).
3. Tester and tester-testee characteristics
   a. Gender of each party.
   b. Rapport.
   c. Features relevant to past life traumas.
4. What is measured
   a. At the present time in psychiatry, we measure only correlates of psychiatric disorders; until the pathogenesis is understood and demonstrated, we will not know whether or not we are assessing causative factors or correlates.

b. Briquet's syndrome, borderline personality disorder, the other group B Axis II disorders, and MPD share many characteristics. They are all early-onset psychiatric disorders that interfere with socialization and modulation of emotional expression and social behavior.
c. At this stage of research, our usual psychometric instruments are all designed to assess other psychiatric disorders. As research and theory progress, better instruments will become available.

5

MPD and the popular media
in history

Patients with MPD have captured the attention of the popular media (Simpson 1988; Thigpen & Cleckley 1984). Putnam and colleagues (1984, p. 174) have noted "the sensational coverage given to well-known cases by the media."

There is no doubt that popularized reports of MPD have widely disseminated knowledge of the disorder in our culture (Spanos 1986; Spanos et al. 1986). According to Hacking (1991, p. 843), "disturbed people have seen multiples on TV, read pulp magazines, heard of sensational trials, have friends who say they are multiples." Popular sources have provided extensive information about the characteristics of the disorder (Bowers 1991; Spanos 1986), and most people are basically aware that patients are considered to be victims of other personalities that take over their bodies. It is common knowledge that MPD is associated with amnesias for the alternate personalities and an assortment of dramatic clues such as changes in voice or physical appearance when the personalities switch. Bianchi's repeated complaints of headaches associated with his MPD symptoms may have been behavior he learned from the movie *The Three Faces of Eve* (Orne et al. 1984).

Interested individuals can easily gain further information about the typical presentation of MPD from books and films. Millions of people are passively educated in their own homes by made-for-television movies and other programs designed for mass entertainment appeal. In a recent television movie about Bianchi, the examiner performed the "circle-touch" test to determine whether Bianchi's response to a "catch-22" instruction was consistent with responses characteristic of bona fide multiples. Viewers learned that real multiples, when blindfolded and touched on a part of their hand that is anesthetic from hypnotic suggestion, are supposed to answer incongruously—that they don't feel being touched. It is believed that malingerers will not respond, acting completely as though they don't feel the touch.

Imitative behavior may follow media coverage of a disorder. This has been alleged to occur, for instance, after media accounts of suicide and homicide (Fahy et al. 1989; Philips 1986). The same might be true of MPD.

Kluft's (1984c) four-factor theory of etiology identifies the media and literature as shaping influences determining the form of clinical dissociation. It has been noted that fictional accounts, like popular biographical reports, are a potent source of material from which patients draw in their adoption of alternate personalities (Cutler & Reed 1975). Kluft (1987b) described a woman complaining of MPD symptoms who upon confrontation admitted that she was faking a version of the disorder she had seen on a television soap opera. Slater and Roth (1969, p. 113) contended that MPD is a product of literary experience.

An historical examination of MPD in the popular media may help determine the degree to which these shaping influences have played a role in the development of MPD over time. This review may shed light on the current relationship of the media and MPD in our culture.

Historical Review of Famous Accounts

Fiction

The most famous account of multiple or dual personality was *The Strange Case of Dr. Jekyll and Mr. Hyde,* which described a chemically induced case of dissociation leading to murder (Stevenson 1886). This novel is also thought to be the first description of the disorder in a man (Allison 1981). Its popularity as a book and movie has survived through the decades, and "Jekyll-Hyde" has become a household term for erratic and pathologic changes in mood or behavior. Not long after its original publication, another portrayal of dual personality appeared, Oscar Wilde's 1890 classic, *The Picture of Dorian Gray* (Decker 1986, p. 34).

Other accounts from the same era included *The Somnambulist,* in 1880, in which an upstanding Protestant minister develops a criminal other self who rapes women and kills children; *The Other,* in 1883, which portrays a judge whose alternate personality is the perpetrator of a crime he is investigating; a novel by Charles Richet, a Novel prize-winning physiologist and pioneer in hypnotism in 1889, who wrote about a hypnotized patient who is a wealthy heiress and in love with the doctor; and a 1908 novel *Obsession: Myself and the Other,* depicting a painter whose alternate personality wreaks havoc on his life (Decker 1986, p. 34). Other popular authors writing on alternate personalities, dissociation, and different facets of personality around the turn of the century and later include Marcel Prevost, Luigi Pirandello, Marcel Proust, James Joyce, and Virginia Woolf. Their writers' appreciation of sophisticated scientific knowledge led them to more subtle literary themes compared with the sensational and lurid stories of dual personalities of earlier times (Decker 1986, p. 36).

Decker (1986, p. 34) pointed out that the case histories in the professional literature of that era bore a remarkable resemblance to characters of the works of the literary masters of their day. Janet's famous patient Irene, who developed "hysterical disturbances, somnambulistic crises, hallucinations, and amnesia" in the year 1900 was "strikingly similar" to the character Pauline in Emile Zola's *La Joie de Vivre* of 1884. The character Elektra created by Hofmannsthal (1909) (Decker 1986, p. 34) was much like Breuer's patient Anna O. Freud's patient Dora could be compared to material in a short story by Arthur Schnitzler (Decker 1986, p. 34). A case described in a less well known paper of Freud (Decker 1986, p. 34), "A Seventeenth-Century Demonological Neurosis," is noted to have displayed striking similarities to the character in William Peter Blatty's book *The Exorcist* (Bozzuto 1975). It is not clear who influenced whom.

Nonfiction

The case of Mary Reynolds in the early 1800s appears to have attracted both lay and medical attention. The case was further popularized by a French version of the account by Macnish (1836) and achieved widespread notoriety as *la dame de Macnish*. Apparently some scholars did not recognize that the case of Mary Reynolds was the same case as the "lady of Macnish" and quoted them separately as two different cases of dual personality (Ellenberger 1970, p. 129). The case of Ms. Beauchamp in 1906 (Prince 1906) broke new ice in public exposure because this widely publicized patient exhibited four personalities rather than the usual dual personalities reported prior to her time. From then on, most reported cases had three or more personalities, and the disorder therefore earned the name "multiple personality disorder" (Fahy 1988).

Widespread public awareness of MPD began with the publication of *The Three Faces of Eve* in 1957; this case is considered the most celebrated MPD case of all time. It was also thought to be the only MPD case in existence at that time. *The Three Faces of Eve* became a best-seller and was made into an Academy Award-winning motion picture. The second most famous popular case was described in the book *Sybil*, published in 1973, and the movie based on this book, starring Sally Field, won four Emmys. The actress who played Eve in the movie based on that account, Joanne Woodward, was cast in the role of the therapist in *Sybil*.

In the last 20 years, the number of book-length reports on MPD has mushroomed, as can be seen from the dates of these accounts listed in Table 6-1. These accounts will also be examined in detail in Chapter 6.

Television talk shows periodically include individuals with multiple personality among their featured guests, and soap operas and weekly evening sit-coms and crime dramas have also included MPD in their segments. Fahy (1989) feels the widespread public awareness of MPD through media exposure has influenced public perception of MPD, as well as of all psychiatric disorders. MPD has been described as "culture-specific" (Aldridge-Morris 1989, p. 109) and "an iatrogenic, largely culture-bound disorder" (Simpson 1988, p. 535). Aldridge-Morris (1989, p. 109) claims that "the diagnosis of multiple personality owes as much to cultural influence as does its ontogeny."

It is surmised that because MPD often develops in histrionic persons, these individuals are not only particularly susceptible to the disorder, but also might be especially prone to draw attention to themselves through their dramatic symptoms and seek the limelight (Thigpen & Cleckley 1984). Individuals who achieve public acclaim through media dissemination of their stories may thus be selected for being dramatic, and this drama may be further enhanced by artistic license in an effort to provide a story that is more interesting and dramatic to make it more salable (Stern 1984). Velek and Balon (1986) asserted that the media depiction of MPD has distorted its clinical picture. Victor (1975, p. 202) commented that popular accounts of psychiatric illness resemble "a fairy tale, and *Sybil* is no exception." Kluft (1985, p. 3) wrote, "Lay accounts which exploit MPD for sensationalistic ends can make this condition appear a subject more fit for a soap opera than for science."

Popular portrayals of MPD typically present the disorder in a relatively attractive light with high drama (Spanos 1986; Spanos et al. 1985). The protagonist in these depictions gains self-esteem and dignity and receives abundant sympathetic attention from significant others, and sometimes from highly recognized experts, as well as from the media. The picture painted by these accounts may be especially compelling for the individuals who are most vulnerable to this disorder.

Benefits to real individuals so portrayed in the media include public acclaim, boosted self-esteem, and financial reward. Simpson (1988) speculates that no other psychiatric or medical condition is as "rewarding" as MPD to those "supposedly 'suffering' from it." He describes patients with "excessive claims" garnering "excessive interest" by the public—and by their therapists, who also seem to enjoy the attention aroused by their association with these cases. Mental health professionals suspect that exaggerated popular images of mental illness offer unstable people—"especially self-dramatizing histrionic persons and sociopathic liars—too many opportunities to deceive themselves and others and deny responsibility for their actions" (Harvard 1985, p. 1).

Fahy (1988) believes that written and cinematic biographies of MPD patients have led to an increased number of patients presenting themselves to experts. This phenomenon was previously observed by Thigpen and Cleckley (1984) in the wake of the extensive public attention their famous case of Eve attracted. Soon after their account was published, these authors were barraged with queries from hundreds of would-be multiples describing symptoms that the authors were convinced were shaped by the descriptions of Eve's symptoms. Of these, they saw only one person they believed had genuine MPD.

As another reflection of the recent popularity of the disorder, a number of "alleged MPD cases" were referred to authors Tozman and Pabis (1989) for evaluation. These clinicians "addressed them otherwise. (Rarely, a case did manifest a degree of dissociation)" (p. 708). The source of the increasing number of cases, according to Thigpen and Cleckley (1984), is uncritical application of the diagnosis during a wave of public attention to the disorder. Hacking (1991, p. 841) states, "pulp publicity in the media conspires with psychiatrists in the multiple personality movement to create the symptoms."

Bowers (1991, p. 170) contends that "the various pathogenic fantasies, inspired by television . . . can result in MPD-type symptoms prior to any therapeutic intervention." Fahy (1988, p. 601) noted that "An individual may learn to enact the MPD role, collecting impressions from popular books and films." Spanos and colleagues (1986) have hypothesized a process by which MPD is manufactured. In it, individuals first learn details about the presentation of MPD from a variety of available sources such as movies, books, or gossip. They then seek legitimation of their own rendition of these symptoms from friends, family, and/or therapists. In time, their own enactments and the endorsement they receive from others may convince them that they truly have these secondary identities that take them over. Bowers (1991, p. 168) states, "a fantasied alter ego—stimulated, perhaps, by media accounts of MPD—can become increasingly complex and differentiated" in therapy. He has observed (p. 168), "The more complex the fantasies, the more complex the suggested effects."

Fahy and colleagues (1989) feel that the popular media portray MPD in a sympathetic light and publicize the condition as a "high-status disorder." This image is then reinforced by sick-role privileges and is subtly encouraged within therapeutic relationships, sanctioned by the widespread acceptance of the nosologic validity of this disorder. Cutler and Reed (1975) described a woman who showed conversion symptoms under stress and entered fugue states in which she exhibited a variety of personalities based on her own past experiences and things she had read. These authors argued that under most circumstances the personalities would have likely occurred only once or twice, but attention from the woman's doctors resulted in persistence and elaboration of her alternate personalities.

MPD and the Media Today

The confusion among psychiatric professionals over the nosologic status of this disorder has filtered into the public domain through the media. The public has inherited the psychiatric profession's historical confusion of MPD with schizophrenia (Harvard 1985; Rosenbaum 1980). The early roots of this misunderstanding grew from Bleuler's link of the splitting he associated with schizophrenia with splitting of the personality. This was an unfortunate association that led to his origination of the term "schizophrenia," literally translated as "split mind," which is still confused with MPD. Bleuler (1924, p. 138) further contributed to the confusion by writing that "it is not alone in hysteria that one finds an arrangement of different personalities one *succeeding* the other: through similar mechanisms schizophrenia produces different personalities existing *side by side.*" Bleuler apparently saw little difference between multiple personality and schizophrenia.

Unfortunately, misunderstandings such as this, once embedded in the culture, tend to persist despite the availability of correct information and continue to be perpetuated by media endorsement. The failure to differentiate schizophrenia from MPD continues to be manifested in gross media misstatements equating anything composed of divided extremes with any term that contains the root "schizo." Blatant examples include the movie *Schizoid,* about a maniac with a murderous side, as well as innocently coined phrases such as "schizophrenic policy," "schizophrenic weather patterns," and "schizophrenic market conditions." This confusion is perhaps best illustrated by a popular T-shirt slogan:

> Roses are red,
> Violets are blue,
> I'm schizophrenic,
> And I am too."

One commendable example of a popular author who is knowledgeable and has taken care to stress the distinction between MPD and schizophrenia, however, is Tom Clancy (1991), who in a recent novel, *The Sum of All Fears,* wrote, "the Soviet Union had developed an instant case of political schizophrenia. Wrong term, Ryan reflected. Multiple-personality disorder, perhaps" (p. 372).

The judicial system is another source of material for media dissemination of ideas about MPD. Several MPD cases have earned public attention through the judicial system when the insanity plea has been invoked to escape responsibility for violent crimes perpetrated by the alternate personalities, usually men. The first MPD patient ever found not guilty by reason of insanity was Paul Miskimen, who allegedly murdered his wife (Allison 1982).

Two celebrated forensic MPD cases have been described in book-length accounts: Milligan, the campus rapist, and Bianchi, the Los Angeles Hillside Strangler. Milligan succeeded in winning a not guilty by reason of insanity (NGRI) verdict on the basis of MPD; he was hospitalized at a maximum-security facility and later released to outpatient treatment. Thigpen and Cleckley (1984, p. 66) referred to Milligan's MPD defense as "a gross miscarriage of justice and denigration of psychiatry." Bianchi did not succeed with his insanity plea. In the process, however, his case received considerable professional and public attention.

Since 1977, at least 18 cases of murder defendants claiming MPD have come to light (Coons 1991). All but two were men. Hypnosis was used in the diagnosis of most of them. Two received NGRI verdicts, two were considered incompetent to stand trial, two had unknown outcomes, and the rest were declared guilty. With the growing popularity of MPD, it is expected that the number of legal cases will also grow.

As a reflection of the burgeoning attention to MPD and the increasing number of cases in the United States, a case with a new twist recently emerged in the national media spotlight during the preparation of this manuscript. A man was convicted of rape because of a sexual act he had performed with an alternate personality of a woman with MPD. The accused was allegedly aware of the woman's psychiatric condition and knowingly invoked the assistance of one of her alternate personalities to permit the act. He received a guilty verdict and is appealing.

In other parts of the world, where the growth of interest in MPD lags behind American trends, the media are seen to have a shaping influence on the development of the disorder as it spreads. In India, the media seem to be shaping a clinical picture slightly different from that in America. Hindi cinema usually depicts any dramatic changes in the personality or behavior of patients it glamorizes as the result of certain characteristic events such as sleep or automobile accidents. Unlike American cases, the transitions from one alternate to another in Indian MPD cases are characteristically mediated by overnight sleep (Adityanjee et al. 1989).

Hacking (1991, p. 857) describes recent American patterns in personality switching in multiples as speeding up, happening "much more suddenly and instantaneously than in the past." He compares the rapidity of switching with the practice of " 'zapping,' of switching channels on television" (p. 857). He writes, "This is no great feat because the alters are typically stock characters with bizarre but completely unimaginative character traits, each one a stereotype or one might say TV-type who readily contrasts with all the other characters" (p. 857).

Spanos and colleagues (1986) point out that clinical details in the presentation of MPD symptoms have roots in personal conceptions of how both MPD and related psychopathology originate. These ideas stem from childhood notions and from cultural conceptions partly derived from information gained throughout a lifetime of media bombardment. Similar mechanisms operate in the formation of conversion symptoms, which take the shape of what the patient believes is the manner in which dysfunction manifests. Such notions are often anatomically or physiologically incongruous, such as the classic presentation of hysterical anesthesia in a glove-stocking distribution or with precise demarcation or "splitting" at the midline of the body (Hier 1982, p. 204).

The widespread media dissemination of information about MPD poses potential problems for research. Ross and colleagues (1990c) have pointed out that one of the advantages of the DDIS in their study was that this instrument assesses diagnoses of somatization disorder, major depressive episodes, borderline personality, and all the dissociative disorders. The authors claimed that this instrument yields few or no false-positive diagnoses of MPD because subjects would have to possess prior knowledge of the MPD profile to produce a convincing picture of the disorder on that interview schedule. The hazard to this plan posed by media education is that the media have contaminated the public awareness with a great deal of specific detail about the presentation of the disorder, which could be inadvertently merged into the symptom picture reported in a research interview. Merskey (1992, p. 337) stated that because of media influence, no modern case of MPD "can be taken to be veridical since none is likely to emerge without prior knowledge of the idea."

It is widely appreciated that physicians are also influenced by the media, and this phenomenon has been invoked in explaining the apparent increase in the incidence of MPD (Velek & Balon 1986). Fahy (1989) specifically cites the profound impact of the account of Sybil that reached both professional and general public audiences. Allison (1974b) described having educated himself by viewing the movie *The Three Faces of Eve* and reading the book it was based upon twice; he also read *Sybil*. Kluft (1987b, p. 364) observed, "Lay interest in celebrated cases of multiple personality disorder and the exploitation of its dramatic potential in innumerable television productions have gradually brought the disorder to the attention of the professional community."

Even busy physicians probably watch enough television to be exposed to this material sooner or later. Education by popular media has probably reached many mental health professionals prior to their exposure to MPD in the academic literature, given the dearth of professional attention to the disorder until very recently. As recently as 1984, Kluft (1984a, p. 22) noted that most clinicians "have never seen MPD apart from its representation in the media", leaving the greater education for many mental health professionals about MPD in the hands of the lay media, as it is for the public.

Media influence on evolving patterns of medical or psychiatric conditions is neither new nor singular to MPD, and clinical fads and fashions are well recognized in medicine. Following the release of the movie *The Exorcist,* Bozzuto (1975) reported four new cases of possession by the devil, the symptoms always beginning within a day of viewing the film, and Aldridge-Morris (1989, p. 101) reported two additional persons claiming sightings of Satan after seeing the movie. A similar case was reported that was precipitated by Alfred Hitchcock's movie *Psycho* (Bozzuto 1975). Bozzuto calls these episodes "cinematic neuroses." Aldridge-Morris, however, believes that the schizophreniform presentation of these cases suggests that they are actually "hysterical psychoses."

Chodoff (1987, p. 124) spoke of "the tendency for certain conditions (i.e. 'shell shock', neurasthenia) to be recognized, rise in popularity, and then decline." The media have played a role in popularizing a number of other medical conditions that specialists encounter in periodic waves of patients requesting investigation of symptoms known to be associated with these conditions (Pearson et al. 1983). Examples of this phenomenon include chronic fatigue syndrome, food allergy, and premenstrual syndrome. These conditions may be most prevalent in higher socioeconomic populations prone to "tendencies to self-diagnosis and the seeking of further medical opinions" (Rix et al. 1984, p. 125). In a study of allergy to foods, over 25% of a series of 23 patients "had identified their 'allergies' after reading the book *Not All in the Mind*" (Mackarness 1976; Pearson et al. 1983; Rix et al. 1984). An additional 50% of subjects in that report had obtained the idea they had the illness through suggestions raised by medical or other health professionals (Pearson et al. 1984).

The recent epidemic of chronic fatigue syndrome in America is probably the best example of a disorder garnering controversial attention in the professional literature and spurring intense media interest (Wessely & Powell 1989). *Newsweek* (Cowley et al. 1990) described chronic fatigue syndrome as the "disease of the '90's," and some physicians who treat the syndrome reported receiving as many as 2000 phone calls about the condition every month. Articles about this syndrome have also appeared in other well-circulated publications aimed at higher socioeconomic audiences such as *Consumer Reports* (1990) and *Runner's World* (Skloot 1990). Of interest, the psychiatric diagnoses associated with chronic fatigue syndrome and environmental allergy are the same ones sharing comorbidity with MPD: somatization disorder, depression, and anxiety disorders (Greenberg 1990; Kruesi et al. 1989; Pearson et al. 1983; Rix et al. 1984; Taerk et al. 1987; Wessely & Powell 1989).

With this background on the history of MPD in the popular media, we will now turn to an in-depth analysis of book-length personal accounts of MPD. Given the escalating number of such accounts in the last two decades, these works may be among the best sources of information on current trends in the popular representation of MPD.

6

Popular biographical accounts of MPD: A detailed analysis of 21 books

Given the potential for print media to affect the spread and character of MPD, it seemed pertinent to examine published accounts of the disorder to find out what the public and mental health professionals are learning from the popular literature. Popular accounts of MPD can be reevaluated in the context of our present understanding of the clinical presentation and natural history of this disorder (material extensively reviewed in Chapter 3).

Publishers have produced an amazing assortment of biographies and autobiographies of MPD patients offering detailed descriptions of their experience. We have collected all of these books and read them. During the course of our reading, we began to notice certain patterns and, as a result, decided to review all the books in a systematic manner in order to quantify their information. The following report on this large, untapped body of literature is part of our effort to explore the nature of the popular portrayal of the disorder.

The value of listening to what patients have to tell us directly has been underscored by Stern (1984, p. 149), who is critical of the conduct of psychiatric research: "Most professional reports have merely fit their findings into a preexisting theoretic framework, rather than making use of the data to explicate the unique human experience of the subject." The validation model of Robins and Guze and colleagues (1970), being atheoretical and empirical, avoids this problem and is thus appropriate to use in studying subjective accounts of MPD. This review should both offer in-depth examination of the personal experiences of patients and tabulated information from these sources that can be examined in parallel with the academic literature.

The chapter contains a critical analysis of all popular English-language books portraying cases of MPD that we could find. We have included only full-length books devoted to a single case each, to allow for sufficient detail about sufficient numbers of symptoms for psychiatric diagnosis. A book describing a male multiple with a history of head trauma (Franz 1933) was excluded from this review because it contained almost no descriptive information about symptoms and because the MPD diagnosis was never established. Several other books were excluded from this review because they shared a large portion of their text with other cases or with other issues (Cohen & Giller 1991; Confer & Ables 1983; Mayer 1988, 1991; O'Brien 1985). Some information from one of these books (O'Brien 1985), however, has been added where relevant to supplement available material about other cases.

One of the books that we excluded because it provided too little psychiatric detail for use as part of the review (Confer & Ables 1983) did contain enough information to suggest that the subject had Briquet's syndrome and may have been alcoholic. The patient came from a family troubled by alcoholism, depression, and suicidality, and she had been severely abused sexually and physically. Her somatoform complaints included headaches, numbness, pains in her hands and other locations, "colitis," weakness, feeling "heavy," blackouts, fainting spells, pseudoseizures, amnesia, difficulty breathing, sleepwalking, fatigue, weight loss, feelings of depression, anxiety attacks, hallucinations, and suicidality. She also had alcoholic blackouts and episodes of aggression while intoxicated.

The list of books included in this review was amassed from two recently published bibliographies (Boor & Coons 1983; Damgaard et al. 1985) and from the Multiple Personality listing in *Books in Print* (1990-1991), as well as from word of mouth. Eighteen cases (14 women and 4 men), described in 21 books (because the Eve story was told in four books) (Lancaster & Poling 1958; Sizemore 1989; Sizemore & Pittillo 1977; Thigpen & Cleckley 1957), were located and included for review in this study (Bliss & Bliss 1985; Castle & Bechtel 1989; Chase 1987; Clark & Roth 1986; Fraser 1988; Hawksworth & Schwarz 1977; Keyes 1981; LaCalle 1987; Lancaster & Poling 1958; Peters & Schwarz 1978; Peterson & Gooch/Freeman 1987; Prince 1906; Schreiber 1973; Schwarz 1981; Sizemore 1989; Sizemore & Pittillo 1977; Spencer 1989; Stoller 1973; Thigpen & Cleckley 1957; Ward & Farrelli 1982; Watkins & Johnson 1982). A list of these books can be found in Table 6-1.

Our methods are similar to medical chart review studies. To extract the relevant data from these lengthy accounts, we examined the books page by page, noting every potentially significant symptom of any kind. Any information provided about family history, severe environmental traumas, diagnoses applied to cases by their therapists, treatments received, and pertinent behavioral clues was also recorded. We recognize that lifting descriptions of symptoms and behaviors from the context of a book is no substitute for careful interview of the patient and review of medical records, but due to the nature of this study, the accounts themselves were the only consistently available source of information. The amount of information yielded by these techniques was amazing. This method has been successfully employed in similar studies of personal accounts of other psychiatric disorders (North & Cadoret 1981; North & Clements 1981).

DSM-III-R criteria were applied to determine diagnoses from the symptoms described in the accounts, except for the diagnosis of Briquet's syndrome, which was made by the criteria of Perley and Guze (1962). For any given symptom to

Table 6-1 List of MPD Accounts, Authors, and Patients

Title	Year	Author	Subject's Name
The Dissociation of a Personality	1906	Prince	Miss Christine Beauchamp
The Three Faces of Eve	1957	Thigpen & Cleckley	Eve
The Final Face of Eve	1958	Lancaster & Poling	Eve
Sybil	1973	Schreiber	Sybil Dorsett
Splitting: A Case of Female Masculinity	1973	Stoller	Mrs. G
The Five of Me	1977	Hawksworth & Schwarz	Henry Hawksworth
I'm Eve	1977	Sizemore & Pittillo	Eve
Tell Me Who I Am Before I Die	1978	Peters & Schwarz	Christina Peters
The Minds of Billy Milligan	1981	Keyes	Billy Milligan
The Hillside Strangler: A Murderer's Mind	1981	Schwarz	Kenneth Bianchi
The Healing of Lia	1982	Ward & Farrelli	Lia Farrelli
We, the Divided Self	1982	Watkins & Johnson	Rhonda Johnson
Prism: Andrea's World	1985	Bliss & Bliss	Andrea Biaggi
Shatter	1986	Clark & Roth	Kathy Roth
When Rabbit Howls	1987	Chase	Truddi Chase and the Troops
Voices	1987	LaCalle	Christopher Kincaid
Nightmare: Uncovering the Strange 56 Personalities of Nancy Lynn Gooch	1987	Peterson & Gooch/Freeman	Nancy Lynn Gooch
My Father's House: A Memoir of Incest and Healing	1988	Fraser	Sylvia Fraser
Katherine, It's Time	1989	Castle & Bechtel	Kit Castle
A Mind of My Own	1989	Sizemore	Eve
Suffer the Child	1989	Spencer	Jenny Walters Harris

qualify as a symptom of Briquet's syndrome, it had to be described in sufficient detail to demonstrate that the symptom met the severity criterion and was medically unexplained. The Perley-Guze criteria for Briquet's syndrome define a more homogeneous and familial disorder than American Psychiatric Association criteria (1987) for somatization disorder criteria (Cloninger et al. 1986). Because the criteria for Briquet's syndrome also encompass additional psychiatric complaints not included in the DSM-III-R criteria for somatization disorder, the Perley-Guze criteria offered greater opportunities to assess symptoms from our limited sources. For these reasons, the Perley-Guze criteria were considered more relevant than somatization disorder criteria to this study, although the results of both will be presented.

In a study of cases presented in books, the findings could feasibly be affected by the orientation of the authors of the accounts. On the other hand, the authors who were mental health professionals might provide symptom descriptions in more coherent psychological frameworks. The professional accounts, however, might contain distortions consistent with the professional bias of the particular author. Nonpartisan professional writers might provide more objective but less immediate accounts, and these also might be subject to biases from their own ideas on the subject. The authors of the accounts varied, some being the patients themselves, others being the therapists, and still others being unrelated professional writers; several of the books had combinations of the different types of authors. The most detailed and immediate raw descriptions of symptoms might intuitively be expected from the patients themselves as authors of their own accounts. Regardless of authorship, the information provided in these accounts was extensive.

Despite the limitations of our methods, we found that in most cases the material presented was comprehensive enough to point to an unequivocal psychiatric diagnosis, or at least to be strongly suggestive of the diagnostic category. Summary tables depicting the relevant diagnoses, as well as additional clinical information, will be presented, along with a textual presentation of the psychiatric conditions and related factors contained in the accounts. For more interested readers, Appendixes A and B at the end of the book contain, retrospectively, a series of case vignettes summarizing all the accounts and tables with specific information extracted from each account. These appendixes provide greater detail and contextual appreciation of case-by-case clinical information not provided in this chapter.

Summary of Results for All the Cases

Thirteen of the 21 books reviewed were published after 1980, and 5 were published in the 5 years from 1985 to 1989; only 3 dated from before 1970 (Table 6-1).

Table 6-2 summarizes the diagnostic findings of all the cases. All the women qualified for a diagnosis of MPD as defined by DSM-III-R. The MPD diagnosis in two of the four men (Milligan and Bianchi), however, was fervently debated by their evaluators, in part because their MPD was being examined in the context of forensic assessment of serious criminal acts including rape, kidnapping, and murder. We will not address this argument in detail, but we agree that there was abundant evidence in both cases arguing against the diagnosis. For the purposes of this review, these cases will be included in our analyses, because they were published as bona fide MPD cases by at least one author. The public would largely accept this presentation and assume that the content of the material in the book represents MPD. General readers would consequently be subject to influence by these accounts as much as by any others.

An experiment has provided preliminary evidence that this was the case. In a graduate-level social work class, approximately 40 students were given the assignment of reading and reporting on the psychiatric illness depicted in biographical accounts of MPD, most of which are presented in this review. All of the students accepted the bias of the author about the validity of the MPD diagnosis. All but one student fully accepted the disorder as described and diagnosed in the accounts without question. The one dissenting student read the book *Two of a Kind* (O'Brien 1985), which discounted the MPD diagnosis in favor of antisocial personality, malingering, and substance abuse, and that student fully accepted these other diagnoses as described by the author. Aside from the substance abuse and depressive disorders presented in the accounts, none of the students detected any other psychiatric disorders. In a second experiment, 76 nursing students were given an assignment of reading and reporting on a book of their own choosing about mental illness. As an indication of the popularity of MPD and fascination with it, 30 of the students chose to read one of the biographical accounts of MPD. Not one nursing student questioned the diagnosis.

Table 6-2 *Definite and Probable Diagnoses*

	Women (N = 14)	Men (N = 4)
Briquet's syndrome	12*	1
Conduct disorder	6	4
Antisocial personality	6†	4
Neither Briquet's syndrome nor antisocial personality	1‡	0
Substance abuse	11ˢ	3

*Includes three probable cases.

†Five of the six women with antisocial personality also had Briquet's syndrome.

‡Meets criteria for substance abuse and borderline personality disorder.

ˢTwo of the 11 substance abusers were iatrogenic.

As seen in Table 6-2, all four men in our review met criteria for antisocial personality disorder. Milligan and Kincaid reported enough somatoform complaints in almost enough categories to qualify them for a diagnosis of Briquet's syndrome, but Hawksworth and Bianchi had only a few somatoform symptoms. Milligan's polysymptomatic and somatoform presentation is consistent with the characteristic profile of MPD presented in Chapter 3. The low number of somatoform symptoms in Bianchi's account, however, do not suggest MPD, although his antisocial personality would be compatible with the presence of MPD.

Among the 14 women subjects, nine definitely met the criteria for Briquet's syndrome and three more were probable. These three probable cases all had a sufficient number of symptoms but were one or two symptom categories short of meeting the criteria. Six of the 14 women and all four men met the criteria for childhood conduct disorder, and all but one of these individuals (Chase) went on to meet the criteria for antisocial personality disorder after the age of 18. Five of the six women with antisocial personality disorder also met criteria for Briquet's syndrome. Only one woman (Johnson) did not meet the probable criteria for either Briquet's syndrome or antisocial personality; this subject, however, met six of the eight DSM-III-R criterion symptoms of borderline personality disorder, definitely qualifying her for this diagnosis.

Eleven of the 14 women and three of the four men (and possibly the fourth man as well) in this series developed drug and/or alcohol abuse; in two of the women the substance abuse disorders were iatrogenic. None of the accounts provided sufficient evidence for DSM-III-R diagnoses of primary major depression, schizophrenia, generalized anxiety disorder, or panic disorder, although many symptoms of these other conditions were described.

The diagnostic findings in these book-length accounts accurately reflect the diagnostic comorbidity described in the academic literature: high rates of somatization (especially in women), sociopathy (especially in men), and substance abuse. These profiles fit the polysymptomatic, polysyndromic pattern described in Chapter 3.

Somatization Disorder

The subject with the highest overall number of somatoform symptoms was Castle, who reported 54. Eve was close with 52 symptoms, but she also had the greatest opportunity to air her symptoms because her case generated four book-length published accounts. The mean number of symptoms of Briquet's syndrome in women was approximately double that of men (34.8 compared with 17.3 symptoms) (Table 6-3). Beauchamp said she didn't like to discuss her physical ailments, yet she reported 41 Perley-Guze symptoms.

Examination of the distribution of medically unexplained symptoms among the 18 cases revealed a pattern of extensive endorsement of symptoms in Groups

Table 6-3 *Number of Symptoms of Antisocial Personality and Briquet's Syndrome*

	Women (N = 14)	Men (N = 4)
Mean no. of symptoms of:		
Briquet's syndrome	34.8	17.3
Conversion	12.1	7.0
Conduct disorder	2.6	6.3
Adult sociopathy	4.2	7.5

2 (conversion symptoms) and 10 (psychiatric symptoms) on the Perley-Guze checklist for Briquet's syndrome. Depressed feelings were the second most frequent symptom acknowledged, with all but one subject reporting this symptom.

Several of the women neglected any mention of sexual or menstrual symptoms in spite of an otherwise loaded Perley-Guze checklist (Beauchamp, Eve, Sybil, Chase, Harris). Chase reportedly had an aversion to sex and could not bring herself to utter words related to sexual functions. In these accounts, the relative paucity of reproductive symptoms compared to other symptoms mentioned may reflect the authors' avoidance of material they perceive as socially unacceptable, especially in the earlier cases from more sexually conservative cohorts. Most of the more recent accounts, however, spared little in the public airing of their female reproductive symptoms. Some were even quite graphic, describing vast quantities of menstrual blood and pain of the severest intensity.

The description of medical and surgical attention to gynecologic complaints belied the absence of gynecologic symptoms in several of the accounts. Eve had a partial hysterectomy for symptoms of endometriosis, as well as an abortion. Fraser had a hysterectomy for pain complaints. Farrelli underwent surgery for gynecological problems and later had a hysterectomy. Harris was hospitalized for gynecologic problems, including once for treatment of a vaginal infection; her surgical history included a hysterectomy for vaginal bleeding and an operation for pelvic relaxation syndrome. Chase was treated for symptoms of premenstrual syndrome, and Castle received medical consideration of this disorder. Mrs. G had to be pregnant to be free of pain. Although Roth did not mention gynecologic procedures, she said she had undergone cosmetic breast reduction surgery.

To learn how the accounts compared diagnostically with different criteria, the somatoform symptoms were also fitted into DSM-III-R criteria for somatization disorder (see Table B-2 in Appendix B). For somatization disorder criteria (13 symptoms required for a diagnosis), women averaged 13 symptoms and men 5; women had a mean of 3 positive screening items and men 1.5. The mean of 13 symptoms in these women with MPD is in line with the 13.5 to 15.2 somatoform symptoms reported in research studies of MPD (Ross et al. 1989a, 1990c).

It appears that the methods of our study were sensitive to somatoform symptoms. All subjects meeting criteria for somatization disorder also met criteria for Briquet's syndrome. Two female subjects with Briquet's syndrome had only probable or possible somatization disorder. One interpretation of these findings might be that the Perley-Guze checklist for Briquet's syndrome is a more sensitive instrument than the DSM-III-R somatization disorder criteria in evaluating these personal accounts, because it picked up two cases not identified by the DSM-III-R criteria. On the other hand, DSM-III-R somatization disorder criteria might be less likely to result in false positive cases whose symptoms might be better accounted for within the framework of MPD.

Conversion Symptoms

All subjects reported at least two conversion symptoms. Beauchamp had 23 conversion symptoms, the highest number reported. The number of conversion symptoms in women was approximately double that of men. The women reported a mean of 12.1 conversion symptoms in Group 2 (range, 2 to 23) and the men had a mean of 7.0 (range, 4 to 15). The most common Perley-Guze symptom overall was in Group 2—amnesia, present in all 18 cases, an observation consistent with academic reports. Although some clinicians may consider amnesia more a part of dissociation than of conversion, we included it under conversion. In part, this is because of the tradition of Perley and Guze (1962), who included amnesia with conversion symptoms on the Briquet's checklist. As explored in greater detail in Chapter 8, the distinction between conversion and dissociation is not entirely clear.

Subjects reported a number of unusual conversion symptoms in their accounts. These included losing the ability to speak English, speaking gibberish, forgetting what a television was, inability to read coins, losing the ability to read, vision closing in, loss of depth perception, forgetting how to drive an automobile, being unable to discern men from women, being unable to recognize one's own reflection in a mirror, forgetting one's name, legs involuntarily jumping and shaking, itching all over and inside, and inability to close one's mouth.

Only two subjects didn't mention hallucinations. Reported hallucinatory experiences included negative hallucinations (not seeing things that are really present) and hallucinations of all five senses. Fourteen subjects reported auditory hallucinations (voices or humming), 12 had visual hallucinations, and 3 had olfactory hallucinations; tactile and gustatory hallucinations were reported by one subject each. Visual hallucinations and illusions included flashes of light, red and green spots, snakes, tarantulas, little men, seeing "images upon images," seeing an earthquake in a store, and seeing the walls closing in.

The weakness of this method of study, in which we were not able to interview subjects personally to probe symptoms in more detail, limited the available information about the quality of the hallucinations reported. For the most part, subjects in the accounts failed to state whether the hallucinations came from inside or outside of their heads, but information from other sources reviewed in Chapter 3 suggests that these experiences were most likely pseudohallucinations, distinct from the psychotic kinds of experiences described by schizophrenics.

Sexual Histories

Adult sexual symptoms were generally related to complaints that their sexual partners were abusive to them. Two subjects (Farrelli and Roth) felt that the only reason men wanted women was for sexual favors. The authors usually related their sexual complaints to childhood sexual abuse.

Several of the female subjects reported deviant sexual behaviors. Both Harris and Mrs. G were sexually promiscuous; Harris was unfaithful to her husband and Mrs. G reported extraordinarily high numbers of both homosexual and heterosexual affairs that started at a young age. Eve's sexual misadventures by contrast were relatively minor, including exhibitionistic dancing and singing and sexual manipulation of her husband.

Fraser, a published novelist, wrote extensively about sexual violence in her fiction. Her account of her MPD focused on her sexuality. Harris and Castle were seductive and flirtatious, and Harris seduced a number of pastors and therapists. Gooch and Harris worked as prostitutes, and Castle and Gooch were employed as strippers.

All four men had highly deviant sexual histories. Hawksworth was an alleged rapist. Milligan kidnapped and raped college coeds and kidnapped homosexual men at gunpoint from roadside restrooms. Bianchi was convicted for brutally raping and murdering at least a dozen women. He owned a library of pornographic literature and films. Kincaid, who was sexually promiscuous, organized a boys' club for the purpose of sexually molesting young boys.

Consistent with academic reports on cases of MPD, these accounts often blamed sexual acting out behaviors on specific alternate personalities.

Histrionic Traits

Subjects were frequently described as histrionic and overdramatic. This is consistent with reports that MPD is frequently related to histrionic personality disorder, which in turn has associations with the proclivity for somatization in this population. Eve, Farrelli, Chase, Milligan, and Harris had well documented temper tantrums. Thirteen subjects (Beauchamp, Eve, Sybil, Mrs. G, Farrelli,

Biaggi, Roth, Chase, Milligan, Kincaid, Fraser, Castle, and Harris) were described as "hysterical," overdramatic, or attention-seeking. Harris was described as the most demanding patient her therapist had ever encountered; she could not get enough attention, draining every possible resource yet remaining unsatisfied.

Therapists often remarked on the theatrical nature of the presentation of the personalities, which closely parallels observations by academicians that these cases may seem acted or theatrical. Beauchamp, Eve, Biaggi, Kincaid, and Castle were described in terms of acting, being on stage, or being theatrical.

Skepticism

The veracity of the symptoms of several of the subjects was at times doubted. These responses are also consistent with reports in the academic literature. (See Chapter 2 for a review of this skepticism.) The skepticism in the accounts ranged from momentary internal hesitations by therapists to descriptions of criticism by colleagues much like the harassment described by Dell (1988a, 1988b).

Expert psychiatric examiners engaged in heated controversies that carried into the psychiatric literature over whether Milligan's and Bianchi's MPD was genuine. Both were eventually pegged as phonies (Coons 1984; Orne et al. 1984).

Several subjects pushed the limits of their therapists' belief in their symptoms. This is perhaps not without reason. For example, both Eve and Sybil claimed that some personalities had blue eyes and others had brown eyes, a phenomenon (changing of eye color) not compatible with human physiology. Harris told elaborate and bizarre stories of extreme childhood physical and sexual abuse by her mother and a satanic cult that several therapists had difficulty believing. Caretakers of Beauchamp, Eve, Mrs. G, Hawksworth, Kincaid, Castle, Harris, and Peters suspected them of faking, exaggeration, conning, or acting. Even the patients themselves sometimes doubted the veracity of their symptoms. Both Roth and Kincaid expressed the concern that their own conditions were faked or unreal.

Antisocial Personality Disorder

Men had approximately double the number of conduct and antisocial symptoms of women (Table 6-3), in agreement with the reports that sociopathy is more typical of male multiples; the women, however, also had considerable antisocial symptomatology, which is also an accurate reflection of the academic literature.

A number of the female subjects had violent tendencies. Biaggi frequently killed cats when she was upset. Harris engaged in property destruction and assault. Fraser and Castle were noted to have problems with physical aggression and violence. Sybil reportedly abused her daughter physically and sexually. Peters beat up her sexual partners and assaulted police officers and hospital personnel, causing serious injuries. Fraser reported that she was preoccupied with sexual violence. Johnson had a violent fantasy life; she also assaulted people, causing severe injuries.

The men were even more violent. Kincaid was physically aggressive and expressed homicidal feelings. Hawksworth was a rough character who engaged in barroom fighting, assaulted police and military personnel, destroyed property, beat and raped women, attempted several murders, and showed no remorse. Milligan was extremely violent. His crimes included assault, robbery, serial rape and kidnapping, armed robbery of pharmacies for narcotics, shooting up a car with a machine gun, and planting a deadly snake in the expected path of an acquaintance.

Bianchi was the most violent and brutal of all the cases. The accounts of his crimes reported by O'Brien (1985) are gruesome and horrifying. He was eventually convicted of raping and murdering 12 women. In the meantime, he physically injured a woman during violent anal intercourse, beat and raped a woman, and threatened a woman with dismemberment and death. He also beat his wife.

Murder was a recurrent theme. Two of the men (Milligan, Bianchi) were convicted murderers; Bianchi was a serial killer. Hawksworth attempted murder, and Mrs. G reported over a dozen murder attempts. Three of the women (Mrs. G, Peters, Farrelli) reported they had attempted to murder their children. Gooch said she had been an accomplice in a gang-related murder of a male friend.

Many of the subjects had trouble with the law. Eve's story described lawbreaking and resisting arrest. Mrs. G spent time in both reform school and jail. Hawksworth escaped prosecution on drunken driving charges through judicial determination of NGRI (on the basis of his MPD). He was also arrested for recklessly causing an automobile accident for which he was sued and lost. He spent considerable time in jail for various charges. Peters spent time in a penitentiary, was released on parole, and violated parole. Milligan was arrested for various crimes, was sentenced to a maximum security prison facility, and broke parole. Bianchi was arrested for smashing a window and eventually went to prison for the series of brutal rapes and murders of which he was convicted. Castle was arrested for her behavior as a stripper.

Three subjects confabulated fantastic stories. In an effort to obtain air transportation back to the United States from Europe, Milligan made up an elaborate story about someone having drugged him. Bianchi fabricated an intricate scheme to cover for his time while he was out committing crimes and murder, telling his wife that he had cancer and was going to the hospital to receive chemotherapy. Bianchi impersonated a psychologist, practicing with a forged license, and even administered inkblot tests to his girlfriend under this ruse. Castle told her boyfriend and other people that she had a brain tumor and was dying, and also made up an elaborate story about her husband and children being tragically killed in a horrible automobile accident.

Other Behavioral, Interpersonal, and Characterological Difficulties

Besides performing antisocial acts and exhibiting histrionic behaviors, the subjects mentioned many other behavioral and interpersonal problems. These reflect the variety of characterological and behavioral problems associated with MPD described in the academic literature.

Near the end of her first account, Eve candidly admitted awareness of her behavior problems. Hawksworth made no efforts to hide his maliciousness. Mrs. G seemed to enjoy boasting about her antisocial acts, especially her homicidal behaviors. Bianchi acted irresponsibly, and frequently missed work, calling in sick when he was not ill. Three subjects (Milligan, Biaggi, Harris) were described as immature and/or unstable; Biaggi occasionally regressed to infancy, and Harris sucked her thumb and exhibited other childish behaviors.

Other characterologic problems identified include unpredictability or impulsivity (Hawksworth, Milligan, Gooch), oversensitivity (Farrelli, Johnson, Biaggi, Kincaid, Harris), self-pity (Castle), irresponsibility (Beauchamp, Eve, Hawksworth, Bianchi, Biaggi, Gooch, Castle, Harris) passivity (Bianchi, Kincaid), manipulation (Sybil, Mrs. G, Milligan, Bianchi, Roth, Kincaid, Harris), demandingness (Milligan, Kincaid, Harris), blaming of others (Eve, Bianchi, Milligan), arrogance and egotism (Milligan), hatefulness (Hawksworth, Johnson), and maliciousness (Hawksworth, Milligan). Additional problems included rage (Beauchamp, Eve, Farrelli), bitterness (Farrelli), feeling the world is against him (Bianchi), obsession with pain and self destruction (Johnson), emptiness and/or feeling lost (Johnson, Roth), loneliness (Roth, Kincaid, Gooch), fear of abandonment (Biaggi, Roth, Gooch), boredom (Roth), identity disturbance (Johnson, Harris), helplessness (Kincaid), poor self esteem (Kincaid, Gooch, Harris), and moodiness (Roth, Castle, Harris).

A number of the subjects had remarkable histories of sometimes severe self mutilation, mirroring information provided in academic reports. Seven subjects (Hawksworth, Mrs. G, Johnson, Biaggi, Gooch, Fraser, and Harris) burned themselves, seven (Mrs. G, Milligan, Johnson, Roth, Gooch, Kincaid, and Harris) cut or stabbed themselves, and four (Milligan, Farrelli, Gooch, and Harris) were headbangers. Gooch ingested a caustic substance and Harris ingested rat poison and turpentine. Two subjects inserted objects into their vaginas including razor blades (Johnson), safety pins, a coat hanger, and caustic drain cleaner (Biaggi). In addition, Peters inserted needles and other sharp objects into her arms to rip open her veins, Milligan attempted to step in the way of moving cars and tried to jump off a roof, Johnson tried to shoot herself, Biaggi binged on food, and Harris bit herself, clawed at her eyes, and set her hair on fire. While recuperating from surgeries in hospitals, Harris purposely tore open her incisions and inflicted caustic burns on her urethra and perineum with drain cleaner. Several subjects reported feeling no pain when doing these things to themselves.

We did not routinely apply borderline personality diagnostic criteria for additional psychiatric diagnoses, because practically all of the subjects met the criteria for Briquet's syndrome and/or antisocial personality disorder on the basis of objective behaviors unequivocally reported in the books. Because the criteria for borderline personality disorder are less objective and not as well agreed upon, we did not attempt systematically to cull out borderline symptoms for this diagnosis as well. We did, however, diagnose one case of borderline personality (Gooch), because she did not meet the criteria for any of the other diagnoses. As the preceding paragraphs show, many of these subjects reported prominent borderline personality symptoms, and some may well qualify for this additional diagnosis. Only Biaggi, Castle, and Harris had been diagnosed by their therapists as having borderline personality. Given the fact that we are already aware that MPD is a polysymptomatic, polysyndromic condition, providing additional personality diagnoses to their already impressive array of other diagnoses did not seem to add much to objective documentation of their symptoms.

Suicidality

Three of the 4 men (Hawksworth, Milligan, and Bianchi) and 7 of the 14 women (Mrs. G, Peters, Johnson, Biaggi, Gooch, Castle, and Harris) had attempted suicide, according to their accounts. Because Harris constantly threatened suicide, her physicians were left in the uncomfortable position of being unable to hospitalize her for every threatened episode. None of the suicide attempts in these cases were medically severe enough to be life-threatening, most having the flavor of manipulative gestures. These findings are also consistent with the academic literature, which describes suicidality as frequent among multiples.

Adult Victimization

Four of the subjects reported a history of victimization. Hawksworth, Farrelli, Biaggi, and Gooch reported that they were raped. For Biaggi, the events were associated with kidnapping and assault with a deadly weapon. Biaggi put herself at risk for victimization by picking up men at night who were likely to brutalize her, resisting advances while engaging in prostitution with unsavory characters, and accepting rides from strangers in bars. In the academic literature, multiples have reported high rates of rape.

Troubled Children

The accounts described troubled childhoods for most of the subjects, consistent with the known juvenile delinquency and behavioral problems described in the histories of multiples. In addition to the criterion symptoms of conduct difficulties, many other childhood behavioral problems were reported.

Eve, Hawksworth, and Fraser were described as malicious, mean, hateful, or hostile children. Eve, Biaggi, and Fraser were said to be disobedient. Juvenile authorities pegged Peters as incorrigible, and she was placed in juvenile institutions. Mrs. G went to reform school. Milligan was placed in a juvenile detention center and was later committed to a state hospital.

Five subjects reported school difficulties. Hawksworth, Milligan, Bianchi, and Harris had poor academic records. Farrelli and Milligan were expelled from school, and Hawksworth was nearly expelled. Harris had prolonged absences from school. Hawksworth and Harris both dropped out of school.

Socialization problems had begun at an early age. Bianchi, Farrelli, Johnson, and Gooch were described as lonely or friendless, and Harris was teased and ridiculed by her peers. Those who had friends sometimes chose deviant ones. Harris hung out with a promiscuous girlfriend and Hawksworth had disreputable friends. Johnson and Milligan had imaginary playmates.

Some of the subjects were quite violent as children. Hawksworth threatened people with guns and attempted to murder friends by shooting them with a bow and arrow or hitting them on the head with a rock. Mrs. G was homicidal from the age of four. Milligan engaged in assault with a weapon, property destruction, and perpetrating a bomb scare. Eve and others were cruel to animals. Peters killed kittens, Chase drowned cats, Bianchi killed cats and dogs, and Harris tortured and killed animals.

Other childhood problems included sexual promiscuity and forcing other juveniles into sexual acts (Hawksworth), daytime (Bianchi) and nocturnal enuresis until age 11 (Kincaid) or 14 (Peters), stuttering (Farrelli), tics (Bianchi), muteness (Farrelli), extreme dieting (Fraser), identity disturbance (Harris), pseudoseizures and multiple somatic complaints (Bianchi), self mutilation (Harris), attention-seeking or self-centeredness (Fraser, Harris, Bianchi), having a negative attitude about the world (Fraser), oversensitivity (Johnson, Harris), moodiness (Harris), and nervousness, passivity, and dependency (Bianchi).

Dysfunctional Families

The families of origin in these accounts were highly dysfunctional and filled with violence. This is consistent with findings reported in studies of multiples and their families. This pattern is also typical of families of patients with Briquet's syndrome, antisocial personality, and borderline personality.

Beauchamp's paternal relatives had violent tempers. Peters' father is believed to have murdered her brother and threatened her mother and grandmother. Peters' brother spent three months in jail for beating his wife. Milligan's parents had frequent drunken brawls. Bianchi's cousin was an accomplice to many of Bianchi's 35 alleged rapes and murders. Farrelli's aunt attempted to murder her mother with a butcher knife. Biaggi's father beat his wife and threatened the lives of others. Biaggi's sister was said to be violent and abusive, and three brothers were allegedly violent. Gooch's grandmother was beaten by one of her husbands. Castle's family life was marked by frequent physical fighting and wife beating. The family became homeless, and the children had to sleep in taverns and cars.

Child abuse was almost a way of life in these families. In line with the classic histories of childhood abuse known to populations of multiples, these accounts provided ample and graphic evidence of this association. As seen in Table 6-4, all of the males reported they had been both sexually and physically abused (also see Table B-6 of Appendix B). Nine of the women reported that they had been child victims of sexual abuse (by a family member in all but one case), and eight reported physical abuse, often brutal and severe, at the hands of one or both of their parents and/or stepparents. Most of the subjects reporting abuse had experienced both physical and sexual abuse; one woman had experienced only sexual abuse. Five of the 14 women made no mention of abuse. This likely represents underreporting as a limitation of this study.

The parents who had been both physical and sexual abusers of subjects in these accounts were Sybil's mother, who abused other children as well as her own daughter; Milligan's stepfather; Bianchi's adoptive mother; Biaggi's father (who reportedly went to prison for charges of incest against his daughter); Chase's stepfather; and Kincaid's stepfather (who went to jail for charges of incest). Harris' cousin also abused children both sexually and physically. Relatives who sexually molested children with no mention of physical abuse included Sybil's father (incestuous abuse); Mrs. G's father, brother, and two uncles; Peters' father and brother; Biaggi's uncle;

Table 6-4 *Abuse History*

	Women		Men	
	N	*(%)*	*N*	*(%)*
Physically abused	8	(57)	4	(100)
Sexually abused	9*	(64)	4	(100)
No abuse reported	5	(36)	0	

*One female subject reported only sexual abuse.

Gooch's father; Fraser's father; and Harris' mother, uncle, and brothers. Relatives who only physically abused children included Hawksworth's father, the mothers of Mrs. G, Roth, and Chase, and both parents of Peters and Castle.

Many of these cases reflected the patterns of intergenerational cycles of abuse. Other family members had reportedly been victims and perpetrators of abuse. Mrs. G's paternal grandfather was a known pedophile. Biaggi's father was himself sexually abused by his own father. Fraser's father had an incestuous relationship with his sister. Harris' mother had been chronically abused sexually by her brothers. Harris' uncle had an incestuous relationship with her mother. Kincaid's mother was physically abused by her husband, and she feared for her life. Gooch's mother was physically abused by her stepfather. Bianchi's biologic father had frequent physical fights with his biological mother. Milligan's mother was beaten by his stepfather. Gooch's aunt and father had an incestuous relationship.

Occasionally subjects openly blamed specific members of their families for their own problems. Milligan personally blamed his father as the cause of his MPD. Sybil's therapist blamed Sybil's disturbed mother. The others who described the initial occurrence or subsequent development of alternates related to physical or sexual abuse by family implicated family members indirectly.

Mothers

The mothers in particular were especially deviant based on the descriptions in the accounts. As mentioned above, several mothers had physically and/or sexually abused the subjects. Sybil's mother stole, acted out sexually and in many other ways, had multiple somatic complaints, and perpetrated depraved forms of sexual and physical abuse on Sybil with sadistic pleasure. Hawksworth's mother's death was suspected to have been a suicide. Peters' mother was alcoholic and sexually promiscuous, and she beat Peters. Milligan's mother had sociopathic behaviors and definite substance abuse, as well as frequent physical fights with his father.

Bianchi's biologic mother was promiscuous and alcoholic (Watkins 1984), very nervous, overly emotional, and had been repeatedly involved in the juvenile court system. She was only 14 years of age when Bianchi was born and she gave him up for adoption at birth. Bianchi was passed around to foster homes until he was adopted at the age of one year. His adoptive mother was felt to be a hypochondriac who was emotionally disturbed and who was accused of abusing him by exposing him to multiple physician examinations for obscure urinary complaints.

Farrelli's mother was emotionally neglectful of Farrelli and had character-ologic problems. Johnson's mother was described as nervous and emotional. Biaggi's nose was bloodied by her mother. Roth's mother may have physically abused her, and Roth had fears that her mother would abandon her. Chase's mother physically abused her by burning her hand.

Kincaid's mother may have had Briquet's syndrome and she exhibited several antisocial behaviors. She had a chronic history of multiple illnesses, pain complaints, and depressions. She was physically and sexually abused by her alcoholic husband. She neglected and finally abandoned Kincaid.

Gooch's mother was physically abused by her own stepfather; the mother was also emotionally abused by her own mother. Castle's mother was physically abused by Castle's father.

Harris' mother, according to Harris, inflicted physical and sexual abuse upon her that was by far the worst described by any subject in this series. Her mother had drunk turpentine when she found out she was pregnant with Harris, a behavior Harris emulated when she herself became pregnant. The mother was "hysterical" and short-tempered. She was constantly sickly with a variety of conditions for which she took to bed. Harris reported extreme physical abuse by her mother including exposure to the elements, extreme cold, and scalding water, being chained up, and being nearly drowned. In addition, the mother violently sexually abused her in association with satanic ritual abuse activities.

Summary of Psychiatric Disorders in Family Histories

Family psychiatric histories (Table 6-5) were positive for behaviors described in biologic relatives suggesting Briquet's syndrome and/or antisocial personality in 10 of the 14 female subjects and in all 4 male subjects. A family history of substance abuse was present in more than half. Five subjects had biologic relatives with possible affective disorder, and six reported suicides in their families. Four subjects had biologic relatives with diagnosed or suspected MPD. Eleven of the 14 had a family history of substance abuse. These family histories are characteristic of the wide variety of psychopathology described in studies of families of MPD patients.

Assortative Mating

Many subjects had deviant spouses and partners. Both of Eve's husbands showed evidence of sociopathy. One of them was sadistic and physically abusive to her, and the other apparently had an alcohol problem. All four of Mrs. G's husbands were said to have characterologic problems. Peters' first husband was physically

Table 6-5 *Family History*

	Subjects with Family History of Behaviors Suggesting:	
	N	(%)
MPD	4	(22)
Briquet's syndrome	5	(28)
Antisocial personality	13*	(72)
Either Briquet's syndrome or antisocial personality	13*	(72)
Affective disorder	5	(28)
Schizophrenia	2	(11)
Other psychosis	3	(17)
Substance abuse	11	(61)
Suicide	6	(33)

*One additional subject had a stepfather who was probably antisocial.

abusive to her and neglectful of the children; her second husband, an alcoholic, committed suicide; her "sadistic" lover beat her. Bianchi's fiance had extramarital affairs and his girlfriend destroyed property. Farrelli's husband was a very strict Catholic with whom Farrelli had sexual conflicts and physical fights. Fraser's husband abused alcohol. Castle's husband threw her out of the house for good.

The abuse went both ways: Roth, Fraser, and Castle struck, kicked, or threw things at their partners.

The difficult marriages and love relationships described by these authors reflect the academic literature (Coons 1980, 1984). The tendency for some multiples to marry sociopaths, drug abusers, sadists, and sexual perverts has been anecdotally reported by Coons (1980). Patients with Briquet's syndrome have similar assortive mating patterns, tending to marry sociopaths and alcoholics and experience marital and sexual discord (Woerner & Guze 1968).

Psychiatric Diagnoses Applied to Cases

All but two of the subjects had received psychiatric diagnoses other than MPD at some time (Table 6-6), including "hysteria" in nine of the 14 women, and in three of the four men. Therapists did not identify four of the women with probable or definite Briquet's syndrome (Chase, Gooch, Fraser, and Harris) but labeled Johnson, who did not meet criteria for Briquet's syndrome or somatization disorder, as having "hysteria." This diagnosis was appropriately applied to Milligan, but neither Hawksworth nor Bianchi had many somatoform symptoms

Table 6-6   *Diagnoses Applied by Mental Health Professionals*

	N	(%)
MPD	18*	(100)
Hysteria	12	(67)
Antisocial personality	6†	(33)
Schizophrenia	9	(50)
Affective disorder	8	(44)
Alcohol abuse	6	(33)
Drug abuse	7	(39)
Others‡	12	(67)

*The MPD diagnosis was hotly debated and subsequently rejected in two cases, both male.

†Four of the six diagnosed as antisocial were males.

‡Neurasthenia, kleptomania, pseudocyesis, egodystonic homosexuality, globus syndrome, rule out premenstrual syndrome, sexual deviation disorder, sexual sadism, phobic disorder, anxiety reaction, anxiety neurosis, mild neurosis, schizophrenic reaction, schizoaffective disorder, unspecified psychosis, schizomanic psychosis, character disorder, borderline personality, hysterical personality, schizoid personality, mixed personality disorder, inadequate personality, unstable personality, dissociated personality, conversion reaction, hysterical dissociation, dissociative reaction, passive-aggressive, somatization, narcissism, anorexia, malingering, conscious faking, Munchausen's syndrome, tic disorder, temporal lobe epilepsy, rule out brain tumor, normal.

suggesting the hysteria label they received. No suspicion of hysteria was mentioned for Kincaid, who reported many somatoform symptoms.

Other disorders were often not identified. Only two of the five women antisocials (Eve and Mrs. G), and three of the four male antisocials (Hawksworth, Milligan, and Bianchi) were diagnosed; the antisocial personalities of Kincaid and three of the women (Peters, Biaggi, and Harris) were not identified. Johnson, whose account did not report compelling evidence of sociopathy, received this diagnosis. The substance abuse problems of Eve, Biaggi, Gooch, Fraser, and Castle were not addressed by their therapists.

Eight of the subjects were classified as having affective disorders. The many other diagnoses applied are also listed in Table 6-6. Six of the subjects collected 10 or more diagnoses each, and the maximum was 19. The mean number of diagnoses besides MPD was 5.5. Often diagnostic impressions of the different clinicians directly contradicted each other. Nine subjects were thought to have schizophrenia and another subject was considered psychotic. Mrs. G was thought to be intermittently psychotic, although her therapist noted that she exhibited no evidence of thought disorder or chronic deterioration, and that her apparent psychotic episodes seemed more like "hysterical psychosis." Johnson's therapist felt that she had evolved from MPD to a "regressed schizophrenic" with hallucinations and delusions arising from childhood memories.

Roth's doctor discounted the diagnosis of hysteria, instead accepting the hypothesis that her MPD syndrome might be covering an underlying schizophrenic condition, although he never actually diagnosed her condition as schizophrenia. Gooch's condition was compared to psychosis and her multiple personality defense system was thought to be a protection from disintegrating into autism or schizophrenia. An evaluation of Harris at a center nationally recognized for specializing in MPD identified an "underlying schizophrenic disorder." Castle's doctor refused to apply a psychiatric diagnosis (other than MPD) due to the concern that it would detract from her story. He did, however, invoke the diagnosis of MPD.

In every account, MPD was reported to be the primary diagnosis, even though most patients accrued several other psychiatric diagnoses. A number of the therapists recognized these other disorders or symptoms of them but chose to consider those other disorders secondary. Cleckley, an expert in antisocial personality disorder, apparently considered this diagnosis either as not present or as secondary to Eve's MPD (Cleckley 1950). Roth's doctor entertained the possibility of hysteria, but discounted the diagnosis because he considered hysteria to be a prevalent, meaningless condition.

The Alternates

Consistent with published studies, the number of alternate personalities of the subjects showed a trend toward increasing numbers by year of publication, as seen in Figure 6-1.

The alternate personalities had often been originally created to help the subject deal with something difficult such as childhood sexual abuse. Some of the subjects blamed their behaviors on the alternate personalities, and in some cases personalities had originally been created to perform acts unacceptable to the subject. For example, Eve had different personalities designed for lying, hiding, and running away. Her alternate personality Eve Black performed behaviors that were unacceptable for her.

Mrs. G found her alternates to be good excuses for her behavioral problems, such as attempting to murder her childhood playmates. Hawksworth's alternate personalities were blamed for his behaviors from the age of four. As an adult, his MPD proved to be a sufficient excuse for a court to declare him NGRI on charges of drunken driving. Milligan's personalities reportedly had first appeared at the age of four, when he blamed an alternate personality for his misbehavior.

Farrelli's first alternates were not recognized until she attempted to choke her baby to death, but as a child Farrelli had been expelled twice from school for apparent actions of her alternate personalities. Johnson's first alternate appeared at age 13 as a response to social rejection and loneliness. Biaggi's first personalities developed at the age of four to protect her from her sexually abusive father. Roth's first alternate personality was created in childhood to help her behave well in order to keep her mother from abandoning her. Roth came to realize that her personalities helped her avoid taking responsibility for her actions.

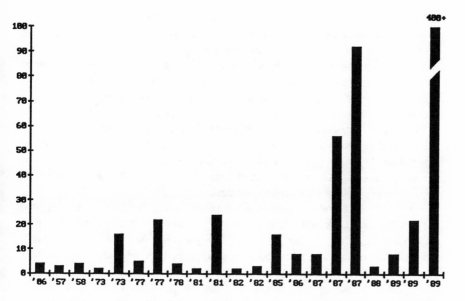

Figure 6–1. Number of alternates by year of publication.

Chase's personalities began early in her childhood to protect her from the experience of physical and sexual abuse by her stepfather. Both Chase's and Sybil's alternates displayed naughty behaviors in childhood for which they were punished, and neither could recall having committed the acts. Each of Sybil's personalities served to take blame for unacceptable behaviors that the original Sybil could not admit to. Kincaid reported that his alternate personalities had developed to help him cope with incest with his father.

According to Gooch's account, her alternate personalities first appeared in response to ritual sexual abuse she experienced as a child, beginning at the age of two. Gooch's personalities always introduced themselves when they came out to make certain that others were informed of their presence. One of her personalities needed her blood for satanic rituals. Each of her alters were specifically created to perform functions otherwise unacceptable to her or to commit acts that she would never attempt, such as taking drugs for her.

Fraser's alternate personalities occurred spontaneously and she learned of them herself without any known assistance from a therapist. Castle said her first alternate appeared during infancy to help her handle her fear of being alone. Castle's doctor was angered when he discovered that she had plagiarized from a children's book to provide the material for her alternates.

Harris' personalities were created when she was three years old in order to help her cope with extreme physical and sexual abuse and to escape from physical and emotional pain. She claimed over 400 alters, and even her alternate personalities had alternates. Her therapist thought she used her personalities to avoid responsibility for her actions. Most of her personalities had a specific purpose in performing activities that were unacceptable to her, such as managing strong emotion, prostituting, and abusing substances.

There were some inconsistencies in the subjects' reports of the occasion of the occurrence of their first alternates. In part, this may be related to the unfolding of memories through progress in therapy. Beauchamp's alters first appeared during hypnosis, but later in the account retrospective mention was made of splitting of her personality during her early childhood. Her alternates were initially mistaken for hypnotic states. Eve's first account described her first alternate personality at the age of six when she had to kiss her deceased grandmother, but in the second account, her first alternate was said to have appeared at age two, when she witnessed a violent accident.

Mrs. G's first alternate personality was reported at age three, telling her that her new baby sister should die, but in another place in her story the first alternate occurred at age four, telling her to kill her playmate. Milligan retrospectively reported that his first alternate personalities had appeared around the age of four, when he was accused of drawing on the wall and breaking a cookie jar; otherwise, there was no apparent presence of the alternates until he was psychiatrically evaluated following his arrest for murder. Bianchi's first alternate personality also appeared during a forensic evaluation after his arrest for several murders, but Bianchi claimed in retrospect that his alternates had first appeared at age nine while his mother was beating him. None of his family or friends had any inkling of any behaviors consistent with MPD prior to his arrest.

The first official appearance of Gooch's personalities occurred as an adult when she was taken by her therapist to a party in order that the guests might see a live case of multiple personality. Roth's account was vague about when her personalities first developed, other than to mention that they first occurred during her childhood. Sybil's account was also vague about when her alternate personalities first appeared. Chase's writing was so vague that it was not possible to determine an age at which her other personalities first appeared, but it may have been at age two.

Treatments Received

Table 6-7 summarizes the treatments the subjects reported receiving in their accounts. All of the subjects received psychotherapy and/or hypnosis. Beyond hypnosis and ordinary psychotherapy, no particular therapy seemed especially important to the long-term outcomes. Several subjects were prescribed multiple medications, including antipsychotics, antidepressants, amphetamines, benzodiazepines, barbiturates, narcotics, unspecified tranquilizers and sleeping pills, lithium, anticonvulsants, and vitamins and tonics. Three subjects received electroconvulsive therapy. Four received treatment for a substance abuse problem.

Table 6-7 Treatments Received

	N	%
Psychotherapy/hypnosis	18	(100)
Antipsychotic Rx	6	(67)
Antidepressant Rx	4	(22)
Lithium carbonate	1	(6)
Amphetamines	1	(6)
"Tranquilizers"	5	(28)
Sleeping pills	3	(17)
Narcotics	4	(22)
Benzodiazepines	3	(17)
Barbiturates	2	(11)
Anticonvulsants	4	(22)
Vitamins/tonics	1	(6)
Substance abuse detoxification/rehabilitation	4	(22)
Electroconvulsive therapy	3	(17)
Lobotomy recommended	2	(11)
Other*	8	(44)

*Chiropractic treatment, relaxation, reparenting therapy, group therapy, marriage encounter, massage therapy, primal therapy, rolfing, bioenergetics, yoga, meditation, straitjacket, other physical restraint, slapping, transcutaneous electrical nerve stimulator (TENS), pain rehabilitation program, halfway house for alcoholics, partial hospitalization, Alcoholics Anonymous.

For two subjects a lobotomy was recommended, and one almost consented to have the procedure. Several of the subjects with polysomatic complaints received a variety of somatic treatments for their symptoms, such as surgery, pain medication, chiropractic treatment, a TENS unit, and pain rehabilitation programs. Unconventional treatments such as primal therapy, massage therapy, rolfing, bioenergetics, yoga, meditation, and slapping and spanking were also tried. Two subjects (Gooch and Johnson) had to be physically restrained, including the use of a straitjacket, and Milligan was placed in seclusion. Untrained therapists occasionally treated the multiples, including a creative writing teacher who used hypnotherapy and caretakers who applied narcotherapy.

Beauchamp, Eve, Farrelli, Biaggi, and Kincaid were found to be very suggestible and easily hypnotized. Personalities were sometimes first discovered under hypnosis; Milligan's and Bianchi's personalities were first recognized during hypnosis as part of their forensic evaluations. Eve, Sybil, Peters, Chase, Gooch, Fraser, and Harris also underwent hypnosis. Eve believes that the use of hypnosis by her therapist aggravated her dissociative tendencies (Sizemore 1989).

The contact with medical and mental health professionals was remarkably extensive in some of the cases. Mrs. G and Biaggi underwent multiple surgical procedures, usually without a cause being found for the physical complaints.

Farrelli had 21 surgeries in 23 years, and 22 physicians were treating her simultaneously. Mrs. G accrued 21 psychiatric hospital admissions, totaling more than five years in the hospital. Harris was hospitalized 27 times in 20 years. Gooch was also repeatedly hospitalized. Castle had been admitted to hospitals and neurological wards across the country, and the possibility of a "professional patient" profile was suggested. As a child, Bianchi was subjected to repeated genitourinary examinations and procedures. Johnson and Biaggi were treated by a succession of therapists, and Gooch was treated by several well known psychiatric experts with no apparent improvement. Biaggi was a frequent emergency room visitor. Harris was well known for seeking help from every possible resource, including medical doctors, mental health workers, and ministers.

The academic literature does not describe this magnitude of utilization of medical services in MPD, although it does in Briquet's syndrome. The literature does, however, suggest that multiples tend to receive excessive inappropriate psychiatric and neurologic treatment.

Transference-Countertransference

The relationships the subjects had with their therapists were often intense, with therapists' responses ranging from fascination and overinvolvement to frustration and aggravation. The accounts provided profuse detail of the difficulties their therapists had with them, fully supporting the variety of responses reported by authors of professional reports in the literature. Eve's doctors were drawn to the fascinating aspects of her disorder (Thigpen & Cleckley 1984). Chase's therapist expressed fascination over having an MPD patient in his practice. This therapist accompanied her during her publicity tour for her book. Biaggi's doctor found treatment of multiples very gratifying, comparing therapy to the use of incantations and spells, sometimes curing MPD in as little as two hours. Harris' therapists, in contrast, reported that because of their work with her, their peers ostracized them and the mental health profession was abusive to them.

Kincaid's account was a story of an intense patient-therapist relationship with strong transference and countertransference between him and his female psychologist. Colleagues accused her of overinvolvement; eventually she developed a social relationship with the patient.

Two subjects (Gooch and Kincaid) received special attention from therapists such as daily sessions, special favors while in the hospital, therapist availability during personal and vacation time, and therapy sessions lasting up to four and even eight hours. Kincaid and Sybil both became very dependent on their therapists; therapy became the central point of Sybil's existence.

Some of the female subjects (Peters, Roth, and Harris) were seductive to their therapists and physicians. Two subjects (Mrs. G and Harris) claimed to have had sexual intercourse with their treating psychiatrists, and Mrs. G also said she smoked marijuana with her psychiatrist. During a therapy session Roth inadvertently exposed her thighs, revealing herself almost up to her waist.

As the published literature would predict, these were not easy patients. Beauchamp, Sybil, and Peters abused or became dependent on medications prescribed for them. Mrs. G, Milligan, Johnson, Gooch, Castle, and Harris were described as extremely manipulative and disruptive patients. Their behaviors included urinating and defecating on the floor of the hospital ward, refusing medications, pretending to take medications and later spitting them out, smuggling alcohol and drugs onto the unit, getting drunk on gate pass, repeatedly escaping from the psychiatric ward and slitting both wrists while in elopement, overdosing and then calling the therapist anonymously to request a rescue response, calling pastors with fake reports of depressions and overdoses, and accusing hospital employees of causing wounds that were actually self-inflicted.

Five subjects were violent in the therapy setting. Violent acts during inpatient stays included property damage (Milligan), rape (Milligan), and assault with injuries to other patients (Peters, Johnson) and staff (Johnson), as well as threats of bodily harm to one's therapist (Milligan). In addition, Harris hit and bit her therapist, and Biaggi assaulted her doctor with a dress pin. Milligan escaped the forensic unit.

These difficulties in treatment are very characteristic of the treatment courses of multiples as described in the professional literature. They are also consistent with the nature of treatment in Briquet's syndrome and borderline personality.

Outcomes

The books ended with complete recoveries from multiplicity in 10 of the cases, with five of the women (Beauchamp, Sybil, Eve, Peters, Johnson, Farrelli) and two of the men (Hawksworth, Kincaid) reporting that they had been free of manifestations of MPD for periods ranging from a brief time to many years. Others were improved but not fully recovered (Biaggi, Gooch, Harris). Some of those whose multiple personalities had been fused required continuing psychotherapy (Peters, Farrelli, Johnson). Two of the men (Milligan, Bianchi) were unimproved. Chase refused to integrate her personalities but remained in therapy. The final status of three of the subjects (Mrs. G, Roth, Fraser) was unclear from the authors' descriptions. Castle was a special case. In the end of the book she was cured, but an afternote written by her therapist indicated that she suffered an unfortunate relapse of MPD just prior to the publication of her book.

Similarly, Eve had several false starts. She was, however, eventually successful in overcoming her MPD. Her three personalities, after their initial fusion, subsequently blossomed to a total of 22. Doctors had declared her cured several times before she finally fused her personalities for the last time many years ago.

Despite Eve's ultimate fusion, however, Velek and Balon (1986) were not convinced of her mental health. Eve's final account is a meritorious and courageous story that describes her successful battle to take responsibility for her behavior and to learn to cope without dissociating.

Professional Knowledge and Aspirations in the Mental Health Field

Several subjects had outside medical, psychiatric, or psychology-related backgrounds, and these findings are summarized in Table 6-8. Beyond this history, a number of the subjects were undoubtedly educated by their therapists, receiving with that information the therapist's particular bias.

Sybil spent considerable time in a university psychology library where she read extensively on psychiatry and case histories. Peters was a registered nurse and had worked at an alcohol treatment facility. Milligan spent many hours reading medical texts. Bianchi had taken college courses in psychology, possessed a number of books on psychology, and had read a great deal on the subject and talked extensively about psychology. Bianchi may have obtained sufficient information about the "correct" presentation of MPD from clues he picked up during the course of his psychiatric examination (Orne et al. 1984; Spanos et al. 1985, 1986). Castle had extensive knowledge, through personal reading, of medicine and psychiatry, and she was well acquainted with diagnostic criteria from reading DSM-III. At one point Castle very successfully impersonated a physician.

After their recovery, a few of the subjects had aspirations to become mental health professionals themselves. Kluft (1989) has commented that "the percentage of MPD patients with alters professing the urge to become therapists appears inordinately high." Eve began to help others overcome MPD and helped educate the public about MPD and mental illness. Roth enrolled in a psychotherapist training program, and Harris took a psychology course. Gooch planned to become a mental health counselor, specifically desiring to study under Dr. Cornelia Wilbur. One of Castle's personalities aspired to a career in internal medicine and was also considering becoming a psychiatrist.

Two subjects, both men, had backgrounds or aspirations in the legal field. Milligan studied law textbooks at great length. Bianchi, who wanted to be a policeman, had taken college courses in police science and had read extensively on the subject.

Several subjects had previous exposure to MPD. Prior to writing her final account, Eve had read the case of Sybil. Bianchi may have read a newspaper article about Milligan in 1984 (Orne et al. 1984). It is likely that Bianchi viewed the film *Sybil* before his first visit with Dr. Watkins. He had also seen the movie *The Three Faces of Eve* and it has been suggested that Bianchi may have incor-

Table 6-8 *Mental Health Background and Aspirations and Occult Experiences*

	N	(%)
Has gained knowledge about MPD through attending lecture on, reading book or article about, or watching movie about Eve, Sybil, or Bianchi	8/15	(53)
Had extensive psychiatric and/or medical knowledge	5	(28)
Trained or worked in mental health field	3	(17)
Aspired to be a mental health professional	3	(17)
Had ties to the occult	9	(50)

porated features of Eve's symptoms into his own clinical presentation. Roth had read about Billy Milligan's 24 personalities in *Penthouse* magazine. Kincaid and Gooch had both read the book *Sybil,* and Biaggi and Chase (the "Oprah Winfrey Show," August 27, 1991) also viewed the movie *Sybil.*

Chase attended a lecture by Chris Sizemore ("Eve"); Harris also met "Eve" and it was felt that this event had an influence on the progress she made toward integration shortly thereafter.

Parapsychology and the Occult

A number of the subjects had inclinations toward the occult as well as toward parapsychological and metaphysical phenomena. This is no surprise given published reports of associations of MPD with these phenomena. Eve, Roth, and Castle claimed to have experiences relating to parapsychology, the occult, and aliens, including mindbending metal, clairvoyance, ESP, psychokinesis, reincarnation, personal recollection of events that happened centuries ago, astral travel, encounters with UFO's and life after death, and visitations by poltergeists.

The subject most extensively tied to satanism and cults was Harris. She described extensive forced cult involvement and extreme abuse from early childhood, which she voluntarily renewed as an adult. Several of her personalities were figures tied into satanism. Other types of involvement in the occult described in the accounts included reading extensively about mysticism and the occult (Hawksworth, Harris), writing about satanic images (Fraser), collecting objects related to the occult (Harris), requesting an exorcism for a complaint of demonic possession (Peters, Harris), practicing spells and rituals to conjure up demons (Harris), participation in voodoo, black magic, and idol worship (Kincaid), attending Pentecostal services and speaking in tongues (Harris), tattooing one's arm with a satanic message (Bianchi), and earning money as a fortune teller (Fraser). Gooch reported recovered memories of being subjected to childhood satanic sexual abuse rituals by her babysitter, recollections that began after she started reading a novel that dealt with satanic abuse.

Misinformation

Several of these books have perpetrated misinformation about schizophrenia, reflecting both professional and public confusion over schizophrenia and MPD. Nine of the MPD subjects were misdiagnosed as schizophrenic, and another subject was considered psychotic.

The subjects of the books, however, were not the only persons demonstrating diagnostic confusion about schizophrenia: family members were also subject to this confusion. In some cases, it appears that family members of subjects were diagnosed in ways other than the symptoms ascribed to them would suggest. Sybil's mother, for example, allegedly engaged in antisocial activities and complained of multiple somatoform symptoms; although no evidence of psychotic symptoms was mentioned, Sybil's therapist invoked a diagnosis of schizophrenia, with no consideration of antisocial personality or Briquet's syndrome. The author then identified the "schizophrenia" as the source of the abusive behaviors. Peters' mother, who evidenced antisocial behaviors and had an alcohol problem, was called "psychotic" in the absence of any identified psychotic symptoms.

Similarly, Biaggi's father was diagnosed paranoid schizophrenic; no psychotic symptoms were noted in the account but he was alcoholic, had amnestic episodes, evidenced multiple antisocial symptoms and overt violence, and had a capacity to be very charming.

The author of the Harris account unfortunately equated MPD with schizophrenia in saying that "split personality" is a schizophrenic condition. On the positive side, however, the Harris account specifically highlighted the unfortunate confusion of "split personality" with schizophrenia.

Authorship

The different accounts had authors with different roles. The accounts of Eve, Beauchamp, Mrs. G, Biaggi, Kincaid, and Harris were written by their therapists. Eve also wrote an autobiographical account of her story, and she coauthored two additional autobiographies with professional writers. Hawksworth, Peters, Farrelli, Gooch, and Castle shared authorship with professional authors in "as-told-to" agreements. The accounts of Roth, Chase, and Fraser were purely autobiographical. The accounts of Sybil, Milligan, and Bianchi were authored by professional writers. Johnson shared authorship with her therapist.

There was some variation in writing style and informativeness of the accounts, depending on authorship of the books. For example, Allison (1974b) noted discrepancies between the therapists' account of *The Three Faces of Eve* and the autobiography *I'm Eve,* which "gave a story quite different from the first two books" written some 23 years earlier (Allison 1981, p. 33). Allison (1974b, p. 15) reported that "when I read Eve's own autobiography (Lancaster, [sic] 1958), there were marked differences in the two stories and just what therapeutic methods other than recovery of early memories really helped was quite unclear." The versions of the case written by the patient herself were more informative and contained many more symptoms, particularly the somatoform symptoms, than the psychiatrist's original version. On the Perley-Guze checklist for Briquet's syndrome the psychiatrists reported 17 symptoms in five categories, insufficient for a diagnosis. Eve, however, described more symptoms in more categories with each passing account, until she eventually had a total of 52 symptoms in 10 categories for a definite diagnosis. All symptoms reported by the psychiatrists were also reported by Eve, adding confidence to the reliability of their symptom reports.

The style of writing in many of the autobiographical accounts was typical of the speech ascribed to individuals with somatization disorder and personality disorders: overdramatic in style (often containing references to blood and violence), often vague in content, and circumstantial (American Psychiatric Association 1987, p. 261; Cloninger & Guze 1970a, 1970b; Drob et al. 1982; Gillstrom & Hare 1988; Kroll 1989, pp. 30–33; Murphy 1982; Purtell et al. 1951; Siomopoulos 1971). Some of the biographical accounts not authored by the actual subjects provided quotations from the subjects illustrating these tendencies in their language.

The accounts of Roth and Gooch in particular described symptoms overdramatically, with the use of violent imagery and similies. These two authors used vivid images such as explosions, blood gushing, fire, and volcanoes in describing their pains. Fraser, a published novelist, had a writing style that was flowery and overdramatic. She mixed passages of fantasies, memories, and dreams so that it was impossible to sort out fact from fantasy. She used extensive demonic and satanic imagery. Kincaid's psychiatrist was also an overdramatic writer. Chase's langauge was so vague that it was difficult to ascertain important historical information, such as when her first alternate personality had appeared.

Public Attention

All of the subjects sought public attention, publishing detailed book-length accounts of their stories. Chase and Sizemore both went on publicity tours with television and radio appearances and national newspaper and magazine interviews, and Sizemore has done extensive speaking nationally. Recently, Chase appeared on the highly popular national talk show, the "Oprah Winfrey Show" (August 27, 1991). *The Three Faces of Eve* became a best-seller and subsequently Sizemore's story was made into an Academy Award-winning movie. The movie based on Sybil's account received four Emmy awards. In 1991, a movie about Bianchi and a made-for-television mini-series about Chase aired on network television, and the case of Milligan was also depicted in a movie. National and foreign presses carried newspaper articles about Gooch's story. Gooch also appeared on the "Oprah Winfrey Show" in 1986 with MPD authority Dr. Bennett G. Braun.

Psychiatrists pointed out that Eve was receiving considerable professional attention for her story and suggested that she might just be acting out her symptoms. The implication of such accusations is that subjects "created" their symptoms to generate public appeal and widespread attention, as well as substantial financial gain. Eve, however, did not receive much financial gain, as reflected by her lawsuit against Fox Studios claiming that they had given her only $7000, a trivial amount considering what her story netted for that company, and an amount she claimed had been invalidly agreed upon because supposedly they knowingly entered into a contract that took advantage of her mentally ill condition.

Bianchi and Milligan achieved extensive public attention due to the brutality of their crimes and the controversy over their MPD. Milligan was described as seeking excessive publicity. A second biography about Bianchi was written and was made into a television motion picture. Milligan's story appeared in *Newsweek* and *Time*.

Harris' therapists indicated that they felt the books *The Three Faces of Eve* and *Sybil* and the movies based on them "had by far the greatest effect in educating the public about multiple personality disorder." They said that *The Three Faces of Eve* account had "introduced the phenomenon of multiple personality to the mental health care community and to the lay public. The disclosure [Eve] allowed gave credence to and popular awareness of the reality of multiple personality."

Afterword

During the final revisions of this manuscript, not surprisingly, given the frequency with which popular accounts of MPD have hit the market, yet another such account was published (Casey 1991). We decided to draw the line on new additions to the list, because at some point the manuscript had to go to press. We have, however, included a summary of the clinical details of this case along with the other vignettes in Appendix A. This subject had many symptoms of Briquet's syndrome and of antisocial personality but failed to meet the criteria for either diagnosis. This may have been due to a myopic focus on the primary features of MPD, with which the author was apparently well acquainted. The subject did, however, easily meet the criteria for borderline personality disorder.

Discussion of the Accounts

We recognize that the method of applying diagnoses to cases in this study is not the standard methodology of epidemiologic studies, although it is similar to a chart review study. If anything, the methods used here would be expected to underdiagnose psychiatric disorders, because we were not afforded the luxury of interviewing the subjects and asking them about criterion symptoms. Instead we had to hope that the authors' descriptions were sufficiently comprehensive to include enough symptoms to rule in or out the diagnoses. There is some evidence that symptoms were underreported. Gooch and Castle, for example, had extensive adult antisocial behaviors but reported few or no childhood conduct symptoms and presented little detail about their childhood conduct. Five women with many somatoform symptoms had an obvious lack of reproductive symptoms on the Perley-Guze checklist for Briquet's syndrome.

Due to the limitations of this study, the diagnoses ascertained may not be an accurate representation of the real disorders in the actual individuals depicted. Rather, they may only reflect the psychiatric conditions as they were reported in the accounts, often by nontherapist authors, or through the direct perceptions of the patients themselves. It is also acknowledged that the cases presented in this review do not represent a random sample. Due to selection bias, the syndromes depicted in these popular accounts may or may not accurately reflect the condition as it occurs in the general population, and in all likelihood represent the far end of the dramatic and remarkable.

Although the therapists in these accounts often acknowledged other disorders, such as "hysteria," sociopathy, and borderline personality, the authors minimized or ignored these other diagnoses and emphasized the more fascinating aspects of the multiple personality syndrome. It is understandable that some of the authors of the accounts may have focused on MPD for the purpose of marketing a book. The reading public would be less likely to be attracted to a book about Briquet's syndrome or personality disorder; hence emphasis on these other disorders, which could be confusing or uninteresting to the lay reader, may have been downplayed.

Nonetheless, symptoms of these other psychiatric disorders were clearly presented in the books, a reflection of the patients' recognition of the importance of these symptoms to their condition. By broadening the focus of the current review to encompass the variety of psychopathology accompanying the more traditional symptoms of MPD, it was seen that somatoform tendencies and/or pervasive characterologic and interpersonal difficulties played a major role in the expression of MPD in these personal accounts. In addition, the accounts of the multiples reflected many other features consistent with somatization disorder—female predominance, early onset, chronicity, histrionic presentation, suicidal gestures (Morrison 1989b), extensive use of medical services, and extraordinary difficulties in treatment—as well as many features of antisocial personality disorder and borderline personality, with histories containing elements of moderate to extreme violence and social deviance, self-mutilation, stormy relationships, and constant crises.

Interestingly, no accounts have been provided by MPD patients who have always been high functioning. Reports such as those by Kluft (1986) of high-functioning MPD patients would predict that these extraordinary cases should be represented among published cases—especially since these published cases would be expected to be biased toward the extraordinary. Of all the patients, Chase, who was described as successful in the real estate business, would be the most likely to be considered high functioning. In a case report the severity of her difficulties could be glossed over, but the results of our study indicate that even she was severely impaired. The high-functioning cases may be the potentially most interesting from a scientific standpoint, but overall these were not present among the published accounts. At any point in time, however, it might have been argued that the current picture of several of them could be construed as high functioning. In the long run, high function did not dominate.

In these accounts of MPD, the frequent family psychiatric histories of Briquet's syndrome, antisocial personality disorder, and substance abuse are like those of persons with Briquet's syndrome and antisocial personality. Briquet's syndrome is associated with a personal and family history of antisocial and delinquent behavior, and vice versa (Cloninger et al. 1975a, 1975b, 1985; Guze et al. 1967, 1971; Liskow 1988; Robins 1966; Woerner & Guze 1968; Zoccolillo & Cloninger 1986), and both disorders have been linked to substance abuse (Cadoret et al. 1985, 1986, 1987; Littrell 1988).

Several of the female MPD subjects had spouses who were alcoholic, antisocial, and/or physically abusive; this is also consistent with known patterns of assortative mating in women with antisocial personality or Briquet's syndrome (Woerner & Guze 1968). The personal history of childhood molestation in the majority of these cases and in MPD in general (Coons et al. 1988; Coons & Milstein 1986; Putnam et al. 1986; Ross et al. 1990c) is also compatible with elevated rates of childhood molestation reported in studies of patients with Briquet's syndrome (Bryer et al. 1987; Morrison 1989a) and in female felons with sociopathy and Briquet's (Cloninger & Guze 1970a).

In summary, the family histories loaded with sociopathy, Briquet's syndrome, substance abuse, and a variety of disorders, the subjects' childhood histories of physical and sexual abuse, and their assortative mating patterns with sociopathic and alcoholic spouses so descriptively presented by these MPD accounts is strikingly consistent with the family histories, childhood abuse histories, and assortative mating patterns of patients with antisocial personality and Briquet's syndrome. The findings from these accounts indicate that these authors reported their stories in a way that accurately reflects current knowledge of MPD. Furthermore, these accounts underscored the intimacy of the relationship between MPD and comorbid disorders that is well documented in the academic literature.

Conclusion

Earlier chapters have documented the effect of published literature on the course of the development of MPD, particularly the effect of popular accounts of MPD on both patients' manifestations of the disorder and on physicians' responses to it. It is clear that the media has had an influential effect on the course of MPD through history that extends into the present. The media has had a role in shaping this disorder in our culture.

While information about the demographics, clinical picture, comorbidity, family history, natural course, and response to treatment in MPD is available in the academic literature, this knowledge has not previously been applied to a systematic review of popular accounts of MPD as provided in this report. Our findings that each of the 18 cases depicted met the criteria for antisocial personality disorder and/or Briquet's syndrome or borderline personality support the contention that further systematic studies of consecutive MPD patients using structured instruments such as the DIS (Robins et al. 1981) with an MPD module or Ross' interview for the dissociative disorders (Ross et al. 1989a) should help to clarify the relationships between these disorders within individuals. The predominance of sociopathy, somatization, and substance abuse in the families of the multiples in the books we reviewed indicates that a carefully designed study might uncover some interesting familial patterns associated with MPD, and could provide important evidence relating to the nosological status of the disorder.

This literature does not include any report from an MPD patient who has been high functioning for most of her life and who does not have any comorbid conditions. Such cases are infrequently described even in the professional literature (Kluft 1986 is one example), and therefore a systematic evaluation of such cases seems crucial. The apparent existence of these cases suggests that the comorbid diagnoses may be mere risk factors for MPD or markers for risk factors rather than being central to MPD. Thus MPD could truly be an independent disorder.

Identification of additional psychiatric diagnoses is of more than theoretical and academic interest to our study of personal accounts of MPD. These other diagnoses help to provide a broader perspective in the context of the patients' overall psychopathology. To point to the subjects' diagnostic comorbidity is not to discount their unusual experience of their multiple personality syndromes, about which they have provided valuable and detailed documentation in their accounts. This comprehensive diagnostic approach should serve to deepen our understanding of the breadth of the distress and disability so vividly expressed in these books.

Many of the individuals described in the accounts obtained treatment years ago, prior to recent developments in psychiatric research allowing precise diagnosis with specific criteria, and prior to systematic studies of large samples of MPD cases describing comorbidity. Because many of these accounts were among the first ever described in such detail, it is understandable that the focus of attention was the obviously fascinating and novel phenomenon of the multiple personalities. Despite their lack of guidance, however, the patients in these accounts did an extraordinary job of painting with their own words their clinical descriptions with great accuracy, reflecting the findings of extensive organized research on the disorder. Considering that these accounts do not represent an unbiased sample of MPD cases, the features they described were remarkably consistent with the professional literature.

Regardless of how a personal description is presented to the public, "serious inferences may . . . be drawn from it" (Victor 1975, p. 202). Unfortunately, the reading public does not have the privilege of being able to read the available accounts with psychiatric knowledge of the comorbidity that is so prevalent in MPD; hence, significant symptoms of other disorders, such as somatization and sociopathy, may be assumed to be an integral part of MPD. The public cannot be expected to be familiar enough with DSM-III-R to know that somatoform symptoms are criterion symptoms of Briquet's syndrome, and that they are not part of DSM-III-R criteria for MPD. Hence the lay reader may not recognize that polysomatic complaints and antisocial behaviors are not necessarily part of the MPD syndrome, and that these symptoms may qualify the individual for additional important diagnoses that might pose more far-reaching problems for the subjects than their MPD. Certainly if students of the mental health professions, as our experiments have shown, fail to recognize additional diagnostic possibilities, the general public, with no mental health background, cannot be expected to be any more alert to alternate possibilities.

Cutler and Reed (1975, p. 18) described the media portrayal of MPD as "a popular, if misleading, concept of mental illness for the layman." Difficulties in the understanding of MPD by the public are especially understandable given the tenuous and controversial placement of MPD in psychiatric nosology at present.

By acknowledging these considerations, the psychiatric profession can be in a stronger position to guide the public to a better appreciation of the disorders represented in these accounts. The recent knowledge that academic research has provided about the polysymptomatic nature of MPD and its high rates of psychiatric comorbidity may enable higher standards of accuracy in reports of psychiatric syndromes, such as MPD, in popular literature in the future.

The effects of more complete information on MPD reaching the reading public could have an impact on the natural course of this disorder in the future. Gruenewald (1977, p. 386) writes, "The sociology of mental disorders suggests that symptoms as well as diagnostic and therapeutic trends tend to change as a function of cultural and societal standards and values as well as the state of extant knowledge." Due to the suggestibility of potentially vulnerable members of this reading audience, the popular media may be playing a substantial role in shaping the manifestations of MPD in a population primed by the media's copious information—some of it substantiated, some of it fanciful. Bowers (1991, p. 168) concurs, writing that "People prone to MPD are very high in hypnotic ability and are, therefore vulnerable to the suggestive impact of ideas, imaginings, and fantasies; what is more, they are high in hypnotic ability because they have learned to use dissociative defenses."

If the publication dates of these books are any indication, the rate of new MPD books appearing in print could be expected to accelerate further in the near future, as it has done in the past decade. Mental health professionals therefore need to keep abreast of popular literature on this disorder as it is prone to affect many people. Media influences left to their own devices may be crucial to the future shaping of the MPD epidemic and represent a resource to be tapped.

Perspectives on MPD

The Nosologic Status of MPD

Two opposing questions have been asked seriously: "How can you believe in multiple personality?" and "How can you ignore all the evidence of MPD?" Some professionals asking these questions act as if the respectability of reputable professionals and scientists is at stake over how they respond to MPD.

Overview of nosologic possibilities

Current knowledge offers at least six ways to conceptualize MPD:

1. MPD is a syndrome that is sufficiently distinct to deserve diagnostic status; comorbid symptoms of other disorders are part of the larger MPD syndrome and therefore do not count in making other comorbid psychiatric diagnoses.

2. MPD is a sufficiently distinct syndrome to deserve diagnostic status, and comorbid disorders are usually secondary conditions.

3. MPD is a severity marker of other disorders such as borderline personality or Briquet's syndrome, identifying an extremely severe variant of those disorders.

4. MPD is a syndrome (perhaps a form of conversion disorder) that is a complication of other disorders, most commonly somatization disorder and personality disorders.

5. MPD is a dissociative symptom with no diagnostic significance created by therapists' suggestions, hypnosis, or autohypnosis.

6. MPD does not exist; it is a form of malingering.

In our opinion, these last two possibilities are untenable. The other four, however, constitute the substance of the persisting controversies.

How can one resolve these controversies in the absence of a known pathophysiologic mechanism for MPD or for any of its comorbid disorders? The time-honored approach of clinical medicine still seems to us the appropriate way to resolve these questions. The validity of a diagnosis is established by clinical description, laboratory findings, exclusion from other disorders, family studies, and follow-up studies. Ross and co-workers (1989c) have pointed out the need for a valid and reliable structured interview for MPD, an instrument necessary if this work is to be carried out in a systematic fashion.

No strong body of genetic, physiologic, or epidemiologic evidence has been advanced to confirm MPD as a psychiatric diagnosis (Fahy et al. 1989). Even some researchers highly invested in the disorder by virtue of the time and effort they have devoted to its study seem disoriented at times regarding the appropriate psychiatric status of MPD. Ross (1989, p. 52) states, "MPD is not a true *disease* entity in the biomedical sense. It is a true psychiatric entity and a true disorder, but not a biomedical disease."

Sutcliffe and Jones (1962) wrestled with the conflict over whether or not MPD exists. They concluded (pp. 251–252):

> There appears then to be no metaphysical or physical basis for asserting that multiple personality is "real". At the same time . . . multiple personality cannot be entirely dismissed as an epiphenomenon of fashion, or of shaping under the prejudices of the therapist, or of hypnosis. Something still remains to be characterized. After speculative explanations and assumptions have been removed, there remain only the observations of behavior classed as "multiple personality disorder" which might serve as a basis for the claim that multiple personality is in some sense real.

To doubt the existence of MPD would require believing that every single patient ever diagnosed with the disorder was consciously malingering; even then it would be an interesting presentation (like Munchausen's syndrome). Attempting to prove the reality or falsity of the symptoms of hysteria or MPD has been called "an impoverished strategy" (S. B. Guze, personal communication, 1991). "Real" in medicine usually means only that an anatomic or physiologic correlate has been identified. The real etiology of a syndrome, however, may reside in arenas outside anatomy or physiology, such as one arising from cultural factors or from deficits of motivation, development, or social skills. Dealing only with the "real"—the documentable physiologic or anatomic parts of ourselves—unnecessarily limits the range of investigation (S. B. Guze, personal communication, 1991).

MPD is a syndrome that cannot simply be considered nonexistent, even if its diagnostic status has not been adequately validated. Aldridge-Morris (1989, p. 53) described the crux of the problem this way:

> The problem is not simply whether or not multiple personality "exists". Clearly, there are a large number of individuals who describe their psyches as being fractured into many disparate selves, and as being amnesic for much of their behavior. The problem is more one of deciding what alternative classifications might be employed to subsume such clinical presentations.

Recognition of the presence of a group of people seeking help from the mental health professions with a common group of complaints and symptoms does not mean that we accept their statements or complaints as literally and scientifically true. Patients with MPD are not fundamentally different from other patients in making statements we might not accept as literally true. One does not have to believe, for example, that the voices schizophrenics hear are really outside their heads, or that psychotic depressives who can smell themselves rotting are really dead. We do not accept the literal truth of the statement of a neurotic depressive that he has never done anything right or that of an anxious, phobic patient that everything frightens her. We accept these statements as an attempt by the patient to share with us his or her inner reality and distress, not as dishonesty.

Just as the recognition of auditory hallucinations as a valid human experience of psychiatric illness is more acceptable to mental health professionals than a blanket acceptance of the face value claim by a patient that aliens from space talk to people, the concept of dissociated parts or aspects of personality may seem more congenial than the possibility of actual multiple personalities presented by MPD patients. But congeniality is not the issue; the issue is how to construe what we are told by the patient about his or her internal reality in trying to help him over his difficulties.

Putman (1986) feels that studies aimed directly at trying to prove the existence of multiple personalities as presented to us by our patients are unlikely to shed much light on MPD. He wisely suggests that we approach MPD in much the same way as we approach other psychiatric disorders, starting with descriptive studies and then moving on to investigations and experimental studies to track down the pathologic mechanisms of the disorder. The best way of doing this, we believe, is within the framework of the five-phase process outlined by Robins and Guze (1970).

In this process of validating a diagnosis (discussed in detail in Chapter 2), the first step is to provide a clinical description. In Chapter 3 we presented an overview of this information. While this phenomenologic information is necessary to establish the validity of a diagnosis, it is not sufficient. Some degree of reliability has been established for the DSM-III-R diagnosis of MPD, an important advance. Reliability, however, does not establish validity—although unreliability does limit validity.

Bowers (1991) complains that many of the authors of the diagnostic criteria for MPD are the same individuals advocating MPD and doing research in dissociation, a situation he finds analogous to the work of T. S. Eliot, who is said to have written his own criteria for good poetry and then written poetry conforming to those standards. This process, however, is typical of developing research in any new area of interest in psychiatry or psychology. The limited acceptance to date of Guze's concept of Briquet's syndrome and the concept of borderline personality in the general domain of psychiatry are similar examples of psychiatric diagnoses being proposed, researched, and evaluated by the whole field. When enough evidence is assembled and the concepts proposed have some useful, well-documented therapeutic implications, a diagnosis becomes generally accepted. If that point is not reached, other diagnostic viewpoints will be proposed to replace the insufficiently supported ones.

The problem of comorbidity

Those who contend that MPD does not warrant diagnostic status emphasize that the disorder overlaps extensively with other disorders. In the Robins and Guze scheme, this means that there is not sufficient evidence of exclusion of other disorders to qualify MPD as a separate disorder. Ross and colleagues (1989c) have recognized the need to establish the features of MPD that reliably differentiate it from other disorders.

Taylor and Martin (1944) stated that MPD is "essentially similar and continuous" with "psychoneuroses." The comorbidity of MPD symptoms with other psychiatric disorders is so great that the condition is frequently mistaken for one of these other disorders (Coons 1984). Kluft (1987b, p. 367) acknowledged this comorbidity:

> MPD rarely presents as a freestanding condition. Almost invariably its manifestations are embedded within a polysymptomatic presentation suggestive of one or more commonplace conditions. Therefore it usually is a superordinate diagnosis that may encompass a plethora of manifestations consistent with other conditions. Symptoms of anxiety and somatoform disorders are common, as are phobic and borderline manifestations. Depressive symptoms are nearly universal, and hallucinations and passive-influence experiences are very common.

Kluft (1985, 1987b) also describes a frequent association of MPD with antisocial personality, substance abuse, and multiple Axis I and II disorders. It seems safe to say that no exclusion criteria have been proposed except in the forensic literature.

The lack of exclusion criteria for MPD is hardly unique to MPD. Diagnoses on Axis II (the axis reserved for personality disorders) seldom have them. Research shows that patients with one Axis II diagnosis frequently meet criteria for four or five personality diagnoses (Widiger & Rogers 1989). The current state of knowledge in personality disorder is quite limited; in that sense, MPD is typical of most Axis II disorders. Cloninger (1987) has proposed a categorical model of personality disorder, but it remains a fascinating research scheme rather than an empirically tested model for clinical purposes.

Much of the MPD literature fails to address adequately the comorbid symptomatology. In some cases these other symptoms are totally ignored. MPD enthusiasts have been criticized for their tendency to focus on the subset of core symptoms defining MPD, oblivious to the multiplicity of attending symptoms (Fahy 1989)—a problem of myopic attention, or tunnel vision. For example, in many articles the alternate personalities command pages and pages of description of their appearance, their character, their likes, dislikes, preferences, and so on, and the many accompanying somatoform, antisocial, and other symptoms receive little attention. If the attending symptoms are mentioned, they may be dismissed as part of the MPD constellation, as manifestations of the different alternate personalities; therefore they are not counted toward making other diagnoses.

Regarding the comorbidity of symptoms in his series of multiples, Bliss (1980, pp. 1391–1392) wrote, "Most cases qualified for the designation of Briquet's syndrome, but they may be diagnosed in other ways, depending on the complaints that capture the attention of the physician." Bliss (1986, p. 158) also believes that "The fact that many multiples qualify by present criteria for such designations as borderline states, schizophrenia, or depression does not indicate that they suffer from two disorders. It simply demonstrates that our criteria are imperfect and our categories heterogenous and arbitrary."

These problems are not unique to psychiatry. It is accepted that some patients with neurologic diseases such as multiple sclerosis may sometimes present in a manner that seems to qualify them for a diagnosis of Briquet's syndrome. Most physicians would say that in the instance of multiple sclerosis initially presenting as Briquet's syndrome, once the multiple sclerosis was confirmed, it would be clear that the original diagnosis of Briquet's syndrome was a plain error likely to result in mismanagement of the case.

A similar situation occurs in psychiatric disorders. It is well known that some patients with schizophrenia initially present with positive symptom reviews for Briquet's syndrome or antisocial personality. Most clinicians would say that schizophrenia is the proper diagnosis because the problems, course, and treatment relevant to schizophrenia are far more pertinent to the immediate management of such patients (i.e., antipsychotic medication) than application of the usual methods of treatment of patients with antisocial personality or Briquet's syndrome.

These last two examples embody the logic of the position that for patients with MPD, previous diagnoses of depression, schizophrenia, or Briquet's syndrome are erroneous. On the other hand, there is no good evidence to direct clinicians to preempt a diagnosis such as Briquet's syndrome or borderline personality in favor of a diagnosis of MPD.

Psychiatrists dealing with a patient with MPD and its usual plethora of coordinate syndromes may resemble the well-known group of blind men around the elephant. Those interested in PTSD detect it, those interested in Briquet's syndrome find that, and so on. The focus on MPD by people interested in MPD is equally understandable, given the dramatic nature of the disorder, the controversy over it, and the inevitable fascination it generates.

The primacy of the MPD diagnosis is a key controversy. It has been claimed that MPD is a superordinate, coordinate, or subordinate diagnosis, a severity marker (an adjective rather than a diagnosis), and a distracting symptom complex. Those skeptical of the validity of MPD as a diagnosis assert that Briquet's syndrome or antisocial personality is the true underlying disorder and that a primary diagnosis of MPD would constitute the mistake of not seeing the forest for the trees. In contrast, the allegation that MPD should be considered the superordinate diagnosis implies that making a big deal out of the other diagnoses would constitute missing the beauty of a particular tree while conceptualizing the forest.

Superordinate diagnosis

The practice of regarding some diagnoses as superordinate to others is well established and well accepted in general psychiatry. For example, alcoholics have secondary depressions and schizophrenics can develop secondary drug problems. In the case of MPD, other experts (Kluft 1985; Ross 1989, p. 3; Ross et al. 1989a) agree with Putnam and colleagues (1984, p. 175), who state that MPD is best considered the "superordinate diagnosis, even when other symptom clusters seem to predominate." By this they mean that MPD patients frequently present symptoms of multiple disorders and could legitimately be said to have those disorders if one applied the criteria for those disorders.

When recognized, comorbid conditions such as somatization disorder, personality disorders, and PTSD, however, are almost invariably considered secondary to MPD (Bliss 1980; Coons et al. 1988; Loewenstein et al. 1987; Nakdimen 1989; Putnam et al. 1984; Solomon & Solomon 1982). Tozman and Pabis (1989, p. 708) wrote, "If PTSD does cause MPD, why is not PTSD emphasized, inasmuch as this is a more significant, ubiquitous, and often unrecognized condition? Similarly, when associated with alcoholism (Ludwig 1984), that, rather than MPD, may be the overriding pathology."

Coordinate diagnosis

Major depression and alcoholism can sometimes be diagnosed in the same patient. Many clinicians say that it is important to diagnose both problems and treat both to help the patient function at a reasonable level. Clinical experience certainly teaches that ignoring a significant aspect of a patient's problems such as alcohol abuse in the face of a major depression is likely to lead to great difficulties for both doctor and patient. This could be called a "coordinate position." An adherent of this position, applying it to MPD, would suggest that all of an MPD patient's problems—multiple personalities, anxiety, depression, psychosis, somatoform and personality disorders, and so on—should be treated carefully and thoroughly.

Subordinate diagnosis—symptom complex

Some deny the primacy of the MPD diagnosis (Fahy 1988; Tozman & Pabis 1989). Fahy and coworkers (1989) strongly urged clinicians not to be distracted from the underlying psychiatric diagnosis by the fascinating presentation of the MPD symptoms. Fahy (1988) stressed the importance of considering "the extent to which MPD may be part of a specific personality disorder" (p. 603) because of the implications for treatment. He further stated that he found "little evidence to suggest that MPD is a distinct diagnosis rather than an intriguing symptom of a wide range of psychological disturbances" (p. 603). He prefers to conceptualize the condition as "a non-specific psychiatric symptom" (p. 604). Velek and Balon (1986) recommend referring to the syndrome as "multiple personality" rather than "multiple personality disorder" because they consider it a syndrome of multiple etiologies.

An appreciation of MPD that does not ignore the disorder, yet does not credit it as a distinct, subsuming diagnosis in the absence of supporting data, is a consideration of MPD as a symptom or a symptom complex complicating another disorder such as somatization disorder (Fahy 1988). Coryell (1983) characterizes MPD as "an epiphenomenon of other illnesses." Just as depression may develop as a secondary condition in the context of another disorder such as somatization disorder, MPD may develop as an accompaniment to other disorders such as somatization disorder, antisocial personality, or borderline personality. By analogy, peripheral vascular disease with gangrene of the extremities is a complication of diabetes, and although the gangrene is not the original diagnosis, the presence of this complication changes the clinical picture considerably and is recognizably associated with serious consequences beyond what was experienced when diabetes was the only problem.

This model recognizes both the reality of the MPD syndrome and the suffering and severe disability associated with it. Individuals with MPD, like patients with somatization disorder and personality disorders, are often socially and economically disabled, sometimes severely so (Rivera 1991; Robins et al. 1991, p. 290; Ross 1989, p. 56; Swartz et al. 1991, p. 254). MPD, like somatization disorder, is no trivial malady, and both result in considerable distress, utilization of expensive medical services, and notorious frustration and difficulty in treatment (Black 1987; Bliss 1980; Dell & Eisenhower 1990; Greaves 1980; Horevitz & Braun 1984; Katon et al. 1991; Kluft 1984d; Monson & Smith 1983; Morrison 1978; Murphy 1982; Quill 1985; Ross 1989, p. 6; Ross et al. 1989e; Schreiber 1973; Slater 1965; Smith et al. 1986; Wilbur 1984a; Zoccolillo & Cloninger 1986a, 1986b).

A severity marker, not a diagnosis

The high degree of comorbidity of other disorders such as borderline personality or Briquet's syndrome with MPD has been used as an argument that the recognition of MPD should be considered an indicator of dysfunction severity of the other disorder rather than as a distinct psychiatric disorder in its own right (Widiger & Rogers 1989). On the other hand, Horevitz and Braun (1984) expressed the reverse idea: that borderline personality disorder in multiples may represent a more severe form of Axis II pathology rather than a genuine difference from MPD. Horovitz and Braun hypothesized a larger multiple personality syndrome with varying manifestations, depending on the individual's disturbance, life history, and course. If this is the case, then MPD and other disorders such as Briquet's syndrome or borderline personality might share a common higher diathesis within this "bigger syndrome" model.

The finding that multiples "are probably the most self-destructive diagnostic group among psychiatric patients" (Ross et al. 1990c, p. 600) and "among the most disturbed individuals who seek the services of mental health professionals" (Ross 1989, p. 56) supports the conclusion that multiple personalities function as a severity marker in borderline personality. In order to satisfy this argument, multiples with borderline personality should be found to have more borderline symptoms than do borderlines without MPD. Similarly, studies determining the severity of somatization in Briquet's patients with and without MPD could be devised to study whether MPD is a severity marker in Briquet's syndrome. If multiples with Briquet's syndrome or borderline personality do not have more symptoms of Briquet's syndrome or borderline personality than do patients who have these disorders in the absence of MPD, this would be evidence against the MPD severity marker hypothesis. These types of questions about one underlying process with markers for different degrees of severity are also ideally suited for family studies.

A spectrum of disorders—but which spectrum?

It is not yet clear how MPD differs nosologically from Briquet's syndrome. Thigpen and Cleckley (1984, p. 66) feel that "it is necessary to keep in mind that multiple personality clearly belongs within the hysteric spectrum of disorders." Kluft (1985, p. 5) counters:

> It might seem parsimonious to suggest the coincidence of MPD with Briquet's syndrome in many cases, or to say this is the "polysymptomatic polyneurosis" of the borderline state, but a close review of this list indicates *symptoms are included from anxiety disorders, somatoform complaints, affective disorders, thought disorders, and borderline states. This is the pragmatic usefulness of the concept of MPD as a superordinate diagnosis.* . . .

This same melange of symptoms is not demonstrably different from those of Briquet's syndrome, which also presents a profusion of symptoms, including polysomatoform symptoms and symptoms of almost every psychiatric diagnosis, such as "pseudohallucinations" and hysterical psychosis, anxiety and depression, substance abuse, and suicide gestures (Bishop & Holt 1980; Goodwin et al. 1971; Woodruff et al. 1972; Zoccolillo & Cloninger 1986b). Patients with antisocial personality disorder and other personality disorders also display many of these other symptoms. An additional link to these other disorders, the remarkable hypnotizability of MPD patients, has also been observed in Briquet's syndrome and in "hysterical psychosis" (Spiegel & Fink 1979). In addition, self-hypnosis, which Bliss (1984b) has attributed to MPD, has also been implicated in conversion, "severe hysterical neuroses," and antisocial disorders (Bliss 1980, 1984c; Bliss & Larson 1985).

The comorbidity and course of MPD are remarkably similar to those of conversion disorders. It has been known for more than 40 years that, like multiple personalities, conversion symptoms are a remitting phenomenon (Carter 1949). Dickes (1974) reported an 81% remission rate for conversion symptoms with conservative treatment, and Black (1987) achieved similar remission rates in the management of conversion symptoms in patients with Briquet's syndrome. Gatfield and Guze (1962) observed a high rate of remission for individual conversion symptoms without concomitant remission from the Briquet's syndrome or personality disorder that it frequently accompanied.

If, after integration of the personalities, a residual chronic Briquet's syndrome or personality disorder persists, the course of MPD could be considered to fit the pattern for conversion syndromes. Then one might hypothesize that the multiple personality phenomenon represents a superimposed condition such as conversion on a backdrop of a few other characteristic disorders. Just as conversion symptoms may arise from multiple origins comorbid with a number of diagnoses, MPD may arise as a complication of a variety of other psychiatric conditions, which, coincidentally or not, happen to be the same ones on which conversion symptoms are most commonly superimposed: Briquet's syndrome, antisocial personality disorder, dissociative disorders (Gatfield & Guze 1962; Woodruff et al. 1969).

This model, while plausible and appreciative of the distress suffered by these patients, may not go far enough in explaining the disorder. The principal evidence currently available to support the argument that this is a halfhearted approach to the problem is the existence of patients with MPD and no apparent comorbid disorder (Kluft 1986). These patients' multiple personalities are not complicating any other condition and thus do not provide support for the model. Conversion symptoms, however, have been documented in persons with no other disorder, suggesting that MPD-only cases are feasible in this model, parallel to the relation of conversion to other disorders.

A number of authors have explored the relationships between conversion and dissociation in trying to illuminate their role in MPD. It is not yet clear how

MPD differs nosologically from other dissociative symptoms and how either of these entities differs from conversion pathology. Aldridge-Morris (1989, p. 107) considers conversion to include dissociative states such as multiple personalities. Conversion is not necessarily confined to somatic symptomatology but may also include psychiatric symptoms such as psychotomimetic and dissociative manifestations (Hollender & Hirsch 1964). Aldridge-Morris (1989, p. 104) has observed the distinction between conversion and "dissociative hysterias" to be blurred. Some authors (Hollender & Hirsch 1964) believe that the concepts of conversion and dissociation may be used interchangeably in some contexts.

Ross (1989, p. 167) noted that conversion disorders are classified as dissociative disorders in the International Classification of Diseases, and he says he does not understand "why North Americans have a problem seeing the correctness of this." He further explains, "A pure, simple dissociation of memory is psychogenic amnesia; a dissociation of motor or sensory function, a conversion disorder." According to Ross, "Freud attempted to make distinctions between repression, conversion, and somatization that are untestable and not clearly thought out."

It has been proposed that dissociation may actually occur as a spectrum of dissociative disorders; DSM-III-R offers a number of diagnostic options supporting this position. Very preliminary studies show that patients with MPD dissociate more (as measured by the DES) than patients with depersonalization or dissociative disorder—NOS (see Table 4-5). This supports the notion of a spectrum. In agreement with Lipton (1943), Rosenbaum and Weaver (1980, p. 602) wrote, "We believe that more progress will be made in the understanding of the syndrome [MPD] by naming it 'dissociated state' as suggested in DSM-III." Cutler and Reed (1975) view MPD as a rare form of fugue state in which an alternate personality is adopted.

Family studies should be readily able to test whether or not two disorders such as MPD and dissociation are heritable and one is a more severe form of the other (Rice & Reich 1985) or whether they are both the product of the same heritable process but express themselves differently due to environmental factors (Cloninger et al. 1978). The relationship between dissociation and hypnotizability could be tested with family studies in a similar way. Family studies might also help to refine measures of dissociation and hypnotizability by identifying items sensitive to environmental, heritable, and both types of factors. Putnam's scale for dissociation is a linear scale (dissociation is greater or lesser); family studies would allow one to test whether there is a threshold one must exceed to manifest a dissociative disorder.

Ross and colleagues (1989a) have reviewed various models of conceptualizing MPD, including the possibility that MPD could be an epiphenomenon of a polymorphous borderline disorder or a disorder sometimes but not always superordinate to another comorbid condition. They concluded that the reciprocal relationship between MPD and borderline personality is complex and not presently understood.

Bowers (1991) recommended reclassifying MPD as an Axis II disorder, which implies that he feels MPD is related to characterologic disorders and is not well conceptualized nosologically. His reasoning is that MPD appears to share origins in childhood physical and sexual abuse, as well as a similar constitutional and historic matrix. Placement of MPD on Axis I recognizes that the alternate personalities are developmentally distinct and complete. But if the alternate personalities have a legitimate claim to being genuine personalities in the developmental sense, and—"By definition, each personality in a multiple personality system has its own unique, stable behavioral, social, and personality patterns" (Horevitz & Braun 1984, p. 76)—then they exist as multiple complete disordered personalities and therefore would belong on Axis II. The extensive overlap of MPD with Axis II disorders would also support its placement on Axis II. Ganaway (1989) suggests classification of MPD as a "Dissociative Character Disorder" (p. 216). Ross (1985) suggests that MPD does not need to appear on Axis I and can usually be subsumed by hierarchically more inclusive Axis II diagnoses such as borderline personality disorder when they are present, citing support for this move from the work of Gunderson and colleagues (Gunderson & Kolb 1978; Gunderson & Singer 1975; Gunderson et al. 1981). On the other hand, the extensive overlap with somatization disorder, depression, and symptoms of other Axis I disorders might argue for Axis I placement. Similar arguments have been made in debates over the best place for Briquet's syndrome on the axes (Pennebaker & Watson 1991).

If MPD were to be moved to Axis II, it would be removed from the dissociative disorders it left behind on Axis I, of which it is a principal character and an anchor. The result would be that the remaining dissociation category left on Axis I would be seriously weakened. In cases where the MPD is an entrenched and stable part of the patient's psychopathology, Ross (1985) feels MPD is such an extraordinary diagnosis that it could stand independently on Axis I. Nosologic understanding of MPD is not yet great enough for a rational decision to be made about the axis to which the diagnosis belongs.

Rates of comorbid diagnoses made by Liskow (1988) in patients with Briquet's syndrome are remarkably similar to those found in MPD (see Table 3-2), and we compare these with the comorbidity rates in studies of MPD. Major depression was reported in 87–94% of hospitalized inpatients with Briquet's syndrome in Liskow's study, compared with rates of up to 91% of MPD patients with depression reported by Ross' group (1990c); alcoholism in 17–32% of Briquet's compared with alcoholism in 10–45% of multiples in other studies (Coons 1984, 1988a; Coons & Milstein 1986; Putnam et al. 1986; Ross et al. 1990c); drug abuse in 21–33% of Briquet's syndrome compared to MPD with 28–55% (Coons 1984, 1988a; Coons & Milstein 1986; Putnam et al. 1986; Ross et al. 1990c); antisocial personality in 17–25% of Briquet's syndrome compared to 20–45% in MPD (Coons 1984; Coons et al. 1988). Anxiety disorders, phobias, obsessive-compulsive disorder, and eating disorders are also reported to be associated with both Briquet's syndrome and MPD (Liskow et al. 1986; Ross et al. 1989e).

172   *Multiple personality disorder*

Table 7-1 summarizes the known comorbidity patterns of five related conditions: MPD, somatization disorder, antisocial personality disorder, borderline personality disorder, and conversion disorder. The overlap in comorbidity with MPD is extensive, more than for any of the other entries in the table. Other features characteristic of patients with MPD, such as female predominance, suicidality, and a history of childhood abuse, have also been described as characteristic of patients with Briquet's syndrome and borderline personality disorders, and many of these characteristics are also seen in antisocial personality disorder (see Table 7-2). MPD is thus not unique in any of these important features.

Table 7-3 shows extensive diagnostic overlap in the familial psychiatric disorders associated with MPD and comorbid disorders. An argument for the lack of specificity of MPD as a diagnosis is its failure to show a clear pattern of psychiatric diagnoses in relatives of MPD patients (Putnam et al. 1986). Sufficient studies to support a characteristic familial pattern of MPD have not been carried out, as they have been for many other disorders. Family studies are an important component of the Robins and Guze process of establishing a diagnosis as a discrete entity. Rice (1986, p. 239) wrote, "Family studies offer a strategy to resolve heterogeneity at two levels. The first is whether heterogeneous subforms represent the same underlying familial process. . . . The other type of heterogeneity results when multiple underlying pathways lead to similar phenocopies."

More can be done to help differentiate MPD from other disorders, another important step in the process of validating a diagnosis. Ross and colleagues (1989a) have compared MPD patients with groups of patients diagnosed with schizophrenia, panic disorder, and eating disorders. They determined that MPD can be differentiated from these other disorders on the basis of clinical features. A similar study comparing MPD with depression, somatization disorder, and the personality disorders with which it frequently occurs would help to determine whether MPD is sufficiently different from these other conditions to afford its own diagnostic status, or whether it represents an extreme form of any of these other disorders.

Studies to differentiate MPD from other conditions could compare the conditions with MPD on natural history, demographic patterns, symptom patterns, family history, course over time, and treatment response. Only if the findings of the Ross study can be extended to document real differences from the disorders most frequently comorbid with MPD can MPD be considered a unique diagnostic entity.

Liskow (1988) has pointed out the possibility that Briquet's syndrome may occur both as a primary illness and as a consequence of another disorder. He also recommends family history studies and follow-up studies of patients with Briquet's syndrome to help answer this nosologic question in Briquet's syndrome. Finding more symptoms of MPD in patients who also have Briquet's syndrome would not prove that it is a complication of MPD, but finding fewer symptoms would argue against the possibility. A study by Coons and Fine (1990)

Table 7-1 Relationship of Diagnoses to Comorbid Disorders Within Individuals*

	Comorbid Disorders within Subjects						
Identified Diagnosis	Somatization Disorder	Antisocial Personality Disorder	Borderline Personality	Conversion Symptoms	Substance Abuse	Affective Disorders	Histrionic and Other Personality Disorders
MPD	X	X	X	X	X	X	X
Somatization disorder	—	X		X	X	X	X
Antisocial personality disorder	X	—	X	X	X		X
Borderline personality disorder		X	—		X	X	X
Conversion disorder	X	X		—	X	X	X

*Akiskal (1981), Bliss (1980, 1986), Coons (1984), Coons and Millstein (1986), Coons et al. (1988), Davis and Akiskal (1986), DeSouza et al. (1988), Gatfield and Guze (1962), Horevitz and Braun (1984), Kluft (1982), Lazare (1978), McGlashan (1983), Peters (1989), Pope et al. (1983), Putnam et al. (1986), Rivera (1991), Ross et al. (1989a, 1990c), Snyder et al. (1982), Widiger and Rogers (1989), Zimmerman and Coryell (1989).

Table 7-2 Gender, Suicidality, and Childhood Abuse History in
MPD and Associated Disorders*

Identified Diagnosis	Percent Female	Suicide Attempts	Childhood Abuse History	
			Physical Abuse	Sexual Abuse
MPD	88	Yes	Yes	Yes
Somatization disorder	≥ 99	Yes		Yes
Antisocial personality disorder	20–30	Yes	Yes	
Borderline personality disorder	62–82	Yes	Yes	Yes
Conversion disorder	84			

*Bliss (1980, 1984), Coons and Millstein (1986), Coons et al. (1988), Gatfield and Guze (1962), Ludolph et al. (1990), Pope et al. (1983), Putnam et al. (1986), Rivera (1991), Robins et al. (1991), Ross and Norton (1989a), Ross et al. (1989a, 1990c), Swartz et al. (1988, 1989), Zimmerman and Coryell (1989).

did suggest that patients with MPD have fewer somatic symptoms than other psychiatric patients.

A similar line of study has been pursued in patients with Briquet's syndrome to determine the nosologic relationship of schizophrenia, which is frequently diagnosable in patients with Briquet's syndrome (Liskow 1988). A small study by Liskow's group (1986) found that the group MMPI profile of schizophrenic Briquet's patients could not be distinguished from that of nonschizophrenic Briquet's patients, and the MMPI profiles of anxiety-disordered Briquet's patients could not be distinguished from those of Briquet's patients without an anxiety diagnosis. Because the presence of Briquet's syndrome affects the same MMPI scales as schizophrenia does, and because the presence of Briquet's affects the same scales as anxiety does (but anxiety and schizophrenia affect different scales), it is not surprising that a lack of difference between Briquet's patients with and without these other diagnoses was noted. A difference might be noted if subscales of the standard clinical scales were used or if a much larger sample size were available, since only differences in severity would be expected.

Consistency over time

Competent follow-up studies must establish a typical prognosis that is uniform and characteristic if the disorder is to conform to the Robins and Guze scheme of diagnostic validation. Thus, if MPD truly is a diagnosis superordinate to Bri-

Table 7-3 Psychiatric Disorders in Biological Relatives of Patients with MPD and Associated Disorders*

Identified Diagnosis	MPD	Somatization Disorder	Antisocial Personality Disorder	Borderline Personality	Substance Abuse	Affective Disorders
MPD	?†	?†	?†	?†	?†	
Somatization disorder		X	X		X	
Antisocial personality disorder		X	X		X	
Borderline personality disorder				X		X

†Not adequately studied to date.

*Akiskal (1981), Akiskal et al. (1985), American Psychiatric Association (1987), Andrulonis et al. (1980), Braun (1986), Coons et al. (1988), Dell and Eisenhower (1990), Loranger et al. (1982), Ludolph et al. (1990), Putnam et al. (1986), Ross et al. (1989c), Stone (1977).

quet's syndrome, the course of patients with MPD, whether or not they also meet the criteria for Briquet's syndrome, should be quite homogeneous and likely different from that of Briquet's syndrome. Conversely, if Briquet's syndrome is the superordinate diagnosis, one would expect the course of MPD patients with Briquet's syndrome to be quite similar to that of Briquet's patients without MPD. Follow-up studies are a sound method for helping to establish which disorder is superordinate.

Kluft (1986) has presented a report of 3 cases of MPD whose outcome was very good, and he claims a total of 12 such high-functioning cases uncovered from a collection of 309 MPD patients. The apparent availability of such cases may provide key data regarding the prognosis. Horevitz and Braun (1984) have suggested that the prognosis relates more to the comorbid diagnoses such as borderline personality disorder. Studies to test this hypothesis can be done. Kluft's report did not provide detailed information on comorbidity. It is unlikely that multiples with full-blown Briquet's syndrome or borderline personality disorder would have a good outcome because of the known courses of these disorders (unless MPD is truly superordinate). If MPD patients with the least comorbidity have the best outcomes, this would not support the validity of MPD as a diagnosis in the Robins and Guze scheme. Our own experience, as described in Chapter 3, is that subjects with florid comorbid disorders such as Briquet's syndrome have poorer outcomes consistent with the natural course of the comorbid disorder.

In a similar vein, diagnostic comorbidity with conversion symptoms was similarly addressed by Gatfield and Guze (1962) in a follow-up study. Conversion in the absence of other disorders was rare, but patients without other disorders tended to have a good prognosis. Those with comorbid disorders (most often Briquet's syndrome) usually remained ill. The conversion symptoms associated with other psychiatric or medical disorders had variable outcomes, often remaining, other times being replaced by different conversion symptoms, and sometimes vanishing.

The full spectrum

It is clear that MPD may be related to a variety of spectra—hysterical, dissociative, and personality. It is important to recognize that the nosologic independence of all these other disorders may be equally affected by MPD. One can easily imagine that there is an n-dimensional space in which these dimensions of conversion hysteria, dissociation, and personality problems exist. What we call MPD is also located in some place(s) in this space. As we study these disorders in relation to each other, we will find more satisfying and useful ways to think about MPD and psychiatric nosology in general.

Etiology

Once the nosologic status of MPD is adequately understood, research can move more easily to determine its etiology, an area of investigation that is not a part of Robins and Guze's five-stage diagnostic validation process. In anticipation of this progress, Cutler and Reed (1975) have derived a three-factor theory of the etiology of MPD. The factors are:

1. Dissociation (either spontaneous or induced by hypnosis)

2. Suggestion, encouragement, and reinforcement by medical attention

3. Role playing

Kluft (1984c) has proposed a four-factor theory of etiology:

1. Dissociation potential and hypnotizability

2. A history of overwhelming life experiences such as childhood abuse

3. External shaping influences and substrates

4. Insufficient social support in helping the individual cope

Without Kluft's first factor, dissociation and hypnotizability, MPD cannot occur or is a result of malingering. As described in earlier chapters, dissociation and hypnotizability have been well documented in MPD. Kluft's second factor, traumatic experiences, especially childhood abuse, have been a consistent finding in studies of MPD to date. Allison's (1974a) paper, entitled "A Guide to Parents: How to Raise Your Daughters to Have Multiple Personalities," includes sexual trauma in childhood and a negative childhood environment as factors contributing to the development of MPD.

Kluft's third factor, external shaping influences and substrates that determine the form taken by dissociative behaviors, includes autohypnosis, elements of a poor childhood environment, errors in interview technique resulting in iatrogenesis, and the media and literature. These have been described extensively, as described in Chapter 2, and substantial evidence has been provided that in some cases these factors can be operative. The fourth factor, insufficient social support, is complex and highly confounded with other personal characteristics and historical features, and will be difficult to study. As previously mentioned, documenting etiologies in psychiatry is difficult if not impossible at this time.

Kluft's four-factor theory easily lends itself to the types of models already developed in genetic epidemiology. Dissociation and hypnotizability, to the extent that they are associated with Briquet's syndrome, are, like Briquet's syndrome, likely to be familially transmitted. In fact, these skills may comprise a substantial part of what is transmitted in families of patients with Briquet's syndrome and borderline personality disorder. The overwhelming life experiences would seem likely to be an environmental, nontransmitted event, although it is conceivable that the experiences could be related to a particularly malignant, transmissible form of antisocial personality in an abusing parent. The third factor, form-shaping experiences, and the fourth factor, countervailing forces, are likely to function as environmental effects as well. Because MPD, like Briquet's syndrome, has a very high female-to-male ratio, currently available statistical models for analyzing sex effects are likely to be informative (Rice 1984).

Because the nosologic status of MPD is in such disarray at the present time, however, efforts to determine the etiology of this disorder are certainly premature. Although theories of posttraumatic stress grounded in childhood abuse, self-hypnosis, and genetic dissociative tendencies are appealing explanations, in the absence of a better nosologic understanding of MPD these ideas are only speculative.

Nosologic Issues Affecting Treatment

Professional agreement on effective treatment cannot occur until MPD has been adequately validated as a disorder. Certainly agreement on the etiology of the disorder will also have some bearing on this subject.

From the logic that MPD is the superordinate diagnosis arises the contention that MPD cannot receive adequate treatment unless the MPD diagnosis is recognized and given priority (Jeppsen 1985; Boor 1982; Greaves 1980; Kluft 1987b; Rivera 1991; Solomon & Solomon 1982; van der Hart & Boon 1989). Treating the comorbid disorders is felt to be ineffective (Bliss 1985; Kluft 1987a, 1987b; Putnam et al. 1984; Rivera 1991; Velek & Balon 1986). Several authors have pointed out that patients diagnosed with Briquet's syndrome, schizophrenia, or other disorders and later determined to have MPD have frequently had a poor response when given the usual treatments indicated by their other diagnoses (Bliss 1985; Kluft 1987a, 1987b; Putnam et al. 1984; Putnam 1989b; Rivera 1991; Velek & Balon 1986). This argument, however, is weakened by the fact that the other disorders most likely to accompany MPD (Briquet's syndrome, borderline personality, antisocial personality) are notorious for chronicity and recalcitrance to all modalities of treatment.

Ross and colleagues (1989a) assert that these other apparent disorders fade away when the personalities are fused, which would not be consistent with the known course of these other diagnoses. A number of authors have reported that a large proportion of multiples they treated have had a complete remission from their multiplicity on follow-up (Boor 1982; Franklin 1990; Herzog 1984; Kluft 1985, 1986, 1987b; Putnam et al. 1984; Ross 1989, p. 3; Ross et al. 1990c).

Those who argue that MPD may be an iatrogenic phenomenon (caused by suggestion, hypnosis, or therapist encouragement to patients with disorders that put them at risk for developing MPD) hold that concentrating on MPD symptoms in therapy may lead to reinforcement and prolongation of MPD-related behaviors (Bowers 1991; Fahy et al. 1989; Simpson 1988). This follows the logic of those who recommend that therapy for patients with Briquet's syndrome should aim at redirecting the patients away from their focus on their somatic symptoms and, in general, follow a conservative, noninvasive approach (Black 1987; Coryell 1983; Morrison 1978; Murphy 1982). This apparently sensible approach to the management of patients with Briquet's syndrome is not supported by any controlled studies with adequate periods of follow-up, to the best of our knowledge. A study of patients with somatization disorder by Smith and colleagues (1986) has provided indications that careful management of this disorder can result in reduction of medical expenses related to its treatment.

Adoption of a strategy for the management of MPD similar to that for Briquet's syndrome has been recommended (Fahy et al. 1989; Simpson 1988). Kluft (1989) disapproves of the use of the "benign neglect" method for discouraging MPD behavior by ignoring it (not rewarding it with attention) in lieu of "active treatment" of MPD. Even if such a strategy in general failed to diminish MPD symptoms, it might still prove advantageous for the management of those MPD patients with Briquet's syndrome. In light of the high rates of somatization in patients with MPD, this method might often prove useful.

Success with this strategy in the management of MPD has been documented in several published case reports (Congdon et al. 1961; Cutler & Reed 1975; Fahy et al. 1989; Hacking 1991; Kohlenberg 1973; Munford & Liberman 1982). This technique was also used successfully in managing an adolescent who claimed he was possessed by Satan (Spiegel & Fink 1979). As described in Chapter 3, the authors' experience with this strategy in the management of MPD has led to some definite therapeutic gains.

The advice that physicians treating somatization disorder would best avoid the temptation to effect a dramatic cure by intense or unconventional therapies (Black 1987; Morrison 1978; Murphy 1982; Quill 1985; Smith et al. 1986) has also been recommended for the management of MPD (Coryell 1983; Cutler & Reed 1975; Fahy et al. 1989). The validity of the conservative management approach to Briquet's syndrome applied to MPD, which has not been validated by research on Briquet's syndrome itself, would depend on the assumption that multiplicity is itself a conversion-like set of symptoms that can be extinguished by nonreinforcement.

The importance of the symptoms of multiplicity in the mind of the therapist dictates his or her choice between the therapeutic strategies of either benign neglect or working toward integration of the personalities. The focus of any therapy is meant to be on what is really important and not the peripheral. The patient does not ordinarily know what is really important other than his or her current degree of distress. Psychotherapists lead patients to talk about their problems in ways and in jargons that the therapists choose. We teach our patients what is important by what we focus on, probe, and reinforce. Because the field does not know, based on appropriately controlled studies, what is important for treatment, how well talking therapies work, what is the natural course of the illness (MPD), or whether multiplicity is a conversion syndrome or the core defect, a call to therapeutic orthodoxy is certainly premature. We do know, however, that we can get patients to avoid talking about the manifestations of multiplicity with us if that is our aim, as has been documented by patients of the authors in Chapter 3. On a cautionary note, Ganaway (1989, p. 217) has pointed out the "potentially deleterious effects of validating unverified trauma memories during the psychotherapy of MPD and its variants."

Once integration of the personalities has been achieved, other problems remain for these patients and therapy is still needed (Bliss 1980, 1986, p. 219; Coons 1986a; Kluft 1982, 1984d). This is understandable to proponents of a coordinate or subordinate position, given the substantial comorbidity of somatization disorder and personality disorder that is undoubtedly still present following integration, if it is achieved at all. Coons and Sterne (1986) found that the MMPI profiles of MPD patients changed little despite therapy, suggesting a stable underlying pathology that goes beyond multiplicity. (Only three patients fused in this intriguing study, and they showed reductions on hypochondriasis and hysteria alone.)

No prospective follow-up studies have been completed on untreated cases to establish the natural course of the disorder (Putnam 1989a), and no controlled studies investigating treatment effects have been done. This lack of systematic research permits development of unrealistic expectations (see Putnam 1989a) and fantasies regarding outcome.

Bowers (1991, p. 171) has observed:

> Another defense of MPD is that when clinicians do not treat MPD patients for the disorder, they do not get better; conversely, accepting the fact that a patient suffers MPD, and treating him/her accordingly, typically leads to improvement or cure. Thus, treatment success validates diagnosis. While I can understand the impetus behind this argument, it simply doesn't hold water.

Treatment response does not necessarily scientifically validate a diagnosis. By analogy, all kinds of headaches may respond to aspirin, and many sources of cardiac arrhythmias may respond to diltiazem; these treatment responses do not validate diagnoses (Bowers 1991) of migraine or atrioventricular block.

Medications have been found ineffective in the treatment of depressive, psychotic, and anxiety symptoms in MPD, and medications are recommended only as palliative treatment and for management of crises (Kluft 1984d). In reality, well-designed, controlled studies of the use of medication in MPD have not been carried out; therefore, "To date, one can use medication only on an empirical-trial basis, with little assurance as to the indications or likely response" (Ross 1989, p. 52). According to Ross (1989, p. 281), "There is no sound basis for any prescription written for an MPD patient and . . . every prescription is an empirical trial without scientific foundation." Moreover, the use of medications in the treatment of MPD involves iatrogenic risks due to the known tendency of these patients to abuse substances and to overdose (Bliss 1980; Kluft 1984d). Because different personalities may respond differently to the same medication, a medication that may seem appropriate might actually be unhelpful or even harmful. Placebo responses are said to be more common than active drug efficacy in these patients (Kluft 1984d).

Psychotherapy is generally agreed to be the best mode of treatment of MPD. According to Kluft (1984a, 1984c), the goal of therapy in MPD is the unification of the patient into one personality, although in some cases this may be only one aspect of treatment or an incidental consideration. This therapeutic aim distinguishes the treatment of MPD from that of any other disorder. Hypnosis is generally recommended, although experts (Bowers et al. 1971; Herzog 1984; Howland 1975) strongly urge caution in using it because of the potential for causing further splitting into alternate personalities.

The relationship of demonic possession to MPD has apparently led some therapists to incorporate elements of this persuasion into patient management, but this has proved largely unsuccessful. Informing MPD patients that their alternate personalities are demonic has met with failure (Fraser 1991; Kluft 1989). Exposure to exorcism is thought to frighten MPD patients and cause further harm (Fraser 1991).

The intensive psychotherapy that is considered the appropriate treatment for MPD functions systematically to uncover memories of early traumatic experiences and work through them with cognitive reprocessing (Rivera 1991). Kluft (1984c) uses a problem-oriented treatment plan, focusing on helping the patient work through the conflicts that resulted in the splitting to begin with. He warns that therapist coercion of the patient to fuse the personalities prematurely, prior to having worked through the conflicts, will doom the fusion to failure, and splitting into personalities will resume.

Once fusion has been accomplished, patients still have many problems and require continued psychotherapy for years (Bliss 1980; Kluft 1982). Ideally, treatment extends for several years (Bliss 1986, p. 219), with two therapy sessions a week (Kluft 1987b). In therapy, difficulties and crises are routine. Relapse is defined as a return to dissociation and splitting into alternates.

The recommended therapy for borderline patients is not very different from that recommended for MPD. In both disorders therapy is described as frustrating and difficult (Groves 1981; Peters 1990; Shea 1991). Like the therapy of MPD, the therapy of borderlines is considered controversial. The goal of therapy for borderlines may include "fundamental personality reorganization," where "regression is promoted" by the therapist (Aronson 1989). Regression may also result in self-mutilative behavior, substance abuse, and damaged interpersonal relationships. For this reason, intensive psychotherapy is considered by some to be potentially dangerous for borderlines (Aronson 1989), although intensive treatment with two or more sessions per week for years has been recommended by others (Groves 1981).

The focus of therapy of borderlines is on "maintaining a positive therapeutic alliance, promoting healthier adaptation, and, in particular, setting limits" (Aronson 1989, p. 520) and is to a large degree behaviorally oriented (Linehan 1987; Shea 1991). Medication for borderlines, as for multiples, is reserved for short-term amelioration of anxious and depressed symptoms (Coccaro & Kavoussi 1991; Groves 1981; Peters 1990), with the recognition of the risk for substance abuse in this group (Groves 1981; Peters 1990).

Outcome studies on the therapeutic experiences of borderlines are notoriously lacking, but available data suggest "very high dropout rates and relatively low rates of improvement" (Aronson 1989, p. 520). Silver (1985, p. 374) has summed up his experience with therapy of borderlines: "Psychotherapy with many of these patients probably still belongs to the area of therapeutic heroics. Hard evidence for good and poor outcome is scarce, with few exceptions."

While these principles of treatment of borderlines have not been systematically applied to MPD patients, it is not known how helpful they would be, especially because it is not even known how helpful these methods are for borderlines. The high frequency of borderline personality associated with MPD suggests that the techniques for managing borderlines would be reasonable to try in multiples: the multiples with borderline personality would be expected to be benefitted, if not the others as well. Horevitz and Braun (1984) suggest that the outcome of multiples is related to the presence of borderline personality; if this can be ameliorated, then perhaps multiples can enjoy a better prognosis, whether MPD or borderline personality is the superordinate disorder.

Conclusion

This review has traced the origins of MPD through history in both academic and popular literature. Clearly, there has been an epidemic of reported cases in the past decade or two. MPD cannot be simply dismissed by those who do not believe. On the other hand, it has not been validated as a diagnostic entity. In the development of this disorder, public sentiment seems to lead academic knowledge. It is up to psychiatrists to clarify MPD in the scientific arena and to the public.

What we call MPD is obviously a heterogenous and complex disorder. In describing psychiatric disorders, Cloninger and Reich (1983, p. 145) suggest that often the "more complex the phenotype, the more steps in the chain of events and the greater the number of loci [genes] and environmental factors that are important to phenotypic variation," so the development of the disorder is likely to be long. They emphasize the importance of ascertaining the dimensionality (via factor analytic studies) and subgrouping of patient types (via cluster analysis).

At present, the nosologic status of MPD cannot be confidently determined. *Current knowledge does not at this time sufficiently justify the validity of MPD as a separate diagnosis.* On the other hand, its diagnostic validity hasn't been disproved.[1] Current information at best can only support MPD as a syndrome or as a conversion-like symptom complicating other disorders.

The recommended course of treatment of MPD is critically dependent on its nosologic placement within psychiatry. It is imperative that research be aimed at clarifying the position of this disorder so that the burgeoning number of cases in our culture can receive optimal treatment. Continued intense conflict within psychiatry regarding this disorder will make the field look foolish and will be a disservice to patients who complain of symptoms of MPD. Without adequate data-oriented studies, psychiatry cannot be unified in its view of MPD. Future research needs to focus on exclusion criteria (comorbid disorders), familial transmission, follow-up studies to determine the natural course of the disorder, and randomized, controlled treatment studies.

---

[1]One of our distinguished colleagues, George Murphy, M.D., at his retirement address covering the changes and developments in psychiatry during his career, suggested that this situation applies to almost all diagnoses listed in DSM-III-R—a position difficult to refute.

Appendix A
Synopses of book-length accounts of MPD

As indicated in Chapter 6, we have read and analyzed all 21 published book-length popular accounts of MPD. Appendix A is a collection of case-by-case synopses of these accounts in the form of clinical vignettes, ordered by year of publication. These synopses include systematically collected information on criterion symptoms of Briquet's syndrome (somatization disorder) and antisocial personality disorder, as well as data relating to other personality disorders, substance abuse, and other psychiatric diagnoses. In addition, material is presented on the family background of psychiatric problems, childhood histories of physical and sexual abuse, treatments received, characteristics of the MPD syndrome, outcomes, authorship, and style of writing. Much of this information is listed in table format in Appendix B. For a summary and discussion of the conglomerate data provided in individual detail in the Appendixes, the reader is directed to Chapter 6. The final entry of this Appendix summarizes a book published during the final preparation of this manuscript that was not included with the original list of 21 books.

The Dissociation of a Personality (Prince 1906)

The subject of the first known book in English describing a case of multiple personality, Christine Beauchamp, exhibited four personalities. The account was written by her psychiatrist. Although she held that she did not like to discuss her physical ailments, she had 41 medically unexplained symptoms of Briquet's syndrome in seven categories on the Perley-Guze checklist, sufficient in number but lacking two categories for qualification for the diagnosis. Her symptoms clustered most heavily in Groups 2 (conversion symptoms) and 10 (psychiatric symptoms), with 23 conversion symptoms and 8 of the 10 possible psychiatric symptoms acknowledged. Her conversion symptoms included blindness, paralysis, anesthesia, aphonia, deafness, visual and auditory hallucinations, ataxia, visual field limitations, and not knowing her own name. Beauchamp's case report lacked any mention of sexual or menstrual symptoms, or of Group 6 symptoms of abdominal pain and vomiting. The account did not mention whether she had ever undergone surgery.

Miss Beauchamp was described as "morbidly impressionable," "extremely suggestive," and prone to "unnecessary emotionalism." She had a "hysterical temperament" and the "general appearance of a hysteric." Her personality switches were likened to a stage comedy, and her therapist wondered if the personalities could be a product of "self-suggestion," "hypnotic acting," or imitating something she had read. She exhibited fits of "nasty temper" with "violent rages which nothing will restrain," resulting in "vandalism."

Childhood conduct problems Miss Beauchamp displayed were truancy and running away. Adult sociopathic symptoms included lying, financial irresponsibility, and irritable and abusive behaviors. She lacked one juvenile and one adult behavior for the diagnosis of antisocial personality. She was reported to be "always experimenting with medications" and requested "morphia" from her doctors. Miss Beauchamp's family history was not described, other than to mention that her father and paternal grandfather both displayed a "violent temper."

Miss Beauchamp was reported to be an excellent hypnotic subject (Sutcliffe & Jones 1962). Her alternate personalities first appeared during hypnosis, and initially they were mistaken for hypnotic states. Later in her account, however, retrospective mention was made of subconscious splitting phenomena during her early childhood. Psychiatric diagnoses applied to Miss Beauchamp were neurasthenia, hysteria, and multiple personality. Her therapy consisted of psychotherapy and hypnosis, though she also received morphine for pain complaints. In the end, Miss Beauchamp was apparently fortunate enough to overcome her multiple personality problem through therapy and was planning to join the Catholic church and enter a convent. Horevitz and Braun (1984) considered Miss Beauchamp's treatment unsuccessful.

Patient Eve (Chris Sizemore) of *The Three Faces of Eve* (Thigpen & Cleckley 1957), *The Final Face of Eve* (Lancaster & Poling 1958), *I'm Eve* (Sizemore & Pittillo 1977), and *A Mind of My Own* (Sizemore 1989)

Eve's psychiatrists observed four personalities (Thigpen & Cleckley 1957), but in Eve's second autobiography (Sizemore & Pittillo 1977), she indicated that she subsequently went on to develop a total of 22 personalities. She said that for years her husband never noticed her other personalities. Prior to writing her final account, Eve had read about the MPD case of Sybil. The accounts written by Eve herself (Lancaster & Poling 1958; Sizemore 1977; Sizemore 1989) were more informative and contained many more symptoms (particularly somatoform symptoms) than the psychiatrists' original version (Thigpen & Cleckley 1957). Allison (1981, 1974b) noted many inconsistencies in her story among her different accounts.

On the Perley-Guze checklist for Briquet's syndrome the psychiatrists reported 17 symptoms in five categories, insufficient for a diagnosis. Eve herself, however, described 28 symptoms in eight categories for a probable diagnosis in her first account (Lancaster & Poling 1958) and 35 symptoms in eight categories in her second account (Sizemore & Pittillo 1977), for a probable diagnosis. In her third account (Sizemore 1989) she reported 26 symptoms in 10 categories for a definite diagnosis, and 16 of these symptoms were still present after she had successfully fused her personalities for the last time. Pooling all the symptoms described in all four accounts, Eve had a total of 52 criterion symptoms in 10 categories, sufficient for a definite diagnosis of Briquet's syndrome.

Eve's somatoform symptoms were most heavily concentrated in the two Briquet's syndrome categories of conversion (Group 2) and psychiatric symptoms (Group 10). She reported 9 of the possible 11 basic conversion symptoms and 9 of the possible 10 psychiatric symptoms. Some of her conversion symptoms were dramatic, including blindness, paralysis, pseudoseizures, aphonia, visual hallucinations, automatisms, speaking gibberish, and not knowing who she was.

Eve made it quite clear in her first two autobiographies that she had lived in a puritanical era in which it was unacceptable to mention problems relating to sexual disorders and female reproduction. This factor might account for the relative lack of sexual symptoms and the absence of menstrual symptoms in her accounts. Eve had undergone a partial hysterectomy for symptoms of endometriosis and had an abortion as well, though she reported that in general she refused her physicians' recommendations for surgery. Eve reported problematic sexual behaviors, including exhibitionistic dancing and singing, and sexually arousing her husband only to then refuse his advances.

At her first psychiatric appointment, Eve was noted as appearing neither histrionic nor overdramatic. But she was later discovered to have "tempestuous emotions and tantrums" and a "mercurial temperament" with "murderous rages"; she was also said to be "self-centered" and lacking a conscience. She was subject to "deep depression." Eve described histrionic episodes such as a fit of tearing off her clothes, screaming, and rolling on the floor half naked; her son then arrived home and "found me crawling along the apartment floor, my mind slipping in and out of consciousness." Her doctor had also observed "la belle indifference." In one instance, Eve behaved in a sexually provocative manner toward her internist.

Near the end of her first account, Eve candidly admitted awareness of personality problems. She also reported that she had resorted to extreme behaviors to get her husband's attention, and once she said that she wanted "to do something drastic to show Don how I feel." At one point, her physician suspected her multiple personality disorder to represent "the greatest leg-pull in history." Eve herself admitted that she was "having fun being a multiple" (Lancaster & Poling 1958). After she was fused, she reported that "the magic had gone out of my life" (Sizemore 1989). Psychiatrists pointed out that Eve was receiving considerable professional (and later public) attention to her case, and she was accused of being just an "actress" who was "on stage." One doctor said that her illness would "no longer be necessary" if she grew in psychotherapy.

Eve described herself as "a constant victim of minor illness." Her autobiographies repeatedly described her as mischievous and disobedient as a child, maliciously destructive and blaming others, and unaccepting of responsibility for her actions. The accounts contain numerous descriptions of juvenile conduct problems, including stealing, lying, property destruction, cruelty to animals, and physical cruelty to people, with her own two first versions mentioning the same five criterion behaviors for conduct disorder. None of these conduct problems, however, were noted in the psychiatrists' account. Eve's juvenile behaviors more than qualified her for a DSM-III-R diagnosis of conduct disorder.

Eve's autobiographies described eight adult antisocial behaviors, including inconsistent employment, lawbreaking and resisting arrest, aggressive and abusive behaviors toward others, financial irresponsibility, lying, irresponsible parenting, sexual promiscuity, and lacking remorse, which definitely qualify her for the diagnosis of antisocial personality disorder. Her psychiatrists noted only two of these behaviors in their account. Her antisocial behaviors were repeatedly ascribed to the MPD, and often a specific alternate personality was blamed for certain actions. One of her personalities had the name "Liar."

Eve claimed to have "psychic experiences" with the ability to mind-bend metal, clairvoyance, reincarnation, and other kinds of "paranormal experience."

Eve's family history was positive for probable Briquet's syndrome in her mother and her maternal grandmother, inferred from symptoms described in the accounts, as well as sociopathic behaviors in both parents.

Her two husbands showed evidence of sociopathy; in addition, one of them physically abused Eve, and the other abused alcohol.

Childhood physical or sexual abuse was not a part of the descriptions provided by Eve or her psychiatrists. However, as a young child, Eve was an eyewitness to a violent and grotesque sawmill accident and another bloody scene when her mother unintentionally cut herself; these events were thought to have triggered her MPD in the absence of any history of child abuse. According to Eve's first autobiography, the first alternate personality occurred at age six, when she was forced to kiss her deceased grandmother. According to the second autobiography, the first alternate personality appeared at age two, when she encountered the dead body of the man who had been mutilated in the sawmill accident.

Therapists who evaluated Eve gave her various other diagnoses over time besides MPD, including "psychopathy," schizophrenia, and depression. A diagnosis of hysteria was suggested by one evaluator and ruled out by another. Her treatment consisted of intensive psychotherapy and hypnosis, and at times she was prescribed sleeping pills and tranquilizers.

It has been reported elsewhere (Coons 1980) that Eve's family "took great delight in the emergence of each successive personality and even helped name some of them." Eve was described as "extremely hypnotizable." Eve eventually came to have a "personal prejudice" against the use of hypnosis, feeling that it had aggravated her dissociative tendencies. She stated that her personality

"Jane" "was an alter created, in part, by Dr. Thigpen's manipulative use of hypnosis" (Sizemore 1989). A subsequent therapist for Eve stated, "I was determined to avoid the pitfall of fascination with the disorder, which has proven so detrimental to the relationships of many MPD patients and clinicians," and he said that he made an effort to avoid giving attention to "switches" in MPD patients. Eve also reported that she uses this same strategy in her own work with MPD patients.

In her final autobiography, Eve stated that she personally accepts responsibility for the behaviors of all her 22 former personalities, because she feels that alternate personalities can discern right from wrong (Sizemore 1989). She further stated that she feels MPD patients should be held responsible for their criminal acts, because the disorder represents "*a willed negligence of responsibility.*"

At the end of her psychiatrists' account and at the end of Eve's first autobiography, Eve was described as having successfully overcome her multiple personality problem. Eve's second personal account, however, described the untimely reappearance of her alternate personalities just before the release of her first autobiography, apparently creating consternation for all parties involved in this publication. Doctors had apparently told Eve that she was cured numerous times over the years. By the end of the second autobiography, Eve and her personalities had again been successfully fused, and by all current reports she has had no symptoms of MPD for many years. Her third autobiography is a courageous work that describes her remarkable efforts to adapt to a mature and productive existence without the option of dissociating under stress. Velek and Balon (1986, p. 72) however, opined that "after reading Mrs. Sizemore's autobiography, one may not be convinced that her health definitely had improved, even some 23 years later." After her final recovery from MPD, Eve continued to experience at least 16 somatoform symptoms in six categories (Sizemore 1989). She wrote (p. 117):

> I was well and famous but facing everyday problems with few normal experiences on which to base my decisions and behavior. Years later, Dr. Kluft would succinctly describe this by observing that, "The cure of multiple personality disorder leaves the patient afflicted with single personality disorder, the state in which most patients seek psychotherapy."

Sybil (Schreiber 1973)

Sybil Dorsett exhibited 16 alternate personalities. It has been written that her personalities "seem to have come about from iatrogenic suggestion in the course of therapeutic action" (Abse 1987, p. 239). The author of her account described "a compendium of physical complaints" and "a variety of psychosomatic illnesses and disturbances in the five senses," including 39 somatoform symptoms in nine Perley-Guze checklist categories, fulfilling criteria for Briquet's syndrome. Sybil's somatoform symptoms clustered heavily in the conversion (Group 2) and psychiatric (Group 10) categories. Her account acknowledged all of the 10 possible psychiatric symptoms, and in the conversion group she had 9 of the 11 possible basic symptoms plus 9 other conversion symptoms. These included blindness, paralysis, anesthesia, aphonia, pseudoseizures, unconsciousness, amnesia, and tunnel vision. As with Eve's case, the text's descriptions shied away from overt descriptions of female reproductive and sexual symptoms, a reporting bias also consistent with Sybil's cultural background. Sybil told Dr. Wilbur that she thought she was "crazy," but Dr. Wilbur disagreed. Sybil's IQ was tested at 170.

Sybil displayed two childhood conduct disorder symptoms, property destruction and physical cruelty to others. She was described as a lonely, moody, nervous child with "emotional problems." In early childhood she developed a routine of being "sick but not sick" that was to become a lifelong pattern. She once said she felt "not at all well" but was told she was "really healthy."

Aside from financial irresponsibility and inconsistent employment, she did not exhibit adult sociopathic behaviors. She was described as manipulative, dependent, vague, and immature, and she created "scenes at home." Once she walked on the furniture and said to her father, "You get out of my way. I might hurt you." During fugues she wanted to act out angry thoughts that nobody loved her by wanting to tear up things, break things, and break glass. During one fugue she broke a window in her psychiatrist's office, and during another she went on a glass-smashing spree on Fifth Avenue in New York, destroying $2000 worth of antique crystal. She also smashed a window in a car and bit its owner's finger.

Sybil "indulged in the ritual of making frequent pilgrimages" to the university's psychology library, where she "steeped herself in psychiatric literature, especially case histories." The rationale given was that she wanted to know all she could about the symptoms of other patients to help her become more adept at concealing her own symptoms; in addition, she was somewhat curious.

Details of Sybil's biological family history suggest probable Briquet's syndrome in her mother and possibly in other relatives, as well as probable sociopathy in both parents. The mother reportedly had a postpartum depression severe enough to render her unable to take care of Sybil for the first six weeks of her life, and Sybil had stayed with relatives during that time. The mother also exhibited "catatonic" behaviors. The mother was described as lonely, unloved, unloving, and angry. She was nervous and had polysomatic complaints. As a girl, Sybil's mother had cut off the sleeves of her father's smoking jacket when she was angry at him. The mother sexually abused the little girls she babysat. She had lesbian sexual affairs with three teenage girls together. The mother liked to walk around town at night with her daughter and defecate with "perverse pleasure" on the lawns and sidewalks of prestigious townspeople she scorned. This behavior was regarded as evidence of psychosis. The mother stole things, with no remorse, and window peeped. She was loud at church functions, danced on a tabletop in a restaurant, and was considered "odd" and "crazy." Despite the presence of these socially deviant behaviors, and citing no clear evidence of definite psychotic symptoms such as delusions or hallucinations, Sybil's therapist stated as fact that her mother was schizophrenic. The "schizophrenia" was said to be the reason for the physical and sexual abuse of Sybil by her mother, and for the subsequent development of Sybil's psychiatric disorder.

The rest of Sybil's family psychiatric history was complicated, with additional mention of other relatives with "schizophrenia" and a variety of relatives who were "neurotic" and had "a variety of psychosomatic illnesses." A maternal aunt had many "physical illness and emotional attitudes" that her son also developed. A "sickly" cousin became a "religious fanatic" and was cured by faith healers, but that cousin's daughter was "a semi-invalid all her life." An uncle and a cousin were also said to suffer from MPD. Sybil's father had an alcohol problem.

Sybil's personal history detailed graphic and horrible scenes of severe sexual and physical abuse at the hands of her mother, beginning at six months of age. The mother kicked her, hit her with a broom handle and a rolling pin, stuffed a washcloth down her throat, "put things inside her, things with sharp edges that hurt," and gave her enemas and told her to "hold the [cold] water inside her." The mother characteristically emitted shrill, sadistic laughter when abusing Sybil, when she locked her in a trunk in the attic, and when she buried her in a wheat crib and nearly smothered her. The mother dislocated Sybil's shoulder on one occasion and fractured her larynx another time. She caused a "serious burn" by pressing a hot iron to Sybil's head, and gave her a black eye and swollen lips. She tied a scarf around Sybil's neck until Sybil gasped for breath, and put cotton in Sybil's nose until she lost consciousness.

The mother had a ritual in which she separated Sybil's legs with a long wooden spoon, tied her feet to the spoon with dish towels, and then strung her upside down to the end of a lightbulb cord suspended from the ceiling. The mother left her crying in space and later returned with an adult-sized enema bag filled to capacity with cold water. She reportedly inserted the enema tip into Sybil's urethra and filled her bladder, which made the mother "scream triumphantly" and then laugh. The mother delighted in giving the child double-sized enemas and huge doses of laxatives and then forcing the child to retain control of her bowels, beating her if she complained. The mother forced a variety of objects into the child's vagina, including a flashlight, a small empty bottle, a little silver box, the handle of a regular dinner knife, a little silver knife, and a buttonhook.

There was also a vague mention of sexual abuse by her father. Sybil slept with her parents until she was nine years old and apparently witnessed her parents having sex regularly. The first appearance of an alternate personality was at the age of three under unclear circumstances. The account reported that when she was punished as a child, she was unaware of having committed the "bad" behaviors that warranted her punishment. Each of her alternate personalities served to take blame for unacceptable behaviors that the original Sybil could not admit to.

Sybil described in detail a number of incidents at a very young age, younger than ordinary brain development would be expected to produce such intact and detailed memory banks. For example, she developed a middle ear infection at six weeks of age, and she associates her recollection of the warmth of the kitchen stove (by which her father sat when holding her during the time of the ear infection) with her father's warmth. Sybil reported in extensive detail the kinds of physical and sexual abuse her mother perpetrated on her as early as six months of age. She recalled her father asking her when she was two years old how she got the black eye and swollen lips, and that she wouldn't tell him.

Diagnoses applied to Sybil by therapists were fairly consistent: "*grande hysterie,*" hysteria, and neurasthenia. Therapy was primarily intensive psychotherapy and hypnosis. She became so involved with her analysis that "she almost literally lived for her Tuesday morning appointments with Dr. Wilbur." She made a great ritual out of trying to decide what to wear when getting ready for appointments. Sybil also received seconal narcosis for a period of time, during which she became dependent on it psychologically, if not physiologically. Once this was recognized, she had to be withdrawn from it—against her will. Sybil fortunately experienced a happy ending to her story: at last report, she had successfully fused her personalities into one through psychotherapy. She now gives lectures and works as a college art professor.

Splitting: A Case of Female Masculinity (Stoller 1973)

Mrs. G's account described two alternate personalities besides her core personality. The account, written by her psychiatrist, consisted in large part of transcriptions of audiotapes of therapy sessions. It described 31 symptoms in nine categories of the Perley-Guze checklist for a definite diagnosis of Briquet's syndrome. The category with the most positive symptoms was Group 10 (psychiatric symptoms), with 9 of the 10 possible symptoms in this category acknowledged. She also had many conversion symptoms, including blindness, pseudoseizures, amnesia, visual and olfactory hallucinations, and slurred speech. Mrs. G was reported to be free of pain only when pregnant. Some of her descriptions were dramatic; for example, on sexual intercourse, a penis felt like a hot wire in her. She claimed to have an erect penis inside her body constantly, a notion she "invented" at age four. Mrs. G recalled that as a child she felt that in order to merit her mother's love she needed to have a penis.

She underwent several surgical procedures, including an appendectomy, where a normal appendix was found, and a second appendectomy (although the surgeons were aware of her prior appendectomy) without findings of significant pathology. Transient cardiopulmonary symptoms led her to have cardiac catheterization and pulmonary angiogram procedures that provided no medical explanation for her complaints. Likewise, a neurologic evaluation including a pneumoencephalogram and an electroencephalogram failed to uncover the cause of the symptoms. Evaluation for complaints of rectal bleeding failed to identify a source. Mrs. G engaged in purposeful cutting and burning of herself to reduce "the pain."

Although Mrs. G's somatoform symptoms were not described in graphic detail, her sociopathic behaviors were. She reported attempting to murder a dozen or more individuals in her lifetime, beginning at the age of four, including her school principal, police officers, her young children in a murder-suicide attempt, her husband, and her mother. From a young age she set fires, and her arsonist behaviors continued into adulthood with frequency. From early childhood she was labeled "mentally ill." She was sexually promiscuous from a young age, claiming over 20 homosexual affairs and "hundreds" of heterosexual encounters; she first became pregnant at age 13 and went on to have five illegitimate pregnancies (one, she claimed, fathered by her "sadistic" and "sexual psychopath" brother). Termed "a difficult child" and clearly meeting criteria for conduct disorder, she was placed in reform school and later spent time in jail. She also accrued 21 psychiatric hospital admissions and boasted that overall she had spent "five years and three months locked up." Her physicians described her as "an outstanding manipulator" and "an unmitigated pain"; she claimed that she once seduced and smoked marijuana with a psychiatrist on the ward.

Mrs. G's crimes included writing bad checks, stealing, six counts of armed robbery, three counts of auto theft, accruing 30 traffic tickets without paying, purposely causing motor vehicle accidents resulting in serious injuries (and without a driver's license), drag racing, riding a motorcycle excessively fast and running the cycle through fences, repeated arson, and the homicide attempts already mentioned. She was described as "a textbook psychopath (antisocial personality)" who "felt no guilt." She seemed to relish reporting that she shot a policeman "in the ass" and shot another man several times in the thighs while aiming at his genitals.

Mrs. G's family psychiatric history, from her description, was positive for sociopathy, probable pedophilia, and alcoholism in her father, who eventually committed suicide. Her brother, who exhibited antisocial behaviors, later became a Christian and "found God." Her paternal grandfather was sexually promiscuous and a known pedophile, and several female relatives were said to be prostitutes.

Mrs. G's four husbands were all said to be "sick" and "neurotic" and showed some sociopathic tendencies. She had been married three times by age 23.

Mrs. G indicated that from the age of six or seven she was sexually abused by her brother, two uncles, her grandfather, and a host of strangers. She also reported that from the age of two, her mother periodically kept her in a box and physically abused her. At the age of nine years, Mrs. G was eyewitness to a bloody and gory suicide of a man she knew. At one point it was reported that Mrs. G's first alternate personality appeared at the age of three years to tell her that her new baby sister should die. In another place in her story, the first alternate was said to have appeared at the age of four, telling her to kill a male playmate, whom she then repeatedly hit in the head with a rock.

Although Mrs. G was thought to be intermittently psychotic, her therapist noted that she exhibited no evidence of thought disorder or chronic deterioration, and that she could "almost instantaneously" turn the psychosis on and off at will. Her psychiatrist noted that her "psychotic episodes seemed self-serving," and instead preferred to think of her condition as "hysterical psychosis." Mrs. G was reportedly "proud of being a nut" and found her alternate personalities to be good excuses for her behavioral problems. She was described as "a text-book psychopath (antisocial personality)." She also collected a variety of hysterical and dissociative labels, as well as antisocial personality, paranoid schizophrenia, and diagnoses of practically every psychiatric category. She abused alcohol, heroin, and LSD and was addicted to amphetamines by age 17; she developed symptoms thought to be complications of amphetamine abuse, including seizures, organic brain syndrome, and psychosis.

Her therapy consisted primarily of psychotherapy, but she was also treated with chlorpromazine and shock treatments. She had 12 psychiatric hospitalizations in 12 years and a total of 21 psychiatric admissions. At the end of the account, her condition was reported as improved (she "was helped" by therapy), yet she remained polysymptomatic and continued in therapy. The writer did not specify whether or not the multiple personalities had resolved. Overall, the writer organized the book in a manner he described as minimizing "scholarship," presenting instead "a book of theories."

The Five of Me (Hawksworth & Schwarz 1977)

As the book's title informs us, Hawksworth claimed five personalities. This book was coauthored by the author of *The Hillside Strangler* (Schwarz 1981), who was also coauthor of the case of Peters (Peters & Schwarz 1978). Hawksworth reported few somatoform symptoms, just eight symptoms in three categories on the Perley-Guze checklist for Briquet's syndrome. Most were in the category of conversion (Group 2) and included pseudoseizures, unconsciousness, amnesia, hallucinations, and disorientation.

Hawksworth admitted to 8 criterion juvenile misbehaviors for a definite diagnosis of conduct disorder, as well as 9 of the 10 possible adult antisocial behaviors for that diagnosis. Juvenile problems included poor academic performance, truancy, and disrespecting his teacher by spitting on him and calling him a "shit-turd" (blaming an alternate for the behavior). He stole blank report cards and sold them to his friends. His father was called to school, and the principal considered expelling the boy. He later became a high school dropout. He beat up boys and girls and was considered "too rough" to play. He threw a rock at another child's head and laughed, expressing disappointment that the child wasn't hurt; he tried to murder a friend with a bow and arrow; he shot at his peers with BB guns; aiming to hit their faces. He beat a peer with a gun and bragged about it but denied it to his father. He threatened his mother's boyfriend with his father's gun and waved the gun at his mother. By eighth grade he was sexually promiscuous and allegedly a date rapist. He ran with friends who were considered wild and disreputable. As a teenager he ran away, disappearing for 10 days with a car.

Hawksworth's father expressed pride at his acting out because he considered it a sign of masculinity. Hawksworth frequently burned his own arm with a cigarette to prove his power. Once he attempted suicide and was admitted to a psychiatric ward. He liked to spend time reading about mysticism and the occult.

As an adult, Hawksworth engaged in barroom fighting. He beat women during wild sexual escapades. He assaulted a police officer and was confined to jail for 28 days. He falsely accused police of stealing his $100 and shouted obscenities in jail. In the Marines he was arrested for hitting a drill instructor. His alleged crimes ranged from driving while intoxicated to felony for robbery, malicious injury, rape, and several attempted murders, and he was frequently in court on charges such as assault and battery, driving while intoxicated, grand theft, resisting arrest, and other charges. He threw a rock through a friend's window. He showed no remorse for hurting others, and instead expressed glee that another driver in a car crash had been seriously injured because that driver had interfered with Hawksworth's race with another car. In another race he purposely ran into another car, running it off the road, and did not stop to see if the driver was injured. He was "out for excitement no matter who got hurt," causing paralysis and other serious injuries to others in his escapades. Once he allegedly zoomed through a police roadblock at 100 miles per hour and was pursued by police, sheriff's deputies, and highway patrolmen. Hawksworth was described as impulsive and unpredictable, prone to extremes of emotion, irresponsible, malicious, without remorse, and "filled with hate and violence" since childhood. He was said to live only for the pleasures of the flesh and the excitement of the moment. He boasted of having casual sex with the governor's daughter and of wild orgies of drinking and sex.

From evidence of behaviors described in the book, Hawksworth's father and possibly his paternal grandmother were sociopathic, and his father was probably alcoholic. His father was unfaithful to his mother, and they fought a great deal. His mother was said to be emotionally unstable and alcoholic. There was some question that his mother's death may have been the result of suicide in an automobile accident that resulted in several deaths.

Hawksworth's father beat him and subjected him to icy showers at the age of one year. Hawksworth reported that his alternate personalities first appeared during his fourth year against this backdrop of physical abuse, and his alternate personalities were blamed for his misbehaviors.

Besides MPD, Hawksworth received psychiatric diagnoses of "manic-depression," sociopathy, hysterical dissociation, and alcoholism. He had brief depressive episodes lasting for one to two seconds. Examiners raised the possibility of conscious malingering with intent to avoid criminal conviction, but a handwriting analyst found "proof" that he really was a multiple. At one point the account clearly described Hawksworth as conveniently changing his personality just before an automobile accident he had caused; he was sued for $11,000 and lost.

Hawksworth was briefly medicated with amphetamines and "tranquilizers." He also received lithium. For a time he attended Alcoholics Anonymous meetings. One doctor told him he was acting out and must turn to God. Another doctor recommended frontal lobotomy, a treatment he did not receive. At the book's end, Hawksworth had experienced a brief remission from his multiple personality syndrome that was expected to be lasting ("cured"), and a court decision had declared him not guilty (on the basis of MPD) on charges of drunken driving.

Tell Me Who I Am Before I Die (Peters & Schwarz 1978)

The account of Christina Peters mentioned four other personalities besides the core personality of Christina. Her biography described few somatoform symptoms, with 10 symptoms in four categories on the Perley-Guze checklist for Briquet's syndrome. Her somatic symptoms were most heavily concentrated in Group 2 (conversion) symptoms, including anesthesia, pseudoseizures, unconsciousness, amnesia, auditory and visual hallucinations, and forgetting what a television was.

She more than met criteria for conduct disorder, scoring eight criterion behaviors, including fighting and injuring others, property destruction, robbery, murdering kittens by drowning and then freezing them, property destruction, and repeatedly running away from juvenile institutions. Juvenile authorities pegged her as "incorrigible." Peters continuously wet the bed until she was 14 years old.

As an adult, she went on to develop antisocial personality disorder with six positive antisocial behaviors. She beat up her boyfriend, causing injuries requiring emergency medical intervention. She also beat and injured her husband. She assaulted police officers, as well as an emergency room doctor and a nurse. In the hospital she stabbed a fellow patient. Her other crimes included burglary, theft of narcotics, child abuse, attempted murder of her daughter, and violation of parole; for her crimes she spent time in a penitentiary. She was considered "capable of killing without emotion."

Peters was trained as a registered nurse and worked at an alcohol treatment facility; she lost her job after being hospitalized for psychiatric treatment. At one point she was addicted to phenobarbital. She attempted suicide in jail by slashing her throat with a wire from hardware in the toilet mechanism.

Her family history was clearly positive for sociopathy. Her father reportedly murdered her brother and "terrorized" her mother and grandmother, lived a life of violence, ran from the law, and perpetrated many serious crimes, including kidnapping, felony, and armed robbery. He died in prison. Peters' mother showed evidence of sociopathy but was described as "psychotic" in the face of sexual promiscuity, abuse of her own child, and alcohol abuse, without mention of psychotic symptoms. The mother was committed to a sanitarium for a year after she was found picking roses in the nude in the middle of the night. Substance abuse was apparent in Peters' father and brother. Peters' brother was jailed for drunkenness and another time spent three months in jail for "felony wife beating"; he also resisted arrest. Peters' father beat her mother.

Peters' first husband was physically abusive to her and irresponsible to the children; her second husband abused alcohol and committed suicide. Her "sadistic" lover beat her.

Peters reported that as a child she was physically abused by both her parents and by nuns who knocked her unconscious, and she was sexually abused by her father and brother. Peters' father reportedly drugged her and her siblings, and beat her until he crippled her so that she was unable to walk. Her first alternate personality appeared at approximately four years of age, reportedly as a reaction to a violent rape by her father.

Psychiatric diagnoses applied to Peters besides multiple personality included depression, alcoholism, substance abuse, and no psychiatric diagnosis. Her psychological test result was reported as normal.

Peters was seductive to her doctor and became angry at him for stopping her drugs. She claimed to have provided oral sex to a physician in exchange for prescription drugs. Treatment was basically psychotherapy and hypnosis, with a brief stay in a substance detoxification program. Peters told her doctor she was possessed and requested an exorcism; he reported that he went through the motions to assist her in believing she was no longer possessed.

At the end of the book she had been successfully fused, was still in group therapy, and was working to put her life back together. The account was written within weeks to months of her recovery; therefore her long-term outcome is not known.

The Minds of Billy Milligan (Keyes 1981)

Billy Milligan claimed 24 personalities. His Perley-Guze checklist score for Briquet's syndrome was very suggestive, but not quite diagnostic, of the disorder. He met 31 symptoms in seven categories, sufficient in the number of symptoms but lacking two positive categories.

Much like the distribution of symptoms in the accounts of the female MPD cases in this study, Milligan's somatoform symptoms clustered in the psychiatric category (Group 10) with 8 of 10 possible symptoms, and also to a lesser degree in the conversion category (Group 2). His most florid conversion symptoms included deafness, amnesia, unconsciousness, hallucinations, periods of color blindness, tunnel vision, periods of "dyslexia," losing the ability to speak English, and not knowing who he was. He made up excuses of physical illness to get out of class, and in the Navy he went to sick bay often and was finally relieved of his job.

Milligan was described as prone to "hysterical reactions" and temper tantrums, and as manipulative and demanding, attention seeking, approval addicted, immature and unstable, uncooperative, impulsive, arrogant, and malicious. He attempted suicide by smashing his head. He also tried to step in the way of moving cars when he felt depressed, attempted to jump off a roof, and stabbed himself in prison. He suffered from "deep depression" and made suicide threats in prison. He said he cried after seeing a television story about him. Milligan was also described as "a fraud and a phony," without remorse ("cold-blooded"), and failing to profit from punishment. He had sadistic fantasies and an "expansive ego." Psychological testing revealed a potential for violent acting out. He engaged in lengthy study of medicine and law textbooks. He studied the martial arts and learned all he could about munitions and demolition.

Milligan's account described seven criterion behaviors of conduct disorder and eight adult sociopathic symptoms, definitely qualifying him for a diagnosis of antisocial personality disorder. As a child, he frequently got into trouble at school for behaviors including lying and making up stories, truancy, poor academic performance, altercations with peers and teachers, threatening his peers with a pocket knife and starting fights with a switchblade knife, and breaking school windows. He created a bomb scare at school that he thoroughly enjoyed; this got him expelled. He received counseling at school for his behavior. As a child, he had an imaginary playmate. Everyone said he was strange. He was placed in a juvenile detention center. At age 14 he hid a knife and threatened to kill his stepfather with it. At age 15 he was committed to a state hospital.

Milligan's adult crimes included three episodes of kidnapping and raping three college coeds, assault, robbery, and kidnapping of homosexual males at gunpoint at roadside restrooms. He used the credit cards he stole, tried to fill an illegal prescription, used fake passports, robbed pharmacies for narcotics, and shot up a car with a machine gun. He dealt drugs on a large scale, collected many guns, and performed the "shotgun" role in organized deliveries of narcotics and guns. He confabulated stories to con others; he made up a story about someone's having drugged him in an effort to obtain air transportation back to the United States from Europe. In erratic acts, he pointed a gun at his head, shot a lamp, put a hole in a wall, and broke a window; he threw a knife at his brother. He threatened to kill his family members and the family members of one of his victims if they talked to the police. He left a cobra in a paper bag on his landlord's door as a warning. Within his maximum security prison facility he abused narcotics and sold drugs, acted out at every opportunity, and threatened the lives of others, and he broke parole. After a judge declared that Milligan lacked accepted moral restraints and embodied a total disregard for human rights, he reported feeling hopeless.

Milligan's family history was marked by sociopathic behaviors ascribed to both parents, as well as definite substance abuse in both parents. His biologic father beat his mother and was hospitalized for depression and alcoholism; he committed suicide during Milligan's childhood. Milligan's stepfather beat his mother, often while drunk, and subjected Milligan to sadistic physical abuse and anal intercourse at age eight or nine. Milligan's alcoholic mother developed alcoholic cirrhosis. She beat Milligan with her arm, and the father threatened to beat her up if she continued. She lived in the fast lane and cultivated relationships with pimps, lesbians, and shylocks. Milligan's family members helped him hide the evidence of crimes he had committed.

Milligan retrospectively reported that his first alternate personalities appeared at around the age of four at moments when he was being accused of drawing on the wall and of breaking a cookie jar, for which Milligan blamed the alternates. Otherwise, alternate personalities were not part of Milligan's behavioral and psychological problems until he was hypnotized as part of the forensic evaluation following his arrest for murders as an adult. The alternate personalities were blamed for his violent criminal acts. Milligan refused to take any responsibility for any of the actions of his alternate personalities. He personally blamed his father as the cause of his multiple personality problem.

Different examiners declared Milligan to have definite MPD, possible MPD, and definitely *not* MPD. Milligan collected diagnoses of hysteria, sociopathy, conversion reaction, psychoneurotic anxiety with depression, passive-aggressive disorder, dissociative disorder, alcoholism, and stimulant abuse. Schizophrenia was ruled out by one evaluator and definitely diagnosed by another. Milligan abused alcohol, marijuana, barbiturates, and amphetamines.

Treatment was psychotherapy, hypnosis, and, on one occasion, antipsychotic medication. On the ward Milligan was attention seeking and manipulative; he demanded special privileges, hid his medication in his cheek, and pitted one staff member against another. He also urinated and defecated on the floor, broke a window, manipulated, cried, and raved, threatened to break his doctor's bones, allegedly raped a patient and escaped from the forensic unit, was placed in the seclusion room for violent behaviors, and self-inflicted wounds, claiming he was beaten by a hospital employee.

At the end of the book, Milligan was unchanged and still in therapy. He was found NGRI (MPD) (*Time* 1979) and was institutionalized until 1984, when he was released (see Orne et al. 1984). Thigpen and Cleckley (1984, p. 65) opined:

> The diagnosis did indeed, wrongfully in our opinion, prevent criminal proceedings in this case. . . . We believe from the material at hand that this deliberate manipulation resulted in a gross miscarriage of justice and denigration of psychiatry. One might reasonably ask to what extent the desire to avoid taking responsibility for his actions motivated him to further dissociate (possibly even after arrest) to the point of exhibiting other sides of himself to the therapists charged to evaluate him.

A major motion picture based on Milligan's story was aired on network television.

The Hillside Strangler: A Murderer's Mind (Schwarz 1981)

Ken Bianchi claimed two alternate personalities. As mentioned, the author of his account was a coauthor of two other books reviewed in this paper (Hawksworth & Schwarz 1977; Peters & Schwarz 1978). Bianchi was fascinated with psychology; he took college courses in psychology and police science and read extensively on these subjects (Orne et al. 1984). He owned half a dozen psychology books, and detectives suspected that he had carefully studied hysterical dissociation and MPD as presented in these books. He reportedly read vast amounts of literature on psychology to help find "explanations—excuses—for his acts and failures." He bought psychology diplomas from diploma mills and planned to set up an office as a psychologist. He took his girlfriend there and administered "inkblot tests" to her. Bianchi had seen the film *Three Faces of Eve* some years previously, and it is likely that he viewed the film *Sybil* in his cell shortly before he first saw Dr. Watkins and revealed his alternate personalities (Orne et al. 1984). He also may have seen a newspaper article about Milligan, and coincidentally Bianchi reported that his first alternate had appeared at the age of nine, the same age reported by Milligan. In addition to any prior knowledge Bianchi had about hypnosis and MPD, it has been suggested that the procedure of his psychiatric evaluation provided him with sufficient information to self-present as multiple personality (Orne et al. 1984; Spanos et al. 1985, 1986).

Bianchi's account reported very few somatoform symptoms, just ten symptoms in three categories of the Perley-Guze checklist for Briquet's syndrome. He did, however, meet criteria for conduct disorder with four criterion symptoms, and also for antisocial personality disorder, scoring positive on 7 of the 10 adult criteria. He had a long history of defaulting on debts, repossessions of his property, unstable employment, compulsive lying, use of aliases, aggressive and abusive behaviors, property destruction, fraud, stealing, robbery, using stolen credit cards, selling drugs, involvement in prostitution, pimping of juvenile prostitutes, and extortion. He posed as a movie agent, a California highway patrolman, and a psychologist.

Bianchi's burning career interest was to do police work, but he could not persist at a junior college program in police science and could not find a police job despite several applications to police departments. He did obtain employment, however, as a security guard, and he stole from the very stores he was hired to protect. He was in the sheriff's reserve program and was always talking about psychology there, although to his listeners his knowledge of the subject reportedly seemed limited.

Bianchi was said to have no self-respect after high school graduation. He frequently missed work, calling in sick when he was not ill. He had at least 12 different jobs during the nine-year period after high school. He was described as having a chronically "irresponsible attitude toward money." His car was repossessed. His pattern of financial responsibility did not change when he fathered a baby. He married his high school girlfriend, but the marriage lasted for less than eight months, ending in annulment. He felt the whole world was against him, and he blamed everyone else for his troubles. His fiancee had extramarital affairs and was herself drawn to excitement. His girlfriend broke things and tore up his apartment. His worst crimes were the brutal, cold-blooded rape and murder of at least 12 women. To cover for his time while he was out committing crimes and murdering, he made up an elaborate scheme, telling his wife that he had cancer and was receiving chemotherapy. He even forged medical reports to "prove" it (Orne et al. 1984), and he had his wife wait in the car while he underwent his "treatments" at the hospital. His home life with her was described as "shattered," and he engaged in wife beating. He frequently bought hard-core sexual literature and had a collection of pornographic movies.

As a child, Bianchi was also described as nervous, passive, and dependent on his mother. He had tics, an eye-rolling habit, and many somatic complaints. He had few friends in school. At age seven he was "manipulative" and "unusually emotionally troublesome." As a child he was prone to falls and head injury. He had what appeared to be petit mal seizures, but epilepsy was ruled out by his physicians, who concluded that his problem was psychological. When hospitalized for genitourinary evaluation, he was noted to have behavior problems and to express many complaints designed to get his mother's attention. He also wet his pants. His medical reports included suspicions that he "might be more of a con artist than deeply troubled." In grade school he was caught with a small group of boys possessing a dangerous array of weapons, including a bat studded with nails, that they were planning to use on their peers (Orne et al. 1984). At age 13 Bianchi was hitting girls. As a child, he killed a cat and put it on a neighbor's porch as a Halloween prank; he also killed rats and a dog. He was sexually active and showed signs of promiscuity beginning at age 16 or earlier.

Bianchi's biologic father was a gambler who had frequent physical fights with his biologic mother. She was described as "extremely nervous" and sexually promiscuous, and she had frequently been involved in the juvenile court system. Only 14 years of age when Bianchi was born, his biologic mother gave him up for adoption at birth. She was described as "a girl of the streets" (Watkins 1984), an alcoholic who spent a great deal of time drinking at the bars. She was a nervous chain smoker who constantly bit her nails. Bianchi was passed around to foster homes until he was adopted at the age of one year. His adoptive mother was described as "easily upset," a "hypochondriac," and "deeply disturbed." She became "severely depressed" when told she needed a hysterectomy. She also spent a good deal of time crying, and, to her caretakers, didn't seem motivated to help herself or her son. She worried excessively about imaginary ailments in her adopted infant, and took him to multiple physicians for repeated invasive genitourinary examinations to an extent called "doctor-shopping"; this eventually led to an investigation by the Society for Prevention of Cruelty to Children. The doctor thought of her as "excitable"; she called him frequently, and he refused to see her or her child unless "absolutely necessary." Bianchi also reported beatings and other physical abuse by his adoptive mother.

Bianchi also had an alcoholic brother. Bianchi's cousin Angelo Buono allegedly was an accomplice to Bianchi in the murders, and he was also named as a partner in several of Bianchi's other deviant acts and crimes.

Bianchi's first alternate personality appeared under hypnosis during a forensic psychiatric evaluation in jail after his arrest for the murders. He claimed in retrospect that the alternate had previously appeared at the age of nine during an episode of a beating by his mother. None of his family or friends were aware of any behaviors suggesting multiple personalities. In fact, family, friends, and neighbors were shocked to hear that Bianchi had been arrested for murder, because they had never observed any deviant behavioral patterns in him and considered him a normal, upstanding citizen. He was so good at covering up for his behaviors that even his wife had no idea.

Bianchi's first evaluator, a psychologist who was an expert in multiple personality and child abuse, diagnosed him as having MPD. Apparently one examiner for the defense lacked key pieces of information about Bianchi's history, such as his history of impersonating a psychologist (Coons 1984). Coons (1984, p. 60) reported that Bianchi had "complete access to his psychiatric record so that he could alter his responses according to what he thought the examiners wanted to know." Subsequent evaluation concluded that he had faked the hypnosis and did not have MPD. After his trial, Bianchi reportedly changed some of the testimony bearing on his diagnosis in the trial of his cousin (Coons 1982).

Other diagnoses Bianchi collected included hysteria, antisocial personality, schizophrenia, sexual sadism, epilepsy, tic disorder, phobic disorder, and a variety of dissociative, psychotic, and personality diagnoses. His MMPI profile reflected psychopathic personality and possible latent schizophrenia (Orne et al. 1984).

Bianchi's treatment is unknown, other than hypnosis and psychotherapy coincident to his psychiatric evaluation. At the end of the book, Bianchi's condition was unchanged; he had confessed to his crimes and was sentenced to prison. His cousin was awaiting trial.

Additional information is provided in the book *Two of a Kind: The Hillside Stranglers* (O'Brien 1985). By age 5½ Bianchi exhibited trance-like states with his eyes rolled back. By age 11 he had angry outbursts and was inattentive to his schoolwork. His IQ was tested at 116, but his school performance was "well below his capacity" and he pled illness to avoid school. His school attendance was poor due to "migraine headaches and other afflictions." He tattooed his arm with the message "Satan's Own M.C." He had a poor job history and was always in trouble and being fired, once when marijuana was found in his desk at work. Another time he stole and used stationery from Universal Studios. On his security job he stole clothing, jewelry, and trinkets; because of this he had to change jobs often, but he was never caught. He was arrested for smashing his girlfriend's window. He was described as having an "unhealthy lust for publicity." He always dated several women at once. He was sexually promiscuous; once he failed to pay a prostitute. He drugged a woman, beat and raped a woman, physically injured a woman with anal intercourse, and threatened a woman with dismemberment and death if she quit prostituting for him.

In 1991, a motion picture based on the O'Brien (1985) account of Bianchi's case was aired on network television. The movie depicted an error Bianchi made in his effort to fake hypnosis; the viewers saw the examiner perform the circle-touch test to determine whether his response to a catch-22 instruction was consistent with responses characteristic of bona fide multiples. The audience learned that when the hypnotist touched him inside a circle drawn on his hypnotically anesthetized hand, he was supposed to say that he didn't feel it (his eyes were closed). He didn't say anything when his hand was touched, which was his slip-up.

The Healing of Lia (Ward & Farrelli 1982)

Lia Farrelli's autobiographical account described three personalities. Her psychiatric history was positive for 40 symptoms in 10 categories on the Perley-Guze checklist for Briquet's syndrome, easily qualifying her for the diagnosis. Like the female multiples in the other accounts in this report, she had many conversion (Group 2) and psychiatric (Group 10) symptoms, but unlike the others, she also scored positive for most of the gastrointestinal symptoms. Her conversion symptoms included blindness, paralysis, anesthesia, amnesia, trouble walking, and "distorted vision" with "images upon images." She also reported that her eyebrows fell out and her face became bald.

She underwent multiple surgical procedures including several gynecologic and abdominal operations. These included operations for a "fallen womb" and a hysterectomy. One listing counted a total of 21 surgeries in 23 years, many for gynecologic problems. She reported that at one point she had 22 physicians treating her simultaneously, and she was paying four hospital bills at once. Descriptions of her medical symptoms were graphically florid, such as menstrual pain so severe that she "hung on the furniture and gasped"; her uterine bleeding ("hemorrhaging" and "pouring blood") "bubbled" through layers of diapers and caused her to "actually fall off the commode," rendering her unable to move her right leg. After a wisdom tooth extraction, she bled for 22 days and required "[blood] transfusions in both arms for days at a time." Her doctor was called upon to remove a fecal impaction after she "had not had a normal evacuation for almost one year." Her pains were repeatedly described as "violent," and descriptions included "pain that ripped from my vagina backward into the rectum." Surgical consultants concluded that this pain was the product of her "imagining the whole condition."

Farrelli was given to "fits of rage," and she repeatedly described herself as "full of rage and anger" and bitterness. She was subject to attacks of tantrums resulting in property destruction, "self-abuse" (e.g., head banging during which she felt no pain), and "violent physical confrontation" with her husband, resulting in injuries. Others said she was "too sensitive" and that she overreacted and exaggerated. Her therapists repeatedly noted that she was "extremely suggestible" and easily hypnotized; she was frequently described as "hysterical" and "near-hysteria."

Farrelli reported few childhood behavioral problems, though she did make vague reference to discipline problems in school and was twice expelled for reasons that were a complete mystery to her. As a child she was "belligerent," reportedly had no friends, stuttered, and at age 10 stopped speaking altogether. As an adult, she attempted to choke her second baby to death, which was also the first clearly described appearance of an alternate personality. Although Farrelli joined a charismatic religious group, her husband was a very strict Catholic, which allegedly created sexual difficulties and marital distress escalating to physical fights. Her view of her husband was that "like all men, they just want women for one reason." From her description, it was unclear whether her husband physically and/or sexually abused her.

Farrelli gave no clear description of major family psychopathology, but an "insane" paternal aunt was committed to an institution after attempting to murder her sleeping mother with a butcher knife. Her mother was said to have a "sour disposition." Her paternal relatives were described as "eccentrics" and "haters" who were unable to get along with anyone. There was no description of childhood sexual or physical abuse, aside from her report of psychological neglect by her parents. She described marital tensions, for which she received marital counseling.

Although Farrelli's "hysterical" and polysymptomatic (and polysurgical) history was recognized by her therapist, her primary diagnosis remained MPD. She was said to have received an "incorrect" diagnosis of "hysterical depression." She was noncompliant with appointments. She claimed to have been "addicted" to tranquilizers *and* antidepressant medication for 11 years under the care of physicians. She also received sleeping pills, neuroleptics, narcotics, and barbiturates during her odyssey, as well as shock treatments that reportedly caused permanent memory loss and loss of her ability to read and write. Her primary therapy consisted of "hypnoanalysis." At the end of her story she was reported to be free of multiple personalities, yet still suffering a vague ennui described as follows: "my mental metamorphosis is not yet complete."

We, the Divided Self (Watkins & Johnson 1982)

Rhonda Johnson reported two personalities in addition to her core personality. Her account was coauthored by herself and her therapist. On the Perley-Guze checklist for Briquet's syndrome, there were only 9 symptoms in two categories, and 8 of the 10 symptoms were in Group 10 (psychiatric symptoms). At one point she described visual hallucinations of demons. The account mentioned no childhood conduct disorder behaviors or adult sociopathic symptoms.

Johnson was described as an individual who was "obsessed with pain" and self-destruction. She entertained fantasies of "ugly butchering" and "brutal beatings" of others. "Part of me is a very violent person," she said. From an early age she was considered "hateful and rebellious," defying authority, and disrespectful. A central component of her psychopathology was recurrent acts of self-mutilation and suicidal gestures. These acts included multiple wrist slashings beginning by age 13, cutting various parts of herself with sharp objects, frequent drug overdoses, burning her extremities with cigarette butts, shooting herself with a rifle at age 16, and inserting razor blades into her vagina.

As a child, Johnson had been oversensitive, friendless, and lonely; she had an imaginary playmate. A central theme during her adolescent and young adult development was disturbance in her self-identity: a "good" student versus a rebellious individual with a violent side. She complained to her doctor that she generally felt "empty and lost." The characteristics described in the above paragraphs satisfy at least five criteria of borderline personality disorder, sufficient to qualify her for this diagnosis. Borderline personality disorder was not among the psychiatric diagnoses she received.

There was no clear description of her psychiatric family history other than mention that her mother was nervous and "emotionally unstable." Johnson did not report physical or sexual abuse as a child. Her first alternate appeared at about age 13 in no apparent relation to specific external circumstances, but the timing of this appearance was described as a response to social rejection and loneliness.

Psychiatric diagnoses she received included MPD, hysteria, "dissociated personality," sociopathy, schizophrenia, schizoaffective disorder, manic-depressive psychosis, psychomotor epilepsy, and anorexia. She also was noted to have abused over-the-counter stimulants at age 13. At one point her doctor reflected, "We didn't have a multiple personality any longer; we now had a regressed schizophrenic, lost in the delusions and hallucinations of her childhood." She was treated with psychotherapy, antipsychotic medication, antidepressants, unknown tranquilizers, anticonvulsant medication, and shock treatments. She claimed that the shock treatments rendered her incapable of reading for the next 16 years. In the hospital, Johnson admitted that "there is a part of me that doesn't want to get well," and she hid her medications in her cheek and smuggled in alcohol and recreational drugs. She attacked another patient, attempting to choke her, and she seriously injured a nurse, who required medical hospitalization for several weeks. Due to her intense anger, poor self-control, and assaultiveness, she was occasionally physically restrained. She went through a succession of therapists, including a prominent medical school psychiatrist, without improvement.

At the end of the story, Johnson had "given birth to wholeness" and was continuing to grow through psychotherapy.

Prism: Andrea's World (Bliss & Bliss 1985)

Andrea Biaggi reported 16 personalities. She related that she had seen the movie *Sybil*. On the Perley-Guze checklist for Briquet's syndrome she met 44 criterion symptoms in nine categories, definitely qualifying her for this diagnosis. She acknowledged all 10 psychiatric symptoms in Group 10. Her more florid pseudoneurologic symptoms included paralysis, anesthesia, aphonia, amnesia, hallucinations, trouble walking, stuttering and babbling, loss of depth perception, and legs involuntarily jumping and shaking.

Biaggi was noted to be prone to having "psychosomatic" symptoms, which reportedly ceased when she gained psychological insight. When she complained to her mother of feeling ill at age 13, her mother told her to "go back to work and stop the foolishness." She told people that she had a brain tumor (which was untrue), and she reported that she imagined fevers. She wrote, a "simple cold had become a major illness in my mind"; "nasal congestion . . . became exaggerated into a conviction that I would soon die"; "my experience [was] that doctors never find anything serious at these times." Biaggi was known to be a "frequent visitor to emergency rooms throughout the Boston area." She underwent gastric stapling surgery for obesity and later had the procedure surgically reversed, along with a cholecystectomy. She had "violent reactions" to physical exams, and she required three injections of Valium to tolerate a pelvic exam, during which her "whole body went into spasms."

Biaggi engaged in self-mutilation, including inflicting second- and third-degree burns on herself and inserting objects into her vagina, including safety pins (requiring medical intervention for removal), a coat hanger, and drain cleaner. She was dismissed from her convent for self-mutilating behaviors. Another behavioral problem was binging on food.

Biaggi was described as "immature" and "neurotic", and she complained of "emptiness inside." One of her alternate personalities characteristically enjoyed being the center of attention at parties. As a child she was unpopular and made poor grades, and was sensitive and moody in a Jekyll-Hyde sense. Her behavior was often called "hysterical," and she had spontaneous "hysterical flights into hypnosis" and "hysterical, inarticulate outbursts." The account described behaviors such as "flipping around on the floor, babbling, crying, curling up in a ball," and "ten minutes of wild gyrations and flailing of arms." Once when her doctor went away on vacation, she reported feeling abandoned and "contemplated hurting herself seriously just to show him how much she was suffering." On at least one occasion she spontaneously regressed to infancy for eight hours and urinated in her bed.

Childhood conduct problems included lying, fire setting, and cruelty to animals. She was described as a "very naughty and disobedient child," causing both parents "a lot of trouble." As an adult she exhibited a poor work history, lying, sexual promiscuity, prostitution, physical aggression, recklessness, financial irresponsibility, and vandalism. These behaviors more than qualify her for diagnoses of conduct disorder and antisocial personality disorder. One of her alternate personalities was described as "capable of real violence." When emotionally upset, she killed cats, which was not an infrequent occurrence. Once she assaulted her doctor with a dress pin.

Biaggi's doctor noted that her father had amnestic episodes and suggested that he too might have suffered from MPD. He had been diagnosed as paranoid schizophrenic and was called "incurably insane." However, his history of a poor work record, chronic financial problems, impersonating a doctor, a capacity to be very charming, child abuse and incest, lying, fighting, wife beating, threatening the lives of others, and alcoholism suggest antisocial personality disorder and substance abuse problems. He was not helped by shock treatments and insulin therapy. Biaggi's sister, who was raped as a child by their father, had temper outbursts and episodes of being "violent and abusive to anyone who got in her way"; she also reported that she believed the Mafia was after her. Three brothers were said to have serious potential for violence; two were alcoholic, and the third was reported to be "troubled" and to have a "ruined" personal life. Biaggi's maternal grandfather committed suicide.

Biaggi came from a family with a tradition of incest going back to her paternal grandfather, who reportedly served time in prison on charges of incest with his daughter. Biaggi's father, who was sexually abused himself, sexually abused Biaggi and her sisters. Biaggi reported that her father put a burning torch up her vagina. She was also sexually abused by an uncle and by multiple non-family members. Biaggi reported that she was physically abused by her mother, who bloodied her nose—"there was a lot of blood." As an adult, Biaggi wandered around at night, picking up men who would brutalize her. Biaggi stated that her first alternate personalities developed when she was four years old to protect her from her sexually abusive father. One of her personalities was a lesbian.

Besides MPD, Biaggi received diagnoses of hysteria, dissociation, psychosis, undifferentiated schizophrenia, acute depression, borderline personality, anxiety neurosis, and temporal lobe epilepsy. She also abused alcohol and used hallucinogenic drugs. Treatment involved a "plethora of drugs" including anti-convulsant medication, major and minor tranquilizers, sedatives, antidepressants, and unidentified pills. She was also restrained in a straitjacket. Two different physicians recommended that she have a lobotomy, and she said that she came very close to consenting to the procedure.

Psychotherapy and hypnosis were the mainstay of Biaggi's psychological treatment. She reported that she had "enough therapists by now to staff a hospital." Her psychiatrist reported that she was "a spectacular hypnotic subject, one of the best he'd ever seen." He reportedly enjoyed working with MPD patients, likening this work to "live theater, part magic," which made him feel "like an ancient thaumaturge, using 'incantations and spells' to cure the sick," sometimes with only "two hours to cure." She had three-hour therapy sessions twice a week. At the end of Biaggi's book, she was not cured but was "stabilized," with some remaining psychological problems that were not clearly specified.

Biaggi was a keynote speaker at a conference in New York City and elicited a standing ovation.

Shatter (Clark & Roth 1986)

Kathy Roth developed eight separate personalities. She reported that she had read about Billy Milligan's 24 personalities in *Penthouse* magazine. Roth's Perley-Guze checklist was positive for 48 symptoms in nine categories, qualifying her for the diagnosis of Briquet's syndrome. Her pseudoneurologic symptoms included paralysis, anesthesia, blindness, aphonia, amnesia, hallucinations, itching all over outside and inside, being unable to discern men from women, being unable to recognize her own reflection in a mirror, being unable to read coins, and losing the ability to read. Her surgical history consisted only of a cosmetic breast reduction procedure, but she had also requested cosmetic surgery on her nose as a present for her 16th birthday.

Her symptoms were presented dramatically; for example, her headaches were described as follows: "her head was going to split open," "the top of her head felt like it was about to explode," and "her head felt as though a bomb had gone off, the pain was so severe." Her doctor admonished her: "Don't be so dramatic about it" when she complained of physical symptoms and he also asked her, "Will you look at me instead of closing your eyes and getting dramatic?" She was frequently described in the book as being "near hysteria," "almost hysterical," "having hysterics," and "sobbing hysterically." She described uncontrollable mood swings with episodes where she "felt as though she was on the brink of a volcano, and that the only solution was to give into the fire, to throw herself over the edge," and "I feel like a blender inside." Once she dramatically "dashed out of the door and collapsed on [her therapist's] threshold."

A central issue of Roth's life in her account was her conflict over her sexuality. She maintained that she did not like men, saying that they "are only after one thing and they're bastards"; "I *hate* men! I want to cut their balls off!" When her husband approached her sexually, she cried, " 'No, don't!'. . . she began sobbing, her breath coming in heaves. She was hysterical, kicking and hitting and weeping. . . . 'A typical man,' she snorted silently. All he wants to do is fuck." The last 50 pages of the book build to a very dramatic climax as her therapy turns to focus on sexual issues. During a therapeutic massage session that was a key component of her therapy, as the masseuse began to rub her thighs she reportedly started bleeding spontaneously from her vagina; simultaneously she had a flashback to a childhood sexual abuse trauma, reliving a rape scene.

Roth reported cutting her arms with a razor blade. She complained of a chronic "terrible emptiness inside," boredom, and loneliness. She reported that she often felt abandoned and rejected by her doctor—for example, when he went away on vacation. She was also described as being frequently "seductive" to her physician. At a therapy session during one of her emotional writhing episodes, her skirt rode up and exposed her thighs almost to the waist. In one such episode, she reportedly "sobbed, twisting and turning on the sofa, wringing her hands together."

The only symptom of conduct disorder or antisocial personality reported by Roth was lying, and possibly sexual promiscuity. Roth claimed that she had ESP and parapsychology experiences such as clairvoyance, as well as reincarnation experiences and the ability to remember events that happened centuries ago.

Roth's maternal grandfather had committed suicide. Otherwise, Roth did not describe any history of psychiatric problems in family members aside from a brief mention of conduct problems and obesity in her daughter. Roth may have been physically abused by her mother, and her father sexually abused her and "raped" her with an ice pick; she was also sexually abused by nonrelatives. Her first personality was created at an unknown age during her childhood as an effort to help her behave well, which she thought was necessary to keep her mother from abandoning her.

Roth first came to psychiatric attention at age 15. The only formal diagnosis applied to Roth was MPD. He doctor suggested that she might be "a hysteric" but then discounted this diagnosis, saying that half of her female peers were hysterics. He also suggested that she might just be "a spoiled brat . . . coming here for attention," another idea that he rejected. He also speculated that her MPD syndrome might be covering an underlying schizophrenic condition, although she was never diagnosed as schizophrenic.

Roth expressed a persistent worry: "I'm scared I'm a phony. I want to be real." She later came to believe that her "splitting is a copout of responsibility." Her doctor explained, "Multiple and manipulate are the same thing."

For her pain complaints Roth was given narcotic analgesics; she also described "living on aspirin every three hours." She did not mention any use of psychotropic medication other than sleeping pills. Treatment was primarily psychotherapy in conjunction with therapeutic massage.

At the end of the book, it appeared that Roth's personalities were either fused or at least in the process of fusing. A note at the end of the book informed the reader that "After continuing her therapy, working toward successfully fusing the personalities, Kathy Roth began her education to become a psychotherapist. There, she hopes she will be able to use her unique personal experience in helping others."

When Rabbit Howls (Chase 1987)

Elsewhere Eve has reported that Truddi Chase attended one of her public lectures about MPD (Sizemore 1989). Chase also reported that she had seen the movie *Sybil* some time after she had been diagnosed with MPD ("Oprah Winfrey Show," August 27, 1991).

Chase and her 92 personalities reported 29 somatoform symptoms in eight categories on the Perley-Guze checklist, making her a likely candidate for a diagnosis of Briquet's syndrome. Sexual and other female reproductive symptoms were generally not mentioned, which is consistent with the lack of mention of these symptoms in Eve's and Sybil's accounts. Chase apparently had an aversion to sex and was unable to utter words associated with sexual function. If this were not the case, she would probably qualify for the diagnosis of Briquet's syndrome. Her overall description of her physical problems, however, suggests that she may well have the disorder:

> ". . . things got so bad that I was treated for Premenstrual Syndrome. The same doctor who had delivered Page [her daughter] prescribed Valium and when that

didn't work, he gave me Librium. The tests seemed to go on forever. I'd never seen so many doctors and needles and pills. No illness was found. But before it was over, they tested me for epilepsy and even though the tests were negative, Dilantin was prescribed. It's supposed to slow the rush of blood through your head. It didn't work. I couldn't stop being a bitch to Norman—that's my ex-husband; I couldn't stop feeling dizzy, or just blacking out.

Chase's somatoform symptoms tended to fall most heavily into the psychiatric (Group 10) and conversion (Group 2) categories. Her conversion symptoms included blindness, anesthesia, amnesia for her entire childhood, hallucinations of snakes, trouble walking, forgetting her name, and forgetting how to drive an automobile.

Chase was described as "hysterical," overdramatic, and prone to "wide emotional swings" and "uncontrollable tantrums." The writing style of her autobiographical account was overdramatic, vague, and circumstantial (consistent with the style of speech said to be characteristic of patients with somatization disorder [American Psychiatric Association 1987, p. 261]), and it contained an overabundance of superlatives.

Chase reported childhood conduct problems of stealing, running away, biting her teacher, and drowning cats, sufficient to qualify her for a diagnosis of conduct disorder. She did not mention any adult sociopathic behaviors.

Chase's maternal grandmother reportedly stole and may have abused alcohol. Her biologic family was not described in sufficient pertinent detail to allow determination of any particular psychiatric syndrome. Her mother beat her and burned her hand. Her stepfather repeatedly raped and sodomized her, beginning at age two. He played a "game" in which he lowered her into a well and threw in live snakes on top of her. The stepfather was violent and severely beat Chase's brother. Their mother had to hold him off with a rifle.

Due to the vagueness of the writing style, it is difficult to ascertain the exact occasion of the initial appearance of Chase's alternate personalities. From the therapist's comments in the book's introduction, it appears that the multiples may have first appeared when Chase was two years old, to protect her from the experience of physical and sexual abuse by her stepfather. Chase reported receiving punishment during her childhood for the acts of her alternate personalities, claiming no knowledge of her behaviors.

The only psychiatric diagnosis Chase received was MPD, as her first mental health contact was with the therapist who made the diagnosis. Of note, an earlier neurologic evaluation ruled out a seizure disorder, though in spite of this she was treated with Dilantin, and the specific symptoms precipitating this evaluation and treatment were not mentioned. She was also treated for premenstrual syndrome, though the symptoms related to this consultation were not described. Her psychiatric treatment consisted primarily of intensive psychotherapy and hypnosis. At one point, she was medicated with benzodiazepines including diazepam and chlordiazepoxide. By the end of her book Chase had not fused her personalities, but had instead resigned herself to living with them and remaining in therapy, aimed at continued "growth and exploration." Chase's therapist accompanied her on a publicity tour for her book. In 1991 a made-for-television miniseries based on her story was aired, and she appeared on the nationally televised "Oprah Winfrey Show" with her therapist.

Voices (LaCalle 1987)

Christopher Kincaid reported eight personalities. He had read the book *Sybil*. On the Perley-Guze checklist for Briquet's syndrome he had 20 symptoms in seven categories, suggestive of the disorder but short of diagnostic. He was noted to have many "psychosomatic" symptoms. His conversion symptoms were amnesia and hallucinations.

Kincaid was described as "attention-seeking," "theatrical," and having a "dramatic nature." He was chronically lonely, "helpless," very passive, and "overly sensitive." It was said that he "structured his relationships to capture attention and motivate people to please him or rescue him"; and "like the coy and provocative hysterical female, Christopher had a quality that said, 'I am a frail and fragile person and I am at your mercy'." He was "in a constant search for gratification of his needs for affection and attention," and "no lover was ever capable of giving him the self-worth he needed."

Kincaid reported feeling that he had a manipulative side, "the whole thing [seeming] so unreal that he fears he must be making it up." At one point his psychologist began to disbelieve his MPD symptomatology, suspecting that he was just conning her. In the hospital he was described as "demanding too many special favors" and creating general turmoil on the ward. Kincaid reported that he was bothered by "homicidal revenge feelings" and that he felt he could be violent. He had a female personality who carved on her arms and "slashed her wrists just to watch the blood flow."

Kincaid reported six positive criteria for a diagnosis of conduct disorder as a child. These behaviors included breaking and entering, stealing, arson, sexual assault on a minor, and physical cruelty to people. He wet the bed until he was 11 years of age. He went on to exhibit seven adult sociopathic behaviors, including sexual molestation of young boys (having formed a boys' club to provide him access to boys), physical aggression, recklessness, conning others, and sexual promiscuity. He reported that he participated in voodoo, black magic, and idol worship.

The account of Kincaid's story, written by his psychologist, was also an account of this psychologist's own struggle with this patient and his problems. It is a story of an intense patient-therapist relationship with strong countertransference of the female psychologist toward her male patient. Persons around her suggested therapist overinvolvement, which evolved to the point where it began to threaten her marriage and her professional standing. This patient became very dependent on her, and she provided lavish attention to him in the form of four-hour therapy sessions, daily therapy, and time otherwise devoted to her personal and family life and holidays.

Kincaid's family history was positive for alcoholism and probable socio-pathy in his father, and descriptions of his mother are compatible with Briquet's syndrome and possible depression with some evidence of sociopathy. His mother, a cocktail waitress, had many illnesses, "aches and pains" through the years, and severe depression. Her husband raped her and beat her until she feared for her life. Kincaid's mother neglected him and finally abandoned her children in the middle of the night. Her life was unfulfilling, and she was "fanatical in her religious beliefs." Kincaid reported that he was physically and sexually abused by his father, and his personalities had developed in an effort to cope with the incest. Kincaid said he was also sexually abused by nonrelatives. Kin-caid's stepfather went to jail for sexually abusing Kincaid's sister.

Aside from Kincaid's known history of drug and alcohol abuse, his only official psychiatric diagnosis was MPD. He was also described as having ego-dystonic homosexuality and a schizoid personality. The only treatment men-tioned in the account was psychotherapy, and he was said to be "easily hypno-tized." Kincaid's condition apparently improved, and upon termination of treatment he developed a social relationship with his therapist. His lover died of AIDS, as reported at the end of the book.

The overall tone of the writing in this book was overdramatic, with frequent references to the therapist's own problems, including frequent crying episodes during therapy with Kincaid, several somatic complaints including nausea, a lump in her throat, insomnia, and a history of hysterectomy.

Nightmare (Peterson & Gooch/Freeman 1987)

Nancy Lynn Gooch reported 56 different personalities. She had read the book *Sybil*. Gooch's book was authored by a professional writer "as told to" by the patient and her "therapist," who was her creative writing teacher.

Gooch had 32 somatoform symptoms in nine categories on the Perley-Guze checklist, meeting full criteria for the diagnosis of Briquet's syndrome. She re-ported all 10 possible psychiatric symptoms in Group 10. She also described a number of conversion symptoms, including blindness, paralysis, anesthesia, aphonia, amnesia, and deafness. She had frequent fugues that began at age seven.

Gooch's surgical history was not described, but the account did mention a two-year period prior to her 16th birthday when she had been "in and out of hospitals for physical problems," which the doctors said was "strange for some-one [her] age." She claimed that when she got upset she bled from stomach ulcers, but it is not clear how closely related this symptom might have been to her ethanol abuse and her habit of swallowing caustic substances such as rust remover and ammonia-based household cleaning solutions. Psychological symptoms were sometimes presented dramatically: "I feel like I can't hold my head together. It's going to explode and everything is going to smash to smithereens"; "I think my brain is bleeding because if I am sad, or cry, I throw up blood"; "I slowly cut both wrists. I watched the blood spurt almost to the bushes."

Gooch reported considerable difficulty with loneliness by age 15 or earlier, and her fear of being alone continued to be a problem for her throughout the rest of her account. Temporary departures of significant persons in her life were interpreted as abandonment and caused her to "regress to . . . self destructive behavior in protest." She had chronic problems with low self-esteem. When she felt depressed or frustrated she would bang her head on a wall, refuse to eat, starve herself, burn herself, and drink caustic substances. She made several suicidal gestures, by cutting her wrists and by ingesting overdoses and toxic substances. Once she called her therapist 'anonymously" to tell her that "someone" (herself) had overdosed and where; she was dutifully rescued. With these behaviors, she met all criteria for borderline personality disorder.

Little is described of her early childhood. According to Gooch, her IQ was tested as 166 in seventh grade, but later testing at a clinic produced an IQ score of 128. At age 15, Gooch joined a gang that was engaged in dealing drugs and was allegedly affiliated with the Mafia. She sneaked out at night from her mother's house to be with the gang. Although Gooch threatened to run away from home, she did not describe actually doing so. She sold drugs for money, and a urine test was positive for heroin. She became sexually promiscuous and was irresponsible about birth control, considering herself lucky that she did not get pregnant. She also engaged in prostitution. It appears that all these behaviors had occurred by her 15th year. Insufficient criterion symptoms are reported, however, to make a diagnosis of conduct disorder.

As an adult, Gooch continued to engage in prostitution and dealing drugs. She abused uppers, downers, speed, angel dust, heroin, and anything she could get her hands on. One of her personalities stole to support her drug habit. She worked as a go-go dancer at a strip bar. Some of her personalities threw temper tantrums and destroyed property. One of her personalities set fires and burned down an abandoned house. Another personality took part in street fights. Gooch was involved in the gang-related murder of a friend, who was reportedly the first and perhaps the only "boy" she had ever loved.

Gooch got into several dangerous situations. The Mafia was said to have a $10,000 price on her head for her alleged role as a police informant. She described being kidnapped from a park and raped at knifepoint at the age of 15. A customer with whom she was engaging in prostitution tried to sodomize her, and when she resisted he stabbed her in the chest. Another time a bar customer with whom she had accepted a ride kidnapped her and attempted to rape her.

Little detail of Gooch's family history was presented. Her paternal grand-father was reportedly alcoholic. Her maternal grandmother married five times; one of the husbands beat her, and one of them also physically abused himself and threatened to sexually abuse his daughter (Gooch's mother). The grand-mother had emotionally abused Gooch's mother. Gooch's stepfather was de-scribed as alcoholic, a playboy, and a charmer.

Gooch first came to psychiatric attention as a child when she entered psy-chotherapy for "bleeding ulcers." As a high school sophomore she had a "fugue" and was taken to a psychiatric ward in a straitjacket. She was hospital-ized a number of times and escaped on at least three occasions, once slitting both her wrists while on elopement. She was treated by a "well known psychiatrist," an expert in fugue states. The first official appearance of her alternate person-alities was to him and some guests at a tea party where she had been taken by her therapist so that these people could see a live case of multiple personality. New personalities always announced themselves upon emergence, for example:

1. "Her first words were, 'I am not Nancy. I am Sarah'."
2. "One late afternoon Nancy/John walked into my empty classroom . . . [and] told me who it was."
3. "Hello, I'm Laureal.". . . I greeted her, "I'm glad to meet you, Laureal."

Gooch was also treated by multiple personality expert Dr. Cornelia Wilbur and her understudy, with no apparent improvement.

Although Gooch's primary diagnosis was MPD, her condition was com-pared to "the symptoms of a psychotic," and her multiple personality defense system was though to "protect her from the more severe disintegration of autism or schizophrenia." Aside from her polysubstance abuse, no other psychiatric diagnoses were mentioned in her account.

After reading Steven King's book *The Shining*, Gooch uncovered a buried memory of having been the victim of repeated satanic sexual abuse rituals by a babysitter for over two years that had commenced when she was two years old. Her first personality had reportedly surfaced during this period. The author claims that "To this day when Nancy recalls the scenes with [her abuser] she starts to bleed." Gooch had a personality named "Promise" who needed Gooch's blood "for rituals." Gooch recalled that more personalities had emerged when she was six years old during a period of sexual abuse by strangers who repeatedly lured her into their house for milk and cookies and presents when she was six. Her parents were unaware of either of the abusive situations in her childhood.

According to Gooch's account, her personalities were specifically created to perform functions otherwise unacceptable to her: "People who lived within her and came out at certain times to perform acts the 'core' personality, as Nancy was called, would never dare." "That's why she needed them, so they would do the drug-taking for her"; "each [personality] is connected with a wish of Nancy's so intense and threatening she could not consciously face it." The thrust of her therapy was to help her learn that "she no longer needed [the personalities], she could take responsibility for her own feelings, control her own dangerous impulses."

Gooch received considerable notoriety for her psychiatric disorder. National and foreign presses carried newspaper articles about her story. She also appeared on the "Oprah Winfrey Show" in 1986, along with multiple personality authority Dr. Bennett G. Braun.

Treatment included chlorpromazine and other medications for relief of complaints of depression and low energy, but her primary treatment consisted of hypnotherapy and individual and group psychotherapy. Her creative writing teacher, who had elected herself to function as a parent figure as well as a "therapist" for her, had studied hypnotherapy to help Gooch. "Intensive" therapy sessions frequently lasted for up to eight hours. Gooch's "therapist" also disciplined her by physical means such as slapping and spanking to aid in controlling the personalities. A couple Gooch lived with who functioned as "foster" parents learned narcotherapy, which they administered to her. A well-known drug addict and alcoholic, Gooch was also treated for substance abuse.

Near the end of the book, Gooch was not well but was making significant progress in therapy: "Nancy can now head toward becoming a whole self, not needing to split into personalities." Gooch related yearnings to be involved in the mental health field, saying, "Someday I'd like to be a mental health counselor and help people in trouble." Her "therapist"-friend disclosed that "Both Nancy and I dream of starting a clinic for the emotionally deprived."

My Father's House: A Memoir of Incest and Healing (Fraser 1988)

Sylvia Fraser reported three personalities, and she attributed her MPD to the experience of chronic sexual abuse by her father. Overall she reported 26 somatoform symptoms in seven categories, failing to qualify for the diagnosis of Briquet's syndrome only due to an insufficient number of positive categories. She had many conversion symptoms, including spells of paralysis, anesthesia, aphonia, pseudoseizures, inability to close her mouth, and hallucinations of snakes. Fraser's surgical history consisted of a hysterectomy performed for complaints of pain in her womb, and fibroids were found on operation.

Fraser is the author of at least four published novels. Her writing skill may have honed and softened some of her more graphic somatoform symptoms into a more palatable form for the general reader. Her overall writing style, however, was flowery and overdramatic. Her use of italics to set off certain sections consisting of a mix of fantasies, memories, and dreams obfuscated the symptom picture. An example of her writing style in her autobiographical account follows:

> . . . A demon-monster raped her here many years ago by stuffing a giant white larva down her throat. Now it has lodged in her womb, threatening her life. I fetch a priest. . . . Inside the girl's womb the priest finds a fetus, half-human half-animal. He holds it up by one cleft foot. "See Satan's child.". . . It is apelike, about three times human size and covered in shaggy fur.

Also:

> Spasms pass through me, powerful, involuntary—my pelvis contracts, leaving my legs limp. My shoulders scrunch up to my ears, my arms press against my sides with the wrists flung out like chicken wings, my head bends back so far I fear my neck will snap, my jaws open wider than possible and I start to gag and sob, unable to close my mouth—lockjaw in reverse. . . .

Fraser's account was frequently punctuated with the word "hysteria"; for example, she described herself as "near hysteria," having "hysterical weeping," and "slipping down the slimy slope into hysteria." After writing the first draft of the manuscript for this book she said, "Now I have a manuscript over two thousand pages written in the first person hysterical." A critic of one of her novels was quoted as saying, "Your book is typical of the kind of hysterical imaginings we're seeing too much of these days." Fraser's descriptions indeed have a histrionic tone and somatizing flair, for example: "A scream of grief had lodged permanently in my chest. It expanded inside me with the insistence of hemorrhaging blood."

As a child, Fraser was said by her teacher to be mean and to have a chip on her shoulder; her mother complained to her, "you think only of yourself." Fraser described herself as a "bad child," "a hostile little girl, a furious teenager and a frequently bad-tempered adult." Other than these vague references to oppositional behaviors, the only specific conduct problem mentioned was lying. In adolescence she engaged in severe dieting and burning her arms with cigarettes (but didn't feel it). As a young adult, she earned money as a fortune-teller, only privately admitting that her act was a con. She once hit her lover with a champagne glass. Aside from these behaviors, she did not provide sufficient detail in other vague references to deviant behaviors to classify her as having antisocial personality disorder.

Fraser's struggle to deal with her sexuality was a central theme in her account, and the book perseverated on sexual issues. Fraser described her four previously published four novels as each being "rife with sexual violence that offended some critics and puzzled me."

Fraser did not describe her family's psychiatric history other than to mention that her father had an incestuous relationship with his aunt, and that her maternal grandfather and a maternal aunt had committed suicide. Her father also had an incestuous relationship with his sister. Fraser's husband was an excessive drinker. Fraser reported that she first split into personalities at the age of seven in direct response to repeated sexual abuse by her father. She learned of the alternate personalities by herself, without any indication of assistance from a therapist.

Although Fraser consulted a hypnotherapist for her problems, no mention of any psychiatric diagnosis was made. At one point she admitted she was abusing alcohol. Fraser also sought relief from her symptoms via primal therapy, massage therapy, rolfing, bioenergetics, yoga, and meditation. At the end of her account she had succeeded, after a dramatic struggle, in forgiving her father. She no longer mentioned the alternate personalities.

Katherine, It's Time (Castle and Bechtel 1989)

Kit Castle reported that she had eight personalities. She was very knowledgeable about medical and psychiatric information, which she had gained through extensive reading of medical texts. Castle's doctor reported that "she displayed knowledge of internal medicine and psychiatry that was astounding," and "she had the working knowledge of about a fourth-year medical student." "She knew the DSM-III . . . backward and forward. She probably knew it better than most mental health professionals." She had named her two cats Skinner and Freud. One of her personalities, a male adolescent character named Jess, aspired to a career in internal medicine and was also considering becoming a psychiatrist.

On the Perley-Guze checklist for Briquet's syndrome, Castle acknowledged 54 symptoms in 10 categories, more symptoms reported than by any other subject in this review of book-length accounts. Her symptoms clustered most heavily in the conversion (Group 2) and psychiatric (Group 10) groups. She reported all 10 criterion psychiatric symptoms. Her more dramatic conversion symptoms included anesthesia, seizures, paralysis, amnesia, hallucinations, trouble walking, loss of control of her bowels and bladder, uncontrollable shaking of an arm and a leg, falling out of bed, double vision, slurred speech, and seeing an earthquake in a store. Her symptoms were described quite dramatically: "Her guts were exploding—a poisonous mushroom cloud was just blowing it all apart, everything, all of it. The whole thing was coming violently undone."

Castle's story was remarkable for her "very long and complicated medical history, involving multiple admissions to hospitals and neurologic wards all over the country." Her complex medical history was summarized in the following paragraphs describing her physician's thoughts about her problems:

> She'd endured enough medical tests to support a small hospital—since last sum-mer, hardly a week had gone by that Liz Castle was not in his office, or in the hospital for one reason or another. Yet still she was plagued by the strangest array of symptoms he'd ever seen—wave upon wave, like assault troops: disturbing neu-rological problems, seizures, weird rashes on her face and hands, crippling abdom-inal pains, neck pain, hallucinations, blackouts.
>
> She'd suddenly develop crippling back pain, and then lose control of her bladder and bowels. He'd rush her to the hospital for a CT scan of the lumbar spine, it would show nothing out of the ordinary—and then the problem would spontaneously resolve. This kind of thing happened over and over. Ghosts! For months, he felt as if he'd been chasing ghosts!
>
> One by one, tests had ruled out nearly every disease syndrome he could think of: lupus erythematosus, multiple sclerosis, endometriosis, rare enzyme disorders.

Castle was described as "a grasping hypochondriac" who "felt comfortable being an invalid." The authors wrote, "If there was any way she could have become a professional patient, she would have. She fed on sympathy." She racked up hospital bills of $60,000 or $80,000 in one year. It was said that "she got CAT scans like other people would go out to dinner." According to the account, "a new medical problem would surface roughly every 21 days" with "increasingly bizarre physical symptoms." At one point Castle admitted that there was no medical reason for her to be in the hospital. Her doctor said to her, "Are you aware that whenever we try to deal with difficult material, you start talking about your medical problems?"

Castle was described as "flirtatious" and moody, her moods swinging to opposite extremes from day to day. She was described as "filling up with hu-miliation and self-pity, drowning in it, reveling in it." She was said to have "a world-class talent for evading the truth," and "she lived in a hysteria of fear and denial." She was also described as having "hungered for the old drama of the spotlight." As a hospital inpatient she refused to take her medication, got drunk on gate pass, threw things, and had tantrums. A nurse accused her of "faking pain just to get drugs."

Castle reported just one behavior problem in childhood: lying. As an adult, however, she displayed eight criterion antisocial symptoms. Her antisocial be-haviors included property destruction, homelessness and wanderlust, child ne-glect, physical aggression, poor work history, sexual promiscuity, arrest for "loud and lascivious behavior on a public stage" while employed as a stripper, financial irresponsibility, lying, bigamy, writing "bad checks [that] started flying in every direction," and impersonating a physician. The rich sociopathic profile of her adult life, along with the deprived and neglected childhood she described, suggest that there may have been other childhood conduct symptoms not mentioned in her account. It is likely that she had antisocial personality disorder as well as Briquet's syndrome.

Castle made up stories, such as telling her boyfriend and other people that she had a brain tumor and was dying. After her husband threw her out of the house, she started a new life for herself, making up an elaborate story that he and the children had been tragically killed in a horrible motor vehicle accident. Subsequently she encountered a highway automobile accident and helped the victims, who were seriously injured. By successfully impersonating a physician, she persuaded the hospital to release to her the coroner's photos of the grossly mangled bodies of the deceased. She subsequently produced these photos as evidence whenever she recounted her story of the accident that she said killed her husband and children.

The favorite subject of one of her personalities was "astral travel, UFO's, and life after death." She claimed to have metaphysical experiences, ESP, psychokinesis, and visitations by poltergeists.

Castle came from a chaotic family background, reporting that as a child she endured family fights, having to sleep in taverns and cars with her family when they were homeless, and that she suffered parental neglect. Her father was described as having extreme mood swings and "rages" during which he smelled bad; he also abused her mother. Castle said that her father had sex with her and prostituted her at the age of five, and that a nonrelative sexually abused her. She also said her parents beat her and gave her black eyes, causing her to miss school. Her father tied her to a tree like a dog and left her all night. He also tied her up and beat her with a coat hanger, fractured her finger, and split her lip. Castle reported that her first alternate personality had developed at the age of 18 months to help her handle her fear of being alone.

Castle's doctor stated that he did not wish to apply a psychiatric diagnosis to her case because he felt this "would detract from rather than enhance our understanding of this very special story." He wrote, however, that "The case could (and most certainly will) be made that Kit's behavior represented the histrionics of a gifted patient with multiple personality disorder." Other diagnoses applied to Castle included psychomotor seizure disorder, no seizure disorder, schizophrenia, "schizomanic psychosis," premenstrual syndrome, borderline personality disorder, personality disorder with hysterical features, hysteria, globus syndrome, Munchausen's syndrome, and "malingering" ("a charade").

Treatment included anticonvulsant medication, benzodiazepines, neck surgery (which "did not put an end to her problems. Not by a long shot"), and both residential treatment for alcoholism and Alcoholics Anonymous. She obtained psychotherapy, resulting in successful fusion of her personalities at the end of the book. A note at the end of the book said, "Kit Castle is now living a private life and pursuing her own personal adventure." Her therapist, however, reported that just before her book was published, she developed a new wave of alternate personalities.

Her doctor was later angered to discover that she had apparently plagiarized material from a children's book as the basis of for her own symptom content. Castle denied ever having read this book, but it was later determined that one of her alternate personalities might have read it, unknown to Castle herself due to "source amnesia."

Suffer the Child (Spencer 1989)

Jenny Walters Harris' book was authored by a professional writer who is also a pediatric nurse with a master's degree and who functioned as Harris' "primary support person." The author was involved in Harris' therapy almost from the beginning. In the five years of her therapy Harris reportedly revealed more than 400 personalities, but the exact number was not specified. According to Sizemore in a foreward to the book (p. xii), this is the first known full-length account describing a case of MPD resulting from cult practices.

Harris had 32 somatoform symptoms in 10 categories on the Perley-Guze checklist, giving her a definite diagnosis of Briquet's syndrome. She acknowledged most of the psychiatric symptoms in Group 10. Her conversion symptoms included anesthesia, aphonia, amnesia, and hallucinations. She had a variety of visual hallucinations, including snakes, faces, and a little man. She was also treated for numerous pain complaints, including pain in her back, arm, leg, and neck, for which no physical cause could be determined despite numerous medical workups. Little mention was made of sexual functions or of menstrual symptoms directly, although she "seemed to be sick the whole time" during pregnancy.

Harris was chronically ill, and over her husband's vocal objections (he was a member of a strict fundamentalist religion and did not believe in doctors), she had extensive contact with the medical profession. She had "examinations, X-rays, consultants called in, but few physical causes for her problems could be found." She was hospitalized 27 times in 20 years, most commonly for urologic and gynecologic problems and for psychiatric episodes. The hospital bills caused chronic financial strains on her family. One hospital admission for treatment of a vaginal infection culminated in transfer to a psychiatric ward. Her husband noted that she liked being in the hospital too much, and "he made no secret that he thought most of the time she wasn't really sick."

Harris underwent numerous surgical procedures, including a hysterectomy to relieve vaginal bleeding, surgery for bladder dysfunction, and an operation for pelvic relaxation syndrome. Following a bilateral carpel tunnel repair, she purposely tore open her incisions. She inflicted caustic burns on her urethra and perineum with drain cleaner while recuperating from gynecologic surgery in the hospital.

Just as Harris' mother had drunk turpentine to try to kill her in the womb, Harris drank turpentine when she learned of her own unwanted pregnancy. Once Harris consumed rat poison reportedly in an effort to prevent obesity; she also ingested rat poison on other occasions for unknown reasons. She suffered from chronic low self-esteem and displayed "expressions of self hate." She purposely cut and burned herself but reported that she could not feel the pain. She made numerous suicide threats and gestures, beginning at age 12.

As a child Harris was described as "difficult" and "strange." She banged her head and bit herself until she bled; from time to time, she cut herself. She also clawed at her eyes and set her hair on fire. She was described as "sensitive," "sullen," "withdrawn," and a loner. She was constantly teased and ridiculed by her classmates. As she grew older, she became moody and unpredictable and displayed "unbelievable self-centeredness." As an adult, she and her personalities exhibited temper outbursts and sucked her thumb, in addition to other "childish behavior."

Harris stated that from childhood she had overwhelming identity disturbances, feeling that she did not know who she really was. In fact, she said she did not even feel human. She interpreted her interpersonal experiences in "childhood absolutes." In eighth grade she was observed to be attention seeking, and she "wanted badly to be special." Friends moving away precipitated feelings of abandonment and "heartbreak," and her reaction was to vow "never to trust anyone again." She complained of fear of being alone. She was described as "constantly searching for love and constantly doubting love."

As a young child, Harris tortured and killed animals, lied, sassed her Sunday school teacher, didn't pay attention in class at school, and was not willing to apply herself to her studies. She had "prolonged absences" from school for unclear reasons. In fourth grade she exposed her well-developed breasts to her schoolmates. Beginning in at least eighth grade she was frequently seductive to and flirtatious with men, including a number of pastors and therapists, resulting in sexual intercourse with one pastor and with a psychiatrist treating her as an inpatient. In ninth grade, Harris' only girlfriend had the reputation of being "loose, fast, [and a] whore." Harris married at the age of 15 and promptly quit school.

In ninth grade (or earlier), Harris was voluntarily abusing alcohol and street drugs. Specifically mentioned substances of abuse were "bennies," "acid," Everclear, "illegal booze," and "whatever she could get," which included intravenous heroin. She mixed alcohol and illicit drugs with her psychotropic medications. She developed a high physical tolerance for psychoactive substances. To support her habit, she became a drug dealer. She also engaged in prostitution. She went through a series of jobs, but "none of them suited her."

Even as an adult Harris went on rampages, broke things, and put her fists through windows. She hit and bit a therapist. She and her husband were frequent participants in reckless auto races on city streets, with no concern for safety or the possibility of arrest. She was unfaithful to her husband, and she frequently lied to him about her whereabouts and the men she was with in the daytime while he was at work. Once she walked out on him.

Little is known of Harris' father. He refused to marry Harris' mother, though he did voluntarily contribute regular child support. Her mother was "excitable" and "hysterical" and had a short temper. She was constantly sickly, stayed in bed, and feared she would die. Her sickly conditions included chronic severe headaches, nosebleeds, dizziness, weakness, "sinking spells," memory loss, and depression. She was a physical and sexual abuser of children to the worst degree, according to Harris. The mother had also been sexually abused by her own brothers for many years. Harris had a cousin who abused alcohol and drugs and who physically and sexually abused children; he was probably also antisocial. One uncle was a child sexual abuser. A son suffered from hyperactivity.

Harris' mother had started prostituting her to the mother's boyfriends and other men when Harris was seven. When Harris was nine, her sociopathic cousin forced sex and drugs on her. She was raped by a cousin and by an uncle. Harris reported that her mother physically and sexually abused her.

Harris' account contained horrible, often gruesome descriptions of abuses she suffered. The mother beat her, locked her in a potato box with rats that bit her, chained her to a post in the basement, locked her out of the house for hours in the dark, cold, rain, and snow, bathed her in blood, bathed her in both icy and scalding water, and nearly drowned her by holding her upside down underwater in a deeply flooded road. The mother stabbed her in the vagina with a knife, shocked her inside the vagina with an electrical instrument, touched her eye with the end of a whirring drill, and forced the child to watch her mother urinate into a cup, which she then made the child drink.

The mother made her participate in satanic cult activities beginning at age two. This entailed more gruesome and brutal abuse, including rape of the little girl, beginning at age five, by the "high priest," who also put his dagger in her vagina; she underwent ritual beatings and was forced to cut her arms with a dagger and to burn herself with coals. At age 10 she "became the devil's bride." Harris thought she recalled that at the age of 12 she had a baby that she gave to the cult, and it was killed, although she was not certain of this. She was also ordered to kill. On one occasion, she was tied naked in a doorway while several men jammed an opened-out coat hanger into her vagina.

Harris reported that many children took part in this ritual abuse with adult members of their families. In addition, these children reportedly suffered placement of live snakes in all orifices, forced bestiality followed by killing of the animals and requiring the children to eat the carcasses, and forcing them to eat live human flesh thinly cut from ankles and wrists. One snowy night, Harris and "more children than she could count" were tied naked with spread legs to crosses and their hands nailed to the crosses. More than one therapist had trouble believing her stories.

Harris' personalities first began when she was three years old, according to her recollection. They were created to help her cope with the abuse and to escape from physical and emotional pain. Her therapist reported, "By refusing to acknowledge alters as parts of herself, she could avoid accountability for their actions." Many of these were not complete personalities but were "fragments." One of her alternate personalities had its own set of multiple personalities. Other personalities included two witches, a high priest with horns, "a powerful demon with no skin, bloody flesh, horns, cloven hooves, and hair on face, chest, and back," and an "ugly male creature, three feet tall, with one big distorted eye, a long nose, and horns." At the front of Harris' book was an appendix describing 35 of her alternate personalities. Each one had a special purpose, such as for anger or fear, for cult participation, to prostitute, to drink and take drugs, to engage in self-abuse, or to play with her child alternates.

As an adult Harris was very interested in the occult, read extensively about it, collected objects related to the occult, and practiced spells and rituals to conjure up demons. She resumed her prior involvement in the cult. A preacher came to perform an exorcism on her, and he saw "legions of demons encircling her house and lining her driveway." Harris also attended Pentecostal services and spoke in tongues.

Harris first received psychiatric attention at age 14, when she wrote a note at school saying that she was afraid of going crazy. At that point she was hospitalized for the first of many times, receiving a tentative diagnosis of "schizophrenic reaction," and later in her hospital stay the diagnosis of "dissociative reaction." Other diagnostic assessments she received included schizophrenia, drug and alcohol abuse, "depressive neurosis," "acute brain syndrome, confusion . . . with a schizophrenic basis," "schizophrenic reaction, paranoid type," "chronic undifferentiated schizophrenia," borderline personality disorder, possible "inadequate personality," learning disabilities, and a "long list of diagnoses." An evaluation at a center nationally recognized for specializing in MPD described her as "a very disturbed individual who copes with stress through dissociation and multiplicity in the context of an underlying schizophrenic disorder." Her therapist explained to her that "there is a tendency to confuse multiple personality with split personality, a term applied to schizophrenia."

During her most recent hospital stay, she reported that she "liked the hospital and wished she could remain beyond the thirty days insurance coverage allowed." On the ward she met other multiples who reported that they had been abused in satanic cults, as she claimed she had been. Harris was often noted to be extremely manipulative ("she was a master at manipulating") and to require "unlimited attention" from therapists: "It's a bit like having thirty hysterical women have your phone number," as one therapist described it. "As much time as they gave her, whatever resources they found for her, she seemed to need more."

Therapy was not easy: "Her therapy was the most demanding they had ever encountered" and her "need to continue to exploit every available resource from ministers to medical doctors to mental health workers served to scatter energies and frustrate [her therapists'] efforts." She was well known to engage in recurrent "behavior patterns of calling pastors and faking overdose and periods of depression." She was chronically suicidal: "The threat of suicide was constant. . . . The common practice for clients to be hospitalized when they experienced suicidal ideation did not fit for Jenny. It would have meant almost continuous hospitalization."

Treatments received by Harris included antipsychotic agents (which she felt made her symptoms worse), unknown pills and injections, electroconvulsive therapy, physical restraint, psychotherapy with "prolonged daily sessions," hypnosis, relaxation therapy, chiropractic treatment, a TENS unit, services of a pain rehabilitation clinic, and a partial hospitalization program.

After meeting national experts in the field of multiple personality, her therapists reported that "validation by a professional colleague . . . helped to counter the effects of three years of feeling ostracized, or at least being considered mavericks by their peers." Harris wrote, "I hope someday that people will understand us, and that doctors and Mental Health will not be against us and abuse us anymore."

Toward the end of the book, Harris was integrating her personalities through intensive therapy, yet she still had considerable progress to make. Her progress had started suddenly after meeting ex-patient Chris Sizemore of *The Three Faces of Eve*. Harris enrolled in a psychology course, and despite continuing symptoms and another hospitalization, she achieved a grade of A. Her therapists were unable to "gauge how much more time will be needed for Jenny to achieve full integration."

The Flock: The Autobiography of a Multiple Personality (Casey 1991)

Joan Frances Casey reported 24 personalities whom she called "the Flock." Casey had read *Sybil* and had seen excerpts of the movie based on that book. She had apparently read extensively on MPD and seemed to have some knowledge of medical and psychiatric terminology. Her writing periodically used words like "narcissistic," "abreaction," and "ataxic gait."

Casey included in her autobiography excerpts of notes from sessions with her therapist. Much of the story was told from the point of view of one of her alternate personalities. Casey appeared to be a relatively high-functioning multiple. She was said to have a high IQ. She was a high school teacher and was working on a master's degree in political science. In her graduate school classes, however, she complained that she had no friends.

Casey described a number of features suggestive of Briquet's syndrome, although she did not describe enough specific symptoms for a diagnosis (17 symptoms in five categories). She reported that as a child her mother knew "there isn't anything wrong with me. There never is. . . . My mother is a lab technician. She spends her time helping sick people who really need her." As an adult, when Casey's physician informed her that he could find no medical explanation for her symptoms, she wrote, "'I know there's nothing wrong with me . . . there's never anything wrong with me.' Her mother's words— 'You're wasting the doctor's time'—echoed through her mind." Another time she expected her doctor to tell her mother that she was pretending to be sick. As a school child, Casey had considerable contact with the school nurse, and apparently many times a year the nurse hugged Casey while she sobbed.

In high school Casey had a series of three week-long hospitalizations for a "mysterious" and "suspicious" condition that left "neurologists, neurosurgeons, ear, nose, and throat specialists, and her internist puzzled over the symptoms and the test results." She had trouble walking (which she called "ataxia"), headaches, and confusion, and could not follow a light with her eyes. A psychologist who examined her called her "hysterical" and "depressed," and a neurologist felt she had "a factor of hysteria" in her symptoms. A neurosurgeon thought she might have a brain tumor or allergic encephalitis. Despite lack of physical evidence of an operable brain lesion, she "came close to undergoing brain surgery," for which her parents refused consent. Casey wrote, "The hospitalizations protected her from having to deal with the aspects of her parents' separation that she least liked."

Casey had many occasions when she either expected people to say that she was feining illness or when she herself said that she was pretending. Casey spent many pages of the book describing how she told her therapist she was pretending, that she "had been playing that game to release pressure and had deceived her into thinking I had multiple personalities," while the therapist countered with persistent arguments to the patient that she had MPD. For some time, the author frequently returned to that theme. She said she even hated the therapist for allowing her "play-acting" to continue.

Casey did not mention any surgical procedures. Although she never alluded to female trouble or a hysterectomy, she had no children of her own and eventually adopted a child.

Casey had a number of borderline and histrionic personality characteristics and qualified for a diagnosis of borderline personality disorder. She had rages and was described as "volatile." At one point she described her alternate personalities as feeling hysterical. She carved a symbol of death into her breast. She purposefully hurled herself off gymnastics equipment ("in a swan dive from the top bar to the floor"), causing herself injury. On various occasions she threw herself through a glass door, dived at a wall, banged her head on a wall, and scratched her wrist with a razor blade. Once she reported that the scratches on her wrists were made to get people to "pay attention to her and her pain." On another occasion she told her therapist that she had urges to leap to her death from a window in order to get her husband to come back to her. She said, "I don't want to die . . . but I guess I wouldn't mind if I got hurt a little. So Keith would understand how much I need him." She had frequent crises and suicidal ideations, and considered committing suicide on her father's grave. People said she "had a flair for the dramatic."

Reading the book *Sybil* made her "feel empty and aching." She needed constant reassurance that her roommate liked her, and she desired to be loved by her therapist. She struggled with issues of abandonment and rejection by her therapist, with whom she had an explosive and tempestuous relationship. She also had major abandonment issues in her relationship with her mother, and worried that people would care for her for only short periods and then abandon her.

As a child, Casey was described as "too sensitive." At the age of 9 she was picked on by other girls at school, and at age 10 she contemplated jumping out of a window. Many people called her a liar. Her parents said she was very impressionable, moody, and suggestible. She had tantrums during which she flung herself at a wall. In high school she cultivated relationships with her teachers, especially her (male) psychology teacher, her lesbian physical education teacher, and her (female) geometry teacher. She spent considerable time outside of school with these teachers. She said the reason she had thrown herself off the gymnastics equipment was to get her gym teacher's attention. She also had vivid sexual fantasies about this teacher, which she attributed to a lesbian personality. When her geometry teacher married and moved to Mexico, Casey felt abandoned and was terribly hurt. Her psychology teacher (who had just been discharged from a locked psychiatric ward after one of many hospitalizations) took sexual advantage of her, first getting her drunk and then soothing her with hypnotic relaxation techniques and having sex with her before she realized what was going on. These experiences all occurred around the time of her mysterious neurologic illness.

As an adult, Casey admitted to lying, sexual promiscuity, assault (kicking her therapist and cracking two ribs), and being sexually seductive to her therapist's husband.

Casey painted her parents in a very negative light but did not provide any other family history. She said her father provoked brawls in bars and stole money during the brawls, engaged in breaking and entering for purposes of robbery, stole a horse, participated in wild car chases, cavorted with wild women, treated women as objects, and got drunk in every port in the Navy. Casey's mother never knew her own biologic father, had grown up with succession of stepfathers, and was abused by her mother's boyfriends. The mother aspired to join a convent but was turned down twice by the religious order. There is some evidence that Casey's mother may have had Briquet's syndrome; she threw up during all nine months of her pregnancy with Casey, and Casey remarked that her mother had a huge collection of pharmaceutical samples—"enough sample bottles so that we'd [all the personalities] be able to medicate ourselves for years."

Casey's mother worked in the medical office where Casey's health records were stored, and Casey alleged that her mother destroyed them. Casey's mother physically abused her. Her father molested her from a very young age and raped her when she was 12. A paternal aunt was also sexually molested by Casey's paternal grandfather.

Casey's parents had wanted her to be a boy, and her mother allegedly hoped that she would die when she was born a girl. For the first few years of Casey's life, her parents dressed her and treated her like a boy. It was during this period, before the author was a year old, that she recalls her first alternate personality splitting off (and her therapist was "amazed at the completeness of some memories of early childhood").

Casey collected a number of psychiatric diagnoses, at one time or another having been called passive-aggressive, depressed, schizoid, psychotic, and "hysterical." Casey also abused multiple drugs, including LSD, mescaline, and cannabis, beginning before age 15 and continuing heavily through high school.

Casey had a long treatment history, starting with a succession of eight therapists. After one of the therapists told her she was passive-aggressive, Casey reported, "I growled at her when I left." Her pattern was to see therapists for three or four visits at most and then move on. She preferred male therapists. Describing her behavior toward one of them, she wrote, "I grinned, letting my eyes convey that I thought he was sexy." She quit seeing this therapist because "he didn't ask me out, even though I made it clear that I was interested, so I never went back."

The therapist who was instrumental in her recovery was the one who provided the excerpts of her records for the book. This therapist was initially "both intrigued and overwhelmed" by Casey. It was not long before Casey became "quite dependent on evening phone calls," and then she wanted to see her therapist outside the office, which ensued. Eventually the therapist began to keep her therapy notes in private, because she felt threatened by her supervisor and by colleagues who expressed concern about the amount of attention she was giving this one patient. Colleagues said the patient was manipulating her. The therapist reacted defensively to her colleagues after she learned that some of them "didn't believe in MPD."

Even though Casey's therapist knew she was becoming dependent on her, she persisted with the pattern they had already established and her "unorthodox treatment techniques." The therapist and her husband engaged in "parenting" Casey, spending "an average of four hours a day with the Flock, not much of it in anything that looks like in-office psychotherapy. But it is therapeutic nonetheless." The therapist wrote, "It's hard being 'on-call' twenty-four hours a day."

Casey spent weekends with her therapist and her husband at their weekend cottage, and she subsequently lived with them for an entire summer. She became "a family" with them. Many times the therapist had doubts about having taken on the challenge of this "concentrated time" to "work through the pathology" of her patient in this way. Casey had "an endless thirst for parenting" and her therapist called it "a drain." The therapist described problems with the patient's "clinging dependency" and "endless recriminations and dissection of 'our relationship'," which was at times explosive.

It was pointed out to Casey by her boyfriend that she was much better psychologically before she started therapy. Indeed, during the first six months of her therapy the personalities gained considerable control, and for some time the patient's problem "seemed worse, with personalities further apart and acting out more vigorously now than we had been before beginning therapy."

Casey eventually made great improvements in therapy and went to Harvard for graduate school (with the Flock that was still with her). She did well academically but started to feel stressed and developed psychosomatic complaints. Casey subsequently had a number of suicidal crises and sought treatment. A series of three psychiatrists did not work out because they found her manipulative and set firm limits on her behavior within the therapeutic setting, and one found her "dramatic changes hard to believe." Casey continued to be intermittently depressed and suicidal; the Flock persisted, and she maintained contact with her primary therapist at long distance.

Casey's boyfriend told her that he refused to marry her because she was a multiple. At that pivotal point the Flock suddenly began to fuse, a process that was not quite finished over a period of a year. The relationship with the boyfriend did not work out, but Casey was integrated. Things were far from perfect, though. She said, "I was integrated, but far from 'healthy'."

Casey subsequently went through a series of relationships with male partners who were physically abusive to her, alcoholic, drug abusers, and "a con man" who stole her money "to support his habit and his mistress." Casey called these "disastrous relationships. I found abusers and provoked them . . . making myself a deserving victim." A year of "more traditional therapy" with a psychiatrist who "hadn't had much experience with multiples" helped her with her problems with men. Casey finally entered a healthy marriage and adopted a son.

Tragically, Casey's therapist died suddenly with her husband in a boating accident after Casey's apparent recovery near the end of the book.

Appendix B
Summary Tables of Book-Length Accounts of MPD

Table B-1 Checklist for Briquet's Syndrome

Account

Eve: Account #: 1.+ 2.* 3.X 4.^

Criteria Symptoms	Beauchamp	Eve	Sybil	Mrs. G	Hawksworth	Peters	Milligan	Bianchi	Farrelli	Johnson	Biaggi	Roth	Chase	Kincaid	Gooch	Fraser	Castle	Harris
Group 1: headaches	X	+#X^*	X	X	X			X††	X		X	X	X	X	X		X	X
sickly	X	#X	X				X	X†	X	X	X		X		X		X	X
Group 2: blindness	X	+#X^*	X	X					X			X	X		X	X		
paralysis	X	X	X								X	X			X	X	X	
anesthesia	X	X^*	X	X		X			X		X	X	X			X	X	X
aphonia	X	X^*	X						X		X	X			X	X	X	X
fits/convulsions		#	X	X	X	X	X	X†									X	X
unconsciousness		+#X	X	X	X	X	X									X		X
amnesia	X	+#X^*	X	X	X	X	X	X	X	X	X	X	X	X	X	X	X	X
deafness	X	X	X				X								X			
hallucinations	X	+#X^*	X	X	X	X	X	X	X	X	X	X	X	X	X	X	X	X

Symptom																	
urinary retention	X															X	
trouble walking	X	X	X												X	X	
other conversion (number)	15	5/4/5/2*	9	6	1	1	11	2	0	4	2	2	6	3	2	11	2
Group 3: fatigue	#*	#*	X	X					X	X	X	X		X	X	X	X
lump in throat		X	X						X					X	X		
fainting	X	+#X					X				X		X	X	X	X	
visual blurring		X		X	X	X	X			X							
weakness		#X^	X	X					X	X	X		X	X	X	X	
dysuria															X	X	
Group 4: breathing difficulty		X		X					X	X	X	X		X	X	X	X
palpitations	X								X	X					X	X	
anxiety attacks		X^		X					X	X	X	X			X	X	X
chest pain			X						X	X		X		X	X	X	
dizziness		#^	X		X		X		X	X	X	X	X	X	X	X	
Group 5: anorexia	X	#X	X	X						X	X					X	
weight loss		#^*	X						X	X	X		X		X	X	
marked weight fluctuation		X^*		X					X	X							X
nausea	X	#X		X	X	X	X		X	X	X	X	X	X	X	X	X

Table B-1 Checklist for Briquet's Syndrome (cont.)

Account

Eve: Account #: 1. + 2. # 3. X 4. ^

Criteria Symptoms	Harris	Castle	Fraser	Gooch	Kincaid	Chase	Roth	Biaggi	Johnson	Farrelli	Bianchi	Milligan	Peters	Hawksworth	Mrs. G	Sybil	Eve	Beauchamp
abdominal bloating									X									
food intolerances																		
diarrhea									X									
constipation																		
Group 6: abdominal pain	X	X	X	X	X		X	X	X			X		X				
vomiting	X	X	X	X	X		X	X	X			X	—	X			#^	
Group 7: dysmenorrhea			X		—				X				—		X			
irregular menses					—								—					
amenorrhea		X			—								—					
excessive bleeding	X				—				X				—	X				
Group 8: sexual indifference	X	X		X		X	X	X				X					+#X	
frigidity				X			X		X			X					+#X^	
dyspareunia				X					X					X				

	0/0/0/1	1			1	3	2	2	3	2	2	2	3	3	2	2	3
other sexual differences (number)	X							X			X						X	X
hyperemesis gravidarum																		
Group 9: back pain	X	^*	X								X						X	X
joint pain		^*									X						X	X
extremity pain	X	X^*						X			X						X	X
burning sex organs/mouth/rectum													X					
other pain (number)	2		1	1			3	1	3		1	5	1	3	2		3	2
Group 10: nervousness	X	#X^*	X	X		X	X	X	X	X	X	X	X	X	X	X	X	X
fears	X	#X^*	X	X	X		X	X	X	X	X	X	X	X	X	X	X	X
depressed feelings	X	+X^*	X	X	X		X	X	X	X	X	X	X	X	X	X	X	X
sick: disrupt duties	X	X	X				X		X		X	X	X	X	X	X	X	X
crying easily		+#X^	X						X		X	X	X	X	X	X	X	X
hopelessness	X		X				X				X	X	X		X		X	
think about dying	X	#X^*	X						X	X	X	X	X	X	X	X	X	X
want to die	X	#X^*	X			X	X		X	X	X	X	X	X	X	X	X	X
think of suicide	X	+#X	X			X	X	X†††	X	X	X	X	X	X	X	X	X	X
suicide attempts	X	+#X^	X	X	X	X	X	X	X	X	X		X	X	X	X	X	X
No. of positive symptoms	41	17/28/35/26 Com-bined: 52**	39	31	8	10	31	10	40	9	44	48	29	20	32	26	54	32

Table B-1 Checklist for Briquet's Syndrome (cont.)

Criteria Symptoms	Beauchamp	Eve Account #: 1.+ 2.# 3.X 4.^	Sybil	Mrs. G	Hawksworth	Peters	Milligan	Bianchi	Farrelli	Johnson	Biaggi	Roth	Chase	Kincaid	Gooch	Fraser	Castle	Harris
No. of positive categories:	7	5/8/8/10 Combined: 10	9	9	9	3	4	7	3	10	2	9	9	8	7	9	7	10
Can make diagnosis?	Prob	No/ Prob/ Prob/ Yes Comb: Yes	Yes	Yes	Yes	No	No	Prob	No	Yes	No	Yes	Yes	Prob	Poss	Yes	Prob	Yes	Yes

+ -Three Faces; # -Final Face; X-I'm Eve; ^-Mind of My Own.

*Symptom was still present in her final book after her successful integration.

**16 symptoms in 6 categories were still present in her final book after her successful integration.

†Watkins 1984.

††Orne et al. 1984.

†††O'Brien 1985.

Table B-2 Criteria for Somatization Disorder

Account

Legend — Eve: Account #: 1.+ 2.# 3.X 4.^

Criteria Symptoms	Beauchamp	Sybil	Mrs. G	Hawksworth	Peters	Milligan	Bianchi	Farrelli	Johnson	Biaggi	Roth	Chase	Kincaid	Gooch	Fraser	Castle	Harris
Gastrointestinal:																	
** 1. vomiting		#^	X			X		X		X	X			X	X	X	X
2. abdominal pain			X					X		X	X			X	X	X	X
3. nausea	X	#X	X		X			X		X	X	X		X	X	X	X
4. bloating								X									
5. diarrhea								X									
6. food intolerances																	
Pain:																	
** 7. extremity		X^*								X	X					X	X
8. back pain	X	^*	X	X						X	X					X	X
9. joint pain		^*									X	X				X	X
10. dysuria																X	

Table B-2 Criteria for Somatization Disorder (cont.)

Account

Eve: Account #: 1.+ 2.# 3.X 4.^

Criteria Symptoms	Beauchamp	Eve	Sybil	Mrs. G	Hawksworth	Peters	Milligan	Bianchi	Farrelli	Johnson	Biaggi	Roth	Chase	Kincaid	Gooch	Fraser	Castle	Harris
11. other pain	X	X		X	X					X	X	X	X	X			X	X
Cardiopulmonary																		
**12. shortness of breath		X		X	X							X	X		X	X	X	X
13. palpitations	X												X				X	
14. chest pain					X							X	X			X	X	
15. dizziness		#^		X			X	X		X		X	X	X	X	X	X	
Conversion/ pseudoneurologic:																		
**16. amnesia	X	+#X^		X	X	X	X	X	X	X	X	X	X	X	X	X		X
**17. difficulty swallowing			X	X									X				X	
18. loss of voice	X	X*	X*									X	X		X	X	X	X
19. deafness	X	X					X								X			

Symptom																	
20. double vision						X	X				X							
21. blurred vision	X	+#X^*	X	X	X	X	X				X			X		X	X	X
22. blindness	X	+#X^*	X		X		X	X		X		X		X		X	X	
23. fainting/loss of consciousness	X	+#X	X		X	X	X					X		X			X	X
24. seizure/convulsion		#	X	X	X		X	X	X†			X				X	X	X
25. trouble walking	X	X	X						X				X	X		X	X	
26. paralysis/muscle weakness	X	#X^	X		X		X	X	X		X	X		X	X	X	X	
27. urinary difficulty		X	X					X	X†		X							
Sexual:																		
**28. burning sex organs/rectum													X					X
29. sexual indifference		+#X			X		X	X		X	X	X	X	X		X	X	X
30. dyspareunia			X								X		X					
31. impotence		+#X^			X	X	X	X	X		X	X						
Female reproductive:																		
**32. dysmenorrhea			X	—	—	X	—	X	X		X				X			
33. irregular menses				—	—	—	—	—	—						—			
34. excessive bleeding			X	—	—	X	X	X	—		X				—			X

†Watkins 1984.

*Symptom was still present in her final book after integration.

Table B-2 *Criteria for Somatization Disorder (cont.)*

Account

Criteria Symptoms	Harris	Castle	Fraser	Gooch	Kincaid	Chase	Roth	Biaggi	Johnson	Farrelli	Bianchi	Milligan	Peters	Hawksworth	Mrs. G	Sybil	Eve: Account #: 1.⁺ 2.# 3.X 4.^	Beauchamp
35. vomiting throughout pregnancy					—					—	—		—					
≥ 13 symptoms (#)	Yes (13)	Yes (20)	No (12)	Yes (13)	No (4)	No (9)	Yes (18)	Yes (14)	No (1)	Yes (17)	No (3)	No (8)	No (5)	No (4)	No (12)	No (11)	No (5) / No (10) / Yes (14) / No (11) / Combined: Yes (20)	No (11)
Can make diagnosis?	Yes	Yes	Prob	Yes	No	Poss	Yes	Yes	No	Yes	No	Poss	No	No	Prob	Poss	Poss	Poss
No. of positive screening items	5	5	4	4	2	1	5	4	1	3	1	2	1	1	3	3	1/2/3/3	1

⁺ - Three Faces; # - Final Face; X - I'm Eve; ^ - Mind of My Own.

*Symptom still present after successful integration.

**Screening items: ≥ 2 suggests a high likelihood of the disorder (American Psychiatric Association 1987, pp. 263–264).

†Orne et al. 1984.

Table B-3 Checklist for Conduct Disorder (CD) and Antisocial Personality Disorder (ASP)

		3 Faces(#)/ Final Face(+)/ I'm Eve(X)/ Mind of My	Account															
Criterion Symptoms	Beauchamp	Own(^)	Sybil	Mrs. G.	Hawksworth	Peters	Milligan	Bianchi	Farrelli	Johnson	Biaggi	Roth	Chase	Kincaid	Gooch	Fraser	Castle	Harris
Conduct disorder: ≥3 behaviors <age 15 (number)	No (2)	No/Yes/Yes/No (0)/(5)/(5)/(0) Overall: Yes(5)	No (2)	Yes (6)	Yes (8)	Yes (8)	Yes (7)	Yes (4)	No (0)	No (1)	Yes (3)	No (0)	Yes (4)	Yes (6)	No (0)	No (1)	No (1)	Yes (4)
1. stole twice, nonconfronting		+X	X	X	X	X							X	X				X
2. runaway twice or permanently	X*		X	X	X	X	X											
3. lying		+X	X	X	X	X	X	X			X		X			X	X	X
4. fire setting			X								X			X				
5. truancy	X		X	X	X	X												
6. breaking in					X	X								X				
7. property destruction		+X			X	X	X	X			X							
8. cruelty to animals		+X					X				X		X	X				X
9. rape/sexual assault							X							X				
10. weapon in fight twice				X		X	X											
11. initiates fights				X	X	X	X	X						X				

Table B-3 Checklist for Conduct Disorder (CD) and Antisocial Personality Disorder (ASP) (cont.)

3 Faces(#)/Final Face(+)/I'm Eve(X)/Mind of My Own(^)

Criterion Symptoms	Beauchamp		Sybil	Mrs. G.	Hawksworth	Peters	Milligan	Bianchi	Farrelli	Johnson	Biaggi	Roth	Chase	Kincaid	Gooch	Fraser	Castle	Harris
																		Account
12. stole, confronting																		
13. physically cruel to people	+X		X	X	X	X	X	X					X	X				X
Antisocial personality disorder:																		
≥ 4 behaviors ≥ age 15: (number)	No (3)	No/Yes/No/No (2)/(7)/(1)/(4) Overall: Yes(8)	No (2)	Yes (8)	Yes (9)	Yes (6)	Yes (7)	Yes (7)	No (2)	No (1)	Yes (7)	No (1)	No (0)	Yes (7)	Yes (5)	No (2)	Yes (8)	Yes (6)
1. inconsistent employment	+		X	X	X		X	X			X			X		X	X	X
2. illegal activities/arrests	+^		X	X	X	X	X	X			X			X	X		X	X
3. irritable and aggressive/abuse	#+X^		X	X	X	X	X	X	X	X	X			X	X	X	X	X

4. financial problems/nonsupport	X	+		X		X	X	X		X		X		X		X	X
5. impulsive/ wanderlust/ homeless			X			X								X		X	
6. lying/alias/ conning	X	#+^	X	X	X	X	X		X	X	X	X	X		X	X	X
7. reckless			X X	X X	X		X		X	X		X				X	X
8. irresponsi- ble parent		+	X	X	X			X								X	
9. sexual promiscuity		`	X	X	X	X	X**			X		X	X	X		X	X
10. lacks re- morse		+	X	X	X	X	X							X		X	X
Diagnosis:	None	CD/ASP	None CD/ASP	CD/ ASP	CD/ ASP	CD/ ASP	CD/ ASP	None	None	CD/ ASP	None CD	CD/ ASP	Poss. ASP	None	Prob. ASP	CD/ ASP

*Elsewhere it has been reported that she ran away at age 16 and never came back (Prince 1920).

**Orne et al. 1984.

Table B-4 *Psychiatric Diagnoses Made from Symptoms Described in Accounts*

Account	Briquet's Syndrome	Conduct Disorder	Antisocial Personality	Substance Abuse
			Diagnosis	
Beauchamp	Probable (41/7)	No (2)	No (3)	No
Eve	Yes (52/10)	Yes (5)	Yes (8)	Yes
Sybil	Yes (39/9)	No (2)	No (2)	(iatrogenic)
Mrs. G.	Yes (31/9)	Yes (6)	Yes (8)	Yes
Hawksworth	No (8/3)	Yes (8)	Yes (9)	Yes
Peters	No (10/4)	Yes (8)	Yes (6)	Yes
Milligan	Probable (31/7)	Yes (7)	Yes (7)	Yes
Bianchi	No (10/3)	Yes (4)	Yes (7)	No
Farrelli	Yes (40/10)	No (0)	No (2)	(iatrogenic)
Johnson*	No (9/2)	No (1)	No (1)	No
Biaggi	Yes (44/9)	Yes (3)	Yes (7)	Yes
Roth	Yes (48/9)	No (0)	No (1)	Probable
Chase	Probable (29/8)	Yes (4)	No (0)	No
Kincaid	Possible (20/7)	Yes (6)	Yes (7)	Yes
Gooch*	Yes (32/9)	No (0)	Possible (5)	Yes
Fraser	Probable (26/7)	No (1)	No (2)	Yes
Castle	Yes (54/10)	No (1)	Probable (8)	Yes
Harris	Yes (32/10)	Yes (4)	Yes (6)	Yes

*Meets DSM-III-R criteria for borderline personality disorder.

Table B-5 Family Psychiatric History

	Diagnosis						Other Information		Child Abuse:**	
Case	Multiple Personality	Briquet's Syndrome	Antisocial Personality	Schizophrenia	Affective Disorder	Psychosis	Substance Abuse	Suicide	Sexual	Physical
Beauchamp			?F*, ?pGF							
Eve	uncle, cousin	M, mGM	?M, ?F		?M		F, mGF		M, F	M
Sybil		?M, ?mAunt, others	?F/?M	?M, ?mAunt ?pSide						
Mrs. G			F, bro, ?pGF, ?females				F	F	2 uncles, bro, GF, NR	M
Hawksworth	F, ?M		F, ?pGM			?M	M, ?F			F
Peters			F, ?M, bro	?M			bro, F, M	?M	F, bro	F, M, NR
Milligan			?F, ?M		F		M, F, stepF	F	stepF	M, stepF
Bianchi		?Adopt.M	?F, ?M, cousin		?Adopt.M		M, bro		?Adopt.M	Adopt.M
Farrelli						?pAunt				
Johnson										
Biaggi	?F		F, ?3bros, ?pGF	?F		?sis	F, 2bros	mGF	F, uncle, NRs	F, M
Roth									NR	?M
Chase			?mGF				?mGF	mGF	stepF	M, stepF
Kincaid	?M	?M	F		M		F		F, NRs	F

Table B-5 Family Psychiatric History (cont.)

| | Diagnosis | | | | | | Other Information | | Child Abuse.** | |
Case	Multiple Personality	Briquet's Syndrome	Antisocial Personality	Schizophrenia	Affective Disorder	Psychosis	Substance Abuse	Suicide	Sexual	Physical
Gooch			?stepF				pGF, stepF			
Fraser								mGF, mAunt	F, NR	
Castle			.?F						F, NR	F, M
Harris†	?M	?M	?M, cousin, ?uncle		?M		cousin		M, cousin, uncle, NR, cult	M, cult

**Experienced by the patient as a child.

†Hyperactive son.

Abbreviations: M = mother; F = father; sis = sister; bro = brother; GM = grandmother; GF = grandfather; stepF = stepfather; m = maternal; p = paternal; NR = nonrelative; Adopt. = adoptive.

Table B-6 Psychiatric Diagnoses Applied to Cases

Case	Diagnosis							
	Multiple Personality	Hysteria	Antisocial Personality	Schizophrenia	Affective Disorder	Alcohol Abuse	Drug Abuse/ Dependence	Other
Beauchamp	Yes	Yes						neurasthenia
Eve	Yes	Yes, No	Yes	Yes	Yes			neurasthenia
Sybil	Yes	Yes					Yes*	kleptomania, pseudocyesis, hysterical dissociation
Mrs. G	Yes	Yes	Yes	Yes	Yes	Yes	Yes	
Hawksworth	Yes	Yes	Yes		Yes	Yes		
Peters	Yes				Yes	Yes	Yes	normal
Milligan	Yes, No, Possible	Yes	Yes	Yes, No	Yes	Yes	Yes	conversion reaction, passive-aggressive, dissociative disorder, psychoneurotic anxiety
Bianchi	Yes, No, Possible	Yes**	Yes	Yes				sexual deviation disorder, sexual sadism, dissociative reaction, delusional psychotic, insane, somatization, petit mal epilepsy, tic disorder, phobic disorder, mild neurosis**, conscious faking, mixed personality disorder, unstable personality, narcissism

Table B-6 *Psychiatric Diagnoses Applied to Cases (cont.)*

					Diagnosis			
Case	*Multiple Personality*	*Hysteria*	*Antisocial Personality*	*Schizophrenia*	*Affective Disorder*	*Alcohol Abuse*	*Drug Abuse/ Dependence*	*Other*
Farrelli	Yes	Yes			Yes		Yes*	psychomotor epilepsy, psychosis, schizoaffective disorder, dissociated personality, anorexia
Johnson	Yes	Yes	Yes	Yes	Yes			
Biaggi	Yes	Yes		Yes	Yes			dissociation, psychotic episodes, character disorder, borderline personality, anxiety neurosis, temporal lobe epilepsy, ?brain tumor
Roth	Yes	Yes						
Chase	Yes							premenstrual syndrome
Kincaid	Yes					Yes	Yes	egodystonic homosexuality, dissociative disorder, schizoid personality, malingering
Gooch	Yes			Yes				
Fraser								psychotic

Castle	Yes	Yes	?Yes		personality disorder with hysterical features, borderline personality, psychomotor seizure disorder, no seizure disorder, globus syndrome, rule out premenstrual syndrome, malingering, Munchausen's syndrome
Harris	Yes		Yes	Yes	schizophrenic reaction, dissociative reaction, depressive neurosis, acute brain syndrome, character disorder, borderline personality disorder, inadequate personality, learning disabilities

*Iatrogenic only.
**Watkins 1984.

Table B-7 Treatment Received by Cases

	Case																	
Treatment	Beauchamp	Eve	Sybil	Mrs. G.	Hawksworth	Peters	Milligan	Bianchi	Farrelli	Johnson	Biaggi	Roth	Chase	Kincaid	Gooch	Fraser	Castle	Harris
Psychotherapy/hypnosis	X	X	X	X	X	X	X	X	X	X	X	X	X	X	X	X	X	X
Antipsychotics		X	X		X				X	X	X				X			X
Antidepressants		X					X		X	X	X				X			
Lithium				X														
Amphetamines		X	X	X								X						
"Tranquilizers"		X	X		X				X	X	X	X						
Sleeping Pills		X	X	X	X				X									
Narcotics	X								X						X			
Benzodiazepines										X	X	X	X				X	
Barbiturates			X	X					X	X	X						X	
Anticonvulsant										X	X						X	
Substance abuse treatment			X	X	X		X			X			X					
Vitamins/tonic		X							X	X								
Shock treatments			X						X	X								X
Other	chiropractic treatment, relaxation, reparenting therapy		Alcoholics Anonymous*		group therapy		group therapy		"marriage encounter"		physical restraint, straitjacket*	massage therapy			strait-jacket, slapping, group therapy	primal therapy, massage therapy, rolfing, bioenergetics, yoga, meditation, halfway house for alcoholics	Alcoholics Anonymous	physical restraint, relaxation therapy, chiropractic treatment, transcutaneous electrical nerve stimulator (TENS), pain rehabilitation program, partial hospitalization

*Recommended lobotomy.

References

Abse DW. Multiple personality, in Roy A (ed): *Hysteria*. New York, Wiley, 1982, pp 165–184.

Abse DW. *Hysteria and Related Mental Disorders,* ed 2. Bristol, England, IOP Publishing, 1987.

Adityanjee, Raju GSP, Khandelwal SK. Current status of multiple personality disorder in India. *Am J Psychiatry* 146:1607–1610, 1989.

Akiskal HS. Subaffective disorders: Dysthymic, cyclothymic and bipolar II disorders in the "borderline" realm. *Psychiatr Clin North Am* 4(1):25–46, 1981.

Akiskal HG, Chen SE, Davis GC, et al. Borderline: An adjective in search of a noun. *J Clin Psychiatry* 46:41–48, 1985.

Aldridge-Morris R. *Multiple Personality: An Exercise in Deception.* London, Erlbaum, 1989.

Alexander VK. A case study of multiple personality. *J Abnorm Soc Psychol* 52:272–276, 1956.

Allison RB. A guide to parents: How to raise your daughters to have multiple personalities. *Fam Ther* 1:83–88, 1974a.

Allison RB. A new treatment approach for multiple personalities. *Am J Clin Hypn* 17:15–32, 1974b.

Allison RB. Multiple personality and criminal behavior. *Am J Forensic Psychiatry* 2:32–38, 1981.

Allison RB. The multiple personality defendant in court. *Am J Forensic Psychiatry* 3:181–192, 1982.

Allison RB, Schwarz T. *Minds in Many Pieces.* New York, Rawson, Wade, 1980.

Ament A. Rape and multiple personality disorder (letter). *Am J Psychiatry* 144:541, 1987.

American Psychiatric Association. *Diagnostic and Statistical Manual of Mental Disorders,* ed 2. Washington, D.C., American Psychiatric Association, 1968.

American Psychiatric Association. *Diagnostic and Statistical Manual of Mental Disorders,* ed 3. Washington, D.C., American Psychiatric Association, 1980.

American Psychiatric Association. *Diagnostic and Statistical Manual of Mental Disorders,* ed 3, rev. Washington, D.C., American Psychiatric Association, 1987.

Andrulonis PA, Blueck BC, Stroebel CF, et al. Organic brain dysfunction and the borderline syndrome. *Psychiatr Clin North Am* 4:47–66, 1980.

Antens E, Frischholz EJ, Braun BG, et al. The simulation of dissociative disorders on the Dissociative Experiences Scale. Paper presented to the 8th annual meeting of the International Society for the Study of Multiple Personality Disorder and Dissociation, Chicago, November 15–17, 1991.

Anthony JC, Helzer JE. Syndromes of drug abuse and dependence, in Robins LN, Regier DA (eds), *Psychiatric Disorders in America: The Epidemiologic Catchment Area Study.* New York, Free Press, 1991, pp 116–154.

Armstrong JG, Loewenstein RJ. Characteristics of patients with multiple personality and dissociative disorders on testing. *J Nerv Ment Dis* 178:448–454, 1990.

Aronson TA. A critical review of psychotherapeutic treatments of the borderline personality: Historical trends and future directions. *J Nerv Ment Dis* 177:511–528, 1989.

Bahnson CB, Smith K. Autonomic changes in a multiple personality (abstract). *Psychosom Med* 37:85–86, 1975.

Barkin R, Braun BG, Kluft RP. The dilemma of drug therapy for multiple personality disorder, in Braun BG (ed), *The Treatment of Multiple Personality Disorder.* Washington, D.C., American Psychiatric Press, 1986, pp 107–132.

Benner DG, Joscelyne B. Multiple personality as a borderline disorder. *J Nerv Ment Dis* 172:98–104, 1984.

Ben-Porath YS, Butcher JN, Graham JR. Contribution of the MMPI-2 content scales to the differential diagnosis of schizophrenia and major depression. *Psychol Assoc* 3:634–640, 1991.

Bernstein EM, Putnam FW. Development, reliability, and validity of a dissociation scale. *J Nerv Ment Dis* 174:727–735, 1986.

Bishop RE, Holt RA. Pseudopsychosis: A re-examination of the concept of hysterical psychoses. *Compr Psychiatry* 21:150–161, 1980.

Black DW. Somatoform disorders. *Primary Care* 14:711–722, 1987.

Blashfield RK, McElroy RA. The 1985 journal literature on the personality disorders. *Compr Psychiatry* 28:536–546, 1987.

Bleuler E. *Text-book of Psychiatry.* Brill AA (trans). New York, Macmillan, 1924.

Bliss EL. Multiple personalities. A report of 14 cases with implications for schizophrenia and hysteria. *Arch Gen Psychiatry* 37:1388–1397, 1980.

Bliss EL. Multiple personalities, related disorders and hypnosis. *Am J Clin Hypn* 26:114–123, 1983.

Bliss EL. A symptom profile of patients with multiple personalities, including MMPI results. *J Nerv Ment Dis* 172:197–202, 1984a.

Bliss EL. Spontaneous self-hypnosis in multiple personality disorder. *Psychiatr Clin North Am* 7:135–148, 1984b.

Bliss EL. Hysteria and hypnosis. *J Nerv Ment Dis* 172:203–206, 1984c.

Bliss EL. How prevalent is multiple personality? (letter). *Am J Psychiatry* 142:1527, 1985.

Bliss EL. *Multiple Personality, Allied Disorders, and Hypnosis.* New York, Oxford University Press, 1986.

Bliss EL. Professional skepticism about multiple personality. *J Nerv Ment Dis* 176:533–534, 1988.

Bliss J, Bliss EL. *Prism: Andrea's World.* New York, Stein & Day, 1985.

Bliss EL, Jeppsen EA. Prevalence of multiple personality among inpatients and outpatients. *Am J Psychiatry* 142:250–251, 1985.

Bliss EL, Larson EM. Sexual criminality and hypnotizability. *J Nerv Ment Dis* 173:522–526, 1985.

Bliss EL, Larson EM, Nakashima SR. Auditory hallucinations and schizophrenia. *J Nerv Ment Dis* 171:30–33, 1983.

Boon S, Drajier N. Diagnosing dissociative disorders in the Netherlands: A pilot study with the structured clinical interview for DSM-III-R dissociative disorders. *Am J Psychiatry* 148:458–462, 1991.

Books in Print. New York, Reed, 1990–1991.

Boor M. The multiple personality epidemic. Additional cases and inferences regarding diagnosis, etiology, dynamics, and treatment. *J Nerv Ment Dis* 170:302–304, 1982.

Boor M, Coons PM. A comprehensive bibliography of literature pertaining to multiple personality. *Psychol Rep* 53:295–310, 1983.

Bowers KS. Dissociation in hypnosis and multiple personality disorder. *Int J Clin Exp Hypn* 39:155–176, 1991.

Bowers MK, Brecher-Marer S, Newton BW, et al. Therapy of multiple personality. *Int J Clin Exp Hypn* 19:57–65, 1971.

Bozzuto JC. Cinematic neurosis following 'The Exorcist': Report of four cases. *J Nerv Ment Dis* 161:43–48, 1975.

Bramwell JM. *Hypnosis: Its History, Practice, and Theory.* London, Delamore Press, 1906.

Brandsma JM, Ludwig AM. A case of multiple personality: Diagnosis and therapy. *J Clin Exp Hypn* 22:216–233, 1974.

Braun BG. Hypnosis for multiple personalities, in Wain HJ (ed), *Clinical Hypnosis in Medicine.* Miami, Fla, Symposia Specialists, Inc, 1980, pp 209–217.

Braun BG. Neurophysiologic changes in multiple personality. *Am J Clin Hypn* 26:84–92, 1983.

Braun BG. Hypnosis creates multiple personality: Myth or reality? *Int J Clin Exp Hypn* 32:191–197, 1984a.

Braun BG. Towards a theory of multiple personality and other dissociative phenomena. *Psychiatr Clin North Am* 7:171–193, 1984b.

Braun BG. Uses of hypnosis with multiple personality. *Psychol Ann* 14:34–40, 1984c.

Braun BG. The transgenerational incidence of dissociation and multiple personality disorder, in Kluft RP (ed), *Childhood Antecedents of Multiple Personality.* Washington, D.C., American Psychiatric Press, 1985, pp 121–150.

Brende JO. The psychophysiological manifestations of dissociation. *Psychiatr Clin North Am* 7:41–50, 1984.

Breuer J. The case of Anna O, in Breuer J, Freud S., *Studies in Hysteria* (AA Brill trans). Boston, Beacon Press, 1950, pp 21–47.

Briquet P. *Traite de l'Hysterie.* Paris, Bailliere, 1859.

Bryer JB, Nelson BA, Miller JB, et al. Childhood sexual and physical abuse as factors in adult psychiatric illness. *Am J Psychiatry* 144:1426–1430, 1987.

Buck OD. Single case study. Multiple personality as a borderline state. *J Nerv Ment Dis* 171:62–65, 1983.

Cadoret RJ, O'Gorman T, Troughton E, et al. Alcoholism and antisocial personality: Interrelationships, genetic and environmental factors. *Arch Gen Psychiatry* 42:161–167, 1985.

Cadoret RJ, Troughton E, O'Gorman TW. Genetic and environmental factors in alcohol abuse and antisocial personality. *J Stud Alcohol* 48:1–8, 1987.

Cadoret RJ, Troughton E, O'Gorman TW, et al. An adoption study of genetic and environmental factors in drug abuse. *Arch Gen Psychiatry* 43:1131–1136, 1986.

Carlson ET. The history of dissociation until 1880, in Quen JM (ed), *Split Minds/Split Brains: Historical and Current Perspectives.* New York: New York University Press, 1986, pp 7–30.

Carlson ET, Putnam FW, Ross CA, et al. A factor analysis of the dissociative experiences scale using multicenter data. Paper presented to the 8th annual meeting of the International Society for the Study of Multiple Personality Disorder and Dissociation, Chicago, November 15–17, 1991.

Carter AB. The prognosis of certain hysterical symptoms. *Br Med J* 1:1076–1079, 1949.

Casey JF, Wilson L. *The Flock.* New York, Alfred A. Knopf, 1991.

Castle K, Bechtel S. *Katherine, It's Time.* New York, Harper & Row, 1989.

Chase T. *When Rabbit Howls.* New York, EP Dutton, 1987.

Chodoff P. More on multiple personality disorder (letter). *Am J Psychiatry* 144:124, 1987.

Clancy T. *The Sum of All Fears.* New York, GP Putnam's Sons, 1991.

Clark NH, Roth K. *Shatter.* New York, Bantam, 1986.

Clary WF, Burstein KJ, Carpenter JS. Multiple personality and borderline personality disorder. *Psychiatr Clin North Am* 7:89–99, 1984.

Cleckley HM. *The Mask of Sanity.* St Louis, CV Mosby, 1950.

Cloninger CR. A systematic method for clinical description and classification of personality variants. *Arch Gen Psychiatry* 44:573–588, 1987.

Cloninger CR. Establishment of diagnostic validity in psychiatric illness: Robins and Guze's method revisited, in Robins LN, Barrett JE (eds), *The Validity of Psychiatric Diagnosis.* New York, Raven Press, 1989, pp 9–18.

Cloninger CR, Christiansen KO, Reich T, et al. Implications of sex differences in the prevalences of antisocial personality alcoholism and criminality for familial transmission. *Arch Gen Psychiatry* 35:924–951, 1978.

Cloninger CR, Bohman M, Sigvardsson S, et al. Psychopathology in adopted-out children of alcoholics. *Psychiatr Dev* 1:1–22, 1985.

Cloninger CR, Guze SB. Psychiatric illness and female criminality: The role of sociopathy and hysteria in the antisocial woman. *Am J Psychiatry* 127:303–311, 1970a.

Cloninger CR, Guze SB. Female criminals: Their personal, familial, and social backgrounds. *Arch Gen Psychiatry* 23:554–8, 1970b.

Cloninger CR, Martin RL, Guze SB, et al. A prospective follow-up and family study of somatization in men and women. *Am J Psychiatry* 143:873–878, 1986.

Cloninger CR, Reich T. Genetic heterogeneity in alcoholism and sociopathy, in Kety S, Rowland LP, Sidman RL, et al (eds), *Genetics of Neurological and Psychiatric Disorders.* New York, Raven Press, 1983, pp 145–166.

Cloninger CR, Reich T, Guze SB. The multifactorial model of disease transmission: II. Sex differences in the familial transmission of sociopathy (antisocial personality). *Br J Psychiatry* 127:11–22, 1975a.

Cloninger CR, Reich T, Guze SB. The multifactorial model of disease transmission: III. Familial relationship between sociopathy and hysteria (Briquet's syndrome). *Br J Psychiatry* 127:23–32, 1975b.

Coccaro EF, Kavoussi RJ. Biological and pharmacological aspects of borderline personality disorder. *Hosp Community Psychiatry* 42:1029–1033, 1991.

Cohen BM, Giller EW. *Multiple Personality from the Inside Out.* Baltimore, Sidrin Press, 1991.

Condon WS, Ogston WD, Pacoe LV. Three faces of Eve revisited: A study of transient microstrabismus. *J Abnorm Psychol* 74:618–620, 1969.

Confer WN, Ables BS. *Multiple Personality: Etiology, Diagnosis, and Treatment.* New York, Human Sciences Press, 1983.

Congdon MH, Hain J, Stevenson I. *J Nerv Ment Dis* 132:497–504, 1961.

Consumer Reports. Chronic fatigue: All in the mind? October 1990, pp 671–675.

Coons PM. Multiple personality: Diagnostic considerations. *J Clin Psychiatry* 41:330–336, 1980.

Coons PM. The differential diagnosis of multiple personality. A comprehensive review. *Psychiatr Clin North Am* 7:51–67, 1984.

Coons PM. Child abuse and multiple personality disorder: Review of the literature and suggestions for treatment. *Child Abuse Neglect* 10:455–462, 1986a.

Coons PM. The prevalence of multiple personality disorder. *Newsletter Int Soc Study Mult Person Dissoc* 4:6–7, 1986b.

Coons PM. Treatment progress in 20 patients with multiple personality disorder. *J Nerv Ment Dis* 174:715–721, 1986c.

Coons PM. Psychophysiologic aspects of multiple personality disorder. A review. *Dissociation* 1:47–53, 1988a.

Coons PM. Misuse of forensic hypnosis: A hypnotically elicited false confession with the apparent creation of a multiple personality. *Int J Clin Exp Hypn* 36:1–11, 1988b.

Coons PM. Iatrogenesis and malingering of multiple personality disorder in the forensic evaluation of homicide defendants. *Psychiatr Clin North Am* 14:757–768, 1991.

Coons PM, Bowman ES, Milstein V. Multiple personality disorder: A clinical investigation of 50 cases. *J Nerv Ment Dis* 175:519–527, 1988.

Coons PM, Fine CG. Accuracy of the MMPI in identifying multiple personality disorder. *Psychol Rep* 66:831–834, 1990.

Coons PM, Milstein V. Psychosexual disturbances in multiple personality: Characteristics, etiology, and treatment. *J Clin Psychiatry* 47:106–110, 1986.

Coons PM, Milstein V, Marley C. EEG studies of two multiple personalities and a control. *Arch Gen Psychiatry* 39:823–825, 1982.

Coons PM, Sterne AL. Initial and follow-up psychological testing on a group of patients with multiple personality disorder. *Psychol Rep* 58:43–49, 1986.

Coryell W. Single case study. Multiple personality and primary affective disorder. *J Nerv Ment Dis* 171:388–390, 1983.

Cowley G, Hager M, Joseph N. Chronic fatigue syndrome. A modern medical mystery. *Newsweek,* November 12, 1990, pp. 62–70.

Cutler B, Reed J. Multiple personality. A single case study with a 15 year follow-up. *Psychol Med* 5:18–26, 1975.

Dahlstrom WG, Welsh GS, Dahlstrom LE. *An MMPI Handbook: Volume I: Clinical Interpretation,* rev. Minneapolis, University of Minnesota Press, 1972.

Damgaard J, Van Benschoten S, Fagan J. An updated bibliography of literature pertaining to multiple personality. *Psychol Rep* 57:131–137, 1985.

Davis GC, Akiskal HS. Descriptive, biological, and theoretical aspects of borderline personality disorder. *Hosp Community Psychiatry* 37:685–692, 1986.

Davis PH, Osherson A. The concurrent treatment of a multiple-personality woman and her son. *Am J Psychother* 31:504–515, 1977.

Decker HS. The lure of nonmaterialism in materialist Europe: Investigations of dissociative phenomena, 1880–1915, in Quen JM (ed): *Split Minds/Split Brains: Historical and Current Perspectives.* New York, New York University Press, 1986, pp 31–62.

Dell PF. Not reasonable skepticism, but extreme skepticism. A reply from Paul F. Dell. *J Nerv Ment Dis* 176:537–538, 1988a.

Dell PF. Professional skepticism about multiple personality. *J Nerv Ment Dis* 176:528–531, 1988b.

Dell PF, Eisenhower JW. Adolescent multiple personality disorder: A preliminary study of eleven cases. *J Am Acad Child Adolesc Psychiatry* 29:359–366, 1990.

Dercum FX. *A Clinical Manual of Mental Diseases.* Philadelphia, WB Saunders Co, 1913.

DeSouza C, Othmer E. Somatization disorders (letter). *JAMA* 255:404, 1986.

DeSouza C, Othmer E, Gabrielli W, et al. Major depression and somatization disorder: The overlooked differential diagnosis. *Psychiatr Ann* 18:340–348, 1988.

Dickes RA. Brief therapy of conversion reactions: An in-hospital technique. *Am J Psychiatry* 131:584–586, 1974.

Drob S, Stewart S, Bernard H. The problem of reinterpretive distortions in group psychotherapy with borderline patients. *Group* 6:14–22, 1982.

Eaton WM. Epidemiology of schizophrenia. *Epidemiol Rev* 7:105–126, 1985.

Edell WS. Relationship of borderline syndrome disorders to early schizophrenia on the MMPI. *J Clin Psychol* 43:163–176, 1987.

Ellenberger HF. *The Discovery of the Unconscious.* New York, Basic Books, 1970.

Evans RW, Ruff RM, Braff DL, et al. MMPI characteristics of borderline personality inpatients. *J Nerv Ment Dis* 172:742–748, 1984.

Evans RW, Ruff RM, Braff DL, et al. On the consistency of the MMPI in borderline personality disorder. *Percept Motor Skills* 62:579–585, 1986.

Fagan J, McMahon PP. Incipient multiple personality in children. Four cases. *J Nerv Ment Dis* 172:26–36, 1984.

Fahy TA. The diagnosis of multiple personality disorder: A critical review. *Br J Psychiatry* 153:597–606, 1988.

Fahy TA. Multiple personality disorder (letter). *Br J Psychiatry* 154:878, 1989.

Fahy TA, Abas M, Brown JC. Multiple personality: A symptom of psychiatric disorder. *Br J Psychiatry* 154:99–101, 1989.

Fagan J, McMahon PP. Incipient multiple personality in children. *J Nerv Ment Dis* 172:26–36, 1984.

Farber IE. Sane and insane: Constructions and misconstructions. *J Abnorm Psychol* 84:589–620, 1975.

Feighner JP, Robins E, Guze SB, et al. Diagnostic criteria for use in psychiatric research. *Arch Gen Psychiatry* 26:57–63, 1972.

Fine R. *The Development of Freud's Thought.* New York, Jason Aaronson, 1962.

Fink D. The comorbidity of multiple personality disorder and DSM-III-R Axis II disorders. *Psychiatr Clin North Am* 14:547–566, 1991.

Fink D, Golinkoff M. Multiple personality disorder, borderline personality disorder, and schizophrenia: A comparative study of clinical features. *Dissociation* 3:127–134, 1990.

Fleming JAE. Multiple personality disorder (letter). *Br J Psychiatry* 154:877, 1989.

Frances A. The DSM-III personality disorders section: A commentary. *Am J Psychiatry* 137:1050–1054, 1980.

Franklin J. The diagnosis of multiple personality disorder based on subtle dissociative signs. *J Nerv Ment Dis* 178:4–14, 1990.

Franz SI. *Persons One and Three: A Study in Multiple Personalities.* New York, Whittlesey/McGraw-Hill, 1933.

Fraser GA. Exorcism: Clinical effects on multiple personalities exposed to exorcism rites. Paper presented at the 8th International Conference of the Society for the Study of Multiple Personality and Dissociation, Chicago, November 15–17, 1991.

Fraser S. *My Father's House: A Memoir of Incest and Healing.* New York, Ticknor and Fields, 1988.

Freud S. *An Autobiographical Study.* London, Hogarth Press, 1948a.

Freud S. *The defence Neuropsychoses. Collected Papers, 1, 59.* London: Hogarth Press, 1948b. (Original publication 1894.)

Freud S. *The Origins of Psychoanalysis. Letters to Wilhelm Fliess.* New York, Basis Books, 1954.

Friedman HJ. Psychotherapy of borderline patients: The influence of theory on technique. *Am J Psychiatry* 132:1048–1052, 1975.

Ganaway GK. Historical versus narrative truth: clarifying the role of exogenous trauma in the etiology of MPD and its variants. *Dissociation* 2:205–220, 1989.

Gartner J, Hurt SW, Gartner A. Psychological test signs of borderline personality disorder. *J Pers Assess* 53:423–441, 1989.

Gatfield PD, Guze SB. Prognosis and differential diagnosis of conversion reactions (a follow-up study). *Dis Nerv Sys* 23:1–8, 1962.

Gilbertson A, Torem M, Cohen R, et al. Susceptibility of common self-report measures of dissociation to malingering. Paper presented to the 8th annual meeting of the International Society for the Study of Multiple Personality Disorder and Dissociation, Chicago, November 15–17, 1991.

Gillstrom BJ, Hare RD. Language-related hand gestures in psychopaths. *J Pers Dis* 2:21–27, 1988.

Goddard HH. A case of dual personality. *J Abnorm Soc Psychol* 21:170–191, 1926.

Godfried MR, Kent RN. Traditional versus behavioral personality assessment: A comparison of methodological and theoretical assumptions. *Psychol Bull* 77:409–420, 1972.

Goettman C, Greaves GB, Coons PM. *Multiple Personality and Dissociation, 1791–1990: A Complete Bibliography.* Norcross, Ga, Ken Burrow & Co, 1991.

Goodwin DW, Alderson P, Rosenthal R. Clinical significance of hallucinations in psychiatric disorders. A study of 116 hallucinatory patients. *Arch Gen Psychiatry* 24:76–80, 1971.

Goodwin DW, Cheeves K, Connell V. Borderline and other severe symptoms in adult survivors of incestuous abuse. *Psychiatr Ann* 20:22–32, 1990.

Gowers WR. *A Manual of Diseases of the Nervous System.* London, Churchill, 1888, Vol 2.

Greaves GB. Multiple personality. 165 years after Mary Reynolds. *J Nerv Ment Dis* 168:577–596, 1980.

Greden JF, Genero N, Price L, et al. Facial electromyography in depression. *Arch Gen Psychiatry* 43:269–274, 1986.

Greenberg DB. Neurasthenia in the 1980s: Chronic mononucleosis, chronic fatigue syndrome, and anxiety and depressive disorders. *Psychosom* 31:129–137, 1990.

Greene RL. Assessment of malingering and deception by objective personality tests, in Rogers R (ed), *Clinical Assessment of Malingering and Deception.* New York, Guilford Press, 1988, pp 123–158.

Griffin RB Jr. The utility of the Rorschach and the MMPI in identifying dissociative disorders. Dissertation presented to the Virginia Consortium for Professional Psychology, Richmond, Virginia, February 1989.

Groves JE. Borderline personality disorder. *N Engl J Med* 305:259–262, 1981.

Gruenewald D. Hypnotic techniques without hypnosis in the treatment of dual personality. *J Nerv Ment Dis* 153:41–46, 1971.

Gruenewald D. Multiple personality and splitting phenomena: A reconceptualization. *J Nerv Ment Dis* 164:385–393, 1977.

Gunderson JG, Englund DW. Characterizing the families of borderlines: A review of the literature. *Psychiatr Clin North Am* 4:159–168, 1981.

Gunderson JG, Kolb JE. Discriminating features of borderline patients. *Am J Psychiatry* 135:792–796, 1978.

Gunderson JG, Kolb JE, Austin V. The diagnostic interview for borderline patients. *Am J Psychiatry* 138:896–903, 1981.

Gunderson JG, Singer MT. Defining borderline patients: An overview. *Am J Psychiatry* 132:1–10, 1975.

Gustin QL, Goodpaster GA, Sajadi C, et al. MMPI characteristics of the DSM-III borderline personality disorder. *J Pers Assess* 47:50–59, 1983.

Guze SB. The role of follow-up studies: Their contribution to diagnostic classification as applied to hysteria. *Semin Psychiatry* 2:392–402, 1970.

Guze SB. The validity and significance of the clinical diagnosis of hysteria (Briquet's syndrome). *Am J Psychiatry* 132:138–141, 1975.

Guze SB. The future of psychiatry: Medicine or social science? *J Nerv Ment Dis* 165:225–230, 1977.

Guze SB. Nature of psychiatric illness: Why psychiatry is a branch of medicine. *Compr Psychiatry* 19:295–307, 1978.

Guze SB, Cloninger CR, Martin RL, et al. A follow-up and family study of Briquet's syndrome. *Br J Psychiatry* 149:17–23, 1986.

Guze SB, Helzer JE. The medical model and psychiatric disorders, in Cavenar JO (ed), *Psychiatry.* Philadelphia, JB Lippincott Co, 1985, Vol 1, Chap 51, pp 1–8.

Guze SB, Perley MJ. Observations on the natural history of hysteria. *Am J Psychiatry* 119:960–965, 1963.

Guze SB, Wolfgram ED, McKinney JK, et al. Psychiatric illness in the families of convicted criminals: A study of 519 first-degree relatives. *Dis Nerv Syst* 28:651–659, 1967.

Guze SB, Woodruff RA, Clayton PJ. A study of conversion symptoms in psychiatric outpatients. *Am J Psychiatry* 128:643–646, 1971.

Hacking I. Two souls in one body. *Crit Inquiry* 17:838–867, 1991.

Haifeiz HB. Hysterical conversion: A prognostic study. *Br J Psychiatry* 136:548–551, 1980.

Harriman PL. The experimental production of some phenomena related to the multiple personality. *J Abnorm Soc Psychol* 37:244–255, 1942.

Harriman PL. A new approach to multiple personalities. *Am J Orthopsychiatry* 13:638–643, 1943.

The Harvard Medical School Mental Health Letter. Multiple personality. 1:1–4, 1985.

Hawksworth H, Schwarz T. *The Five of Me.* Chicago, Henry Regnery, 1977.

Herzog A. On multiple personality: Comments on diagnosis, etiology, and treatment. *Int J Clin Exp Hypn* 32:210–221, 1984.

Heumann BA, Morey LC. Reliability of categorical and dimensional judgments of personality disorder. *Am J Psychiatry* 147:498–500, 1990.

Hier DB. Neuropsychiatric disorders, in Samuels MA (ed), *Manual of Neurologic Therapeutics*. Boston, Little, Brown, 1982, pp 199–215.

Hilgard ER. Professional skepticism about multiple personality (commentary). *J Nerv Ment Dis* 176:532, 1988.

Hirsch SJ, Hollender MH. Hysterical psychosis: Classification of the concept. *Am J Psychiatry* 120:1066–1074, 1969.

Hollenger MH, Hirsch SJ. Hysterical psychosis. *Am J Psychiatry* 120:1066–1074, 1964.

Holmes SJ, Robins LN. The role of parental disciplinary practices in the development of depression and alcoholism. *Psychiatry* 51:24–36, 1988.

Horevitz RP, Braun BG. Are multiple personalities borderline? An analysis of 33 cases. *Psychiatr Clin North Am* 7:69–87, 1984.

Horton P, Miller D. The etiology of multiple personality. *Compr Psychiatry* 13:151–159, 1972.

Howland JS. The use of hypnosis in the treatment of a case of multiple personality. *J Nerv Ment Dis* 161:138–142, 1975.

Janet P. *La automatisme psychologique*. Paris, Alcan, 1889.

Janet P. *The Major Symptoms of Hysteria*. New York, Macmillan, 1907.

Jeans RF. The three faces of Evelyn: A case report. I. An independently validated case of multiple personality. *J Abnorm Psychol* 85:249–255, 1976.

Johnson W. *An Essay on the Diseases of Young Women*. London, Simpkin, Marshall, 1849.

Johnston T. *The Edge of Evil: The Rise of Satanism in America*. Irving, Tex, Word Books, 1989.

Jung CG. On the psychology and pathology of so-called occult phenomena, in Jung CG, (ed.) *Psychology and the Occult*. Princeton, N.J., Princeton University Press, 1902/1977, pp 6–91. Translated by Hull RFC.

Kampman R. Hypnotically induced multiple personality. *Int J Clin Exp Hypn* 24:215–227, 1976.

Katon W, Lin E, Von Korff M, et al. Somatization: A spectrum of severity. *Am J Psychiatry* 148:34–40, 1991.

Keith SJ, Regier DA, Rae DS. Schizophrenic disorders, in Robins LN, Regier DA (eds), *Psychiatric Disorders in America: The Epidemiologic Catchment Area Study*. New York, Free Press, 1991, pp 33–52.

Keyes D. *The Minds of Billy Milligan*. New York, Random House, 1981.

Kline MV. Multiple personality: Facts and artifacts in relation to hypnotherapy. *Int J Clin Exp Hypn* 32:198–209, 1984.

Kline NA. Multiple personality disorder: The new "royal road"? (letter). *Am J Psychiatry* 147:538–539, 1990.

Kluft RP. Varieties of hypnotic interventions in the treatment of multiple personality. *Am J Clin Hypn* 24:230–240, 1982.

Kluft RP. Hypnotherapeutic crisis intervention in multiple personality. *Am J Clin Hypn* 26:73–83, 1983.

Kluft RP. An introduction to multiple personality disorder. *Psychiatr Ann* 14:19–24, 1984a.

Kluft RP. Multiple personality in childhood. *Psychiatr Clin North Am* 7:121–134, 1984b.

Kluft RP. Treatment of multiple personality disorder: A study of 33 cases. *Psychiatr Clin North Am* 7:9–29, 1984c.

Kluft RP. Aspects of the treatment of multiple personality disorder. *Psychiatr Am* 14:51–55, 1984d.

Kluft RP. Making the diagnosis of multiple personality disorder (MPD). *Directions Psychiatry* 5:1–12, 1985.

Kluft RP. High-functioning multiple personality patients: Three cases. *J Nerv Ment Dis* 174:722–726, 1986.

Kluft RP. More on multiple personality disorder (letter). *Am J Psychiatry* 144:124–125, 1987a.

Kluft RP. An update on multiple personality disorder. *Hosp Comm Psychiatry* 38:363–373, 1987b.

Kluft RP. The simulation and dissimulation of multiple personality disorder. *Am J Clin Hypn* 30:104–108, 1987c.

Kluft RP. Iatrogenic creation of new alter personalities. *Dissociation* 2:83–91, 1989.

Kluft RP. Clinical presentations of multiple personality disorder. *Psychiatr Clin North Am* 14:605–629, 1991.

Kohlenberg RJ. Behavioristic approach to multiple personality: A case study. *Behav Ther* 4:137–140, 1973.

Kramer M. Some problems for international research suggested by observations on differences in first admissions rates to mental hospitals of England and Wales and of the United States, Cleghorn RA, Moll AE, Roberts CA (eds), in *Proceedings of the Third World Congress of Psychiatry.* Montreal, University of Toronto Press and McGill University Press, 1961, p 153.

Kroll J. *The Challenge of the Borderline Patient.* New York, WW Norton, 1989.

Kroll J, Sines L, Martin K, et al. Borderline personality disorder: Construct validity of the concept. *Arch Gen Personality* 38:1021–1026, 1981.

Kruesi MJ, Dale J, Straus SE. Psychiatric diagnoses in patients who have chronic fatigue syndrome. *J Clin Psychiatry* 50:53–56, 1989.

LaCalle TM. *Voices.* New York, Dodd, Mead & Co, 1987.

Lachar D, Wrobel TA. Validating clinicians' hunches: Construction of a new MMPI critical item set. *J Clin Consult Psychol* 47:277–284, 1979.

Lancaster E, Poling J. *The Final Face of Eve.* New York, McGraw-Hill, 1958.

Larmore K, Ludwig AM, Gain RL. Multiple personality—An objective case study. *Br J Psychiatry* 131:35–40, 1977.

Larson B. *Satanism: The Seduction of America's Youth.* Nashville, Tenn, Nelson, 1989.

Lazare A. Hysteria. Hackett TP, Cassem NH (eds), *MGH Handbook of General Hospital Psychiatry.* St. Louis: Mosby, 1978, pp 117–140.

Lazare A. Conversion symptoms. *N Engl J Med* 305:745–748, 1981.

Lewis J, Frischholz EJ, Braun BG, et al. The relationship between the Dissociative Experiences Scale (DES) and other self report measures of dissociation. Paper presented to the 8th annual meeting of the International Society for the Study of Multiple Personality Disorder and Dissociation, Chicago, November 15–17, 1991.

Linehan MM. Dialectical behavior therapy for borderline personality disorder, theory and method. *Bull Menninger Clin* 51:261–276, 1987.

Lipton SD. Dissociated personality: A case report. *Psychiatr Q* 17:33–56, 1943.

Liskow BI. Briquet's syndrome, somatization disorder, and co-occurring psychiatric disorders. *Psychiatr Ann* 18:350–352, 1988.

Liskow BI, Clayton P, Woodruff R, et al. Briquet's syndrome, hysterical personality and the MMPI. *Am J Psychiatry* 134:1137–1139, 1977.

Liskow BI, Penick E, Powell B. Inpatients with Briquet's syndrome: Presence of additional psychiatric syndromes and MMPI results. *Compr Psychiatry* 27:461–470, 1986.

Littrell J. The Swedish studies of the adopted children of alcoholics. *J Stud Alcohol* 49:491–499, 1988.

Livesley WJ. The classification of personality disorder: I. The choice of category concept. *Can J Psychiatry* 30:353–358, 1985a.

Livesley WJ. The classification of personality disorder: II. The problem of diagnostic criteria. *Can J Psychiatry* 30:359–362, 1985b.

Livesley WJ. Trait and behavioral prototypes of personality disorder. *Am J Psychiatry* 143:728–732, 1986.

Livesley WJ, Jackson DN. The internal consistency and factorial structure of behaviors judged to be associated with DSM-III personality disorders. *Am J Psychiatry* 143:1473–1474, 1986.

Loewenstein RJ. Multiple personality disorder: A continuing challenge. *Psychiatr Rev* 2:1–2, 1989.

Loewenstein RJ. An office mental status examination for complex chronic dissociative symptoms and multiple personality disorder. *Psychiatr Clin North Am* 14:567–604, 1991.

Loewenstein RJ, Hamilton J, Alagna S, et al. Experiential sampling in the study of multiple personality disorder. *Am J Psychiatry* 144:19–24, 1987.

Loewenstein RJ, Putnam FW. The clinical phenomenology of males with MPD: A report of 21 cases. *Dissociation* 3:135–143, 1990.

Loranger AW, Oldham JM, Tulis EH. Familial transmission of DSM-III borderline personality disorder. *Arch Gen Psychiatry* 39:795–799, 1982.

Ludolph PS. How prevalent is multiple personality? *Am J Psychiatry* 142:1526–1527, 1985.

Ludolph PS, Westen D, Misle B, et al. The borderline diagnosis in adolescents: Symptoms and developmental history. *Am J Psychiatry* 147:470–476, 1990.

Ludwig AM. Intoxication and sobriety. Symposium on multiple personality. *Psychiatr Clin North Am* 7:161–169, 1984.

Ludwig AM, Brandsma JM, Wilbur CB, et al. The objective study of a multiple personality. Or, are four heads better than one? *Arch Gen Psychiatry* 26:298–310, 1972.

Macnish R. *The Philosophy of Sleep*, ed 3. Glasgow: WR M'Phun, 1836.

Mackarness R. *Not All in the Mind*. London, Pan Books, 1976. American ed: *Eating Dangerously: The Hazards of Allergies*. New York, Harcourt Brace Jovanovich, 1976.

Mai FM, Merskey DM. Briquet's *Treatise on Hysteria. Arch Gen Psychiatry* 37:1401–1405, 1980.

Mallett BL, Gold S. A pseudoschizophrenic hysterical syndrome. *Br J Med Psychol* 37:59–70, 1964.

Marcum JM, Wright K, Bissel WG. Chance discovery of multiple personality disorder in a depressed patient by amobarbital interview. *J Nerv Ment Dis* 174:489–492, 1986.

Martin RL. Problems in the diagnosis of somatization disorder: Effects on research and clinical practice. *Psychiatr Ann* 18:357–362, 1988.

Mathew RJ, Jack RA, West WS. Regional cerebral blood flow in a patient with multiple personality. *Am J Psychiatry* 142:504–505, 1985.

Mayer RS. *Through Divided Minds.* New York, Doubleday, 1988.

Mayer RS. *Satan's Children.* New York, GP Putnam's Sons, 1991.

McCallum KE, Lock J, Kulla M, et al. Dissociative symptoms and disorders in patients with eating disorders. Unpublished manuscript, 1992.

McCurdy HA. A note on the dissociation of a personality. *Character Pers* 10:33–41, 1941.

McDougall W. *Outline of Abnormal Personality.* New York, Scribner, 1926.

McGlashan TH. The borderline syndrome. II. Is it a variant of schizophrenia or affective disorder? *Arch Gen Psychiatry* 40:1319–1323, 1983.

Merskey H. *The Analysis of Hysteria.* London, Bailliere Tindall, 1979.

Merskey H. The manufacture of personalities: the production of multiple personality disorder. *Br J Psychiatry* 160:327–340, 1992.

Mesulam MM. Dissociative states with abnormal temporal lobe EEG. Multiple personality and the illusion of possession. *Arch Neurol* 38:176–181, 1981.

Miller RD. The possible use of auto-hypnosis as a resistance during hypnotherapy. *Int J Clin Exp Hypn* 32:236–247, 1984.

Miller SD. Optical differences in cases of multiple personality disorder. *J Nerv Ment Dis* 177:480–486, 1989.

Mitchell SL. Double consciousness, or a duality of person in the same individual. *Med Repository* 1816, N.S. 3b:185–186.

Mitchell SW. Mary Reynolds, a case of double consciousness. *Trans Coll Phys Philadelphia* 3rd Ser, 10, 366–369, April 4, 1988.

Modestin J. Multiple personality in Switzerland. *Am J Psychiatry* 149:88–92, 1992.

Monson RA, Smith GR. Somatization disorder in primary care. *N Engl J Med* 308:1464–1465, 1983.

Moos R, Moos B. *The Family Environment Scale Manual,* ed 2. Palo Alto, Calif, Consulting Psychologist Press, 1986.

Moriselli GE. Personalities alternate e patologia affecttiva. *Arch Psycol Neurol Psichiatria* 14:579–589, 1953.

Morrison JR. Management of Briquet's syndrome (hysteria). *West J Med* 128:482–487, 1978.

Morrison JR. Childhood sexual histories of women with somatization disorder. *Am J Psychiatry* 1989;146:239–241, 1989a.

Morrison J. Increased suicide attempts in women with somatization disorder. *Ann Clin Psychiatry* 1:251–254, 1989b.

Mulhern S. Embodied alternative identities: Bearing witness to a world that might have been. *Psychiatr Clin North Am* 14:769–786, 1991.

Munford PR, Liberman RP. Behavior therapy of hysterical disorders, in Roy A (ed), *Hysteria.* New York, Wiley, 1982, pp 287–303.

Murphy GE. The clinical management of hysteria. *JAMA* 247:2559–2564, 1982.

Nakdimen KA. Splitting and dissociation, borderline personality and multiple personality (letter). *Am J Psychiatry* 146:1236, 1989.

Nestadt G, Romanoski AJ, Chahal R, et al. An epidemiological study of histrionic personality disorder. *Psychol Med* 20:413–422, 1990.

North CS, Cadoret RJ. Diagnostic discrepancy in personal accounts of patients with "schizophrenia." *Arch Gen Psychiatry* 38:133–137, 1981.

North CS, Clements WM. The psychiatric diagnosis of Anton Boison: From schizophrenia to bipolar affective disorder. *J Pastoral Care* 35:264–275, 1981.

O'Brien D. *Two of a Kind: The Hillside Stranglers.* New York, New American Library, 1985.

Orne MT, Dinges DF, Orne EC. On the differential diagnosis of multiple personality in the forensic context. *Int J Clin Exp Hypn* 32:118–169, 1984.

Osgood CE, Luria Z, Jeans RF, et al. The three faces of Evelyn: A case report. *J Abnorm Psychol* 85:247–286, 1976.

Othmer E. Somatization disorder (editorial). *Psychiatr Ann* 18:330–331, 1988.

Packard RC, Brown F. Multiple headaches in a case of multiple personality disorder. *Headache* 26:99–102, 1986.

Pearson DJ, Rix KJB, Bentley SJ. Food allergy: How much in the mind: A clinical and psychiatric study of suspected food hypersensitivity. *Lancet* 1:1259–1261, 1983.

Pennebaker JW, Watson D. The psychology of somatic symptoms. Kirmayer LJ, Robbins JM (eds), *Current Concepts of Somatization: Research and Clinical Perspectives.* Washington, D.C.: American Psychiatric Press, 1991, pp 21–35.

Pepper LJ, Strong PN. Judgmental scales of the Mf scale of the MMPI, unpublished, 1958. Cited in Dahlstrom WG, Welsh GS, Dahlstrom LE, *The MMPI Handbook, Volume 1: Clinical Interpretation,* ed 2. Minneapolis, University of Minnesota Press, 1972.

Perley MJ, Guze SB. Hysteria—the stability and usefulness of clinical criteria: A quantitative study based on a follow-up period of six to eight years in 39 patients. *N Engl J Med* 266:421–426, 1962.

Peters CP, Schwarz T. *Tell Me Who I Am Before I Die.* New York, Rawson, 1978.

Peters CP. Critical issues in the evaluation and treatment of the borderline patient (Part I). *Psychiatr Rev* 2:1–3, 1989.

Peters CP. Critical issues in the evaluation and treatment of the borderline patient (Part II). *Psychiatr Rev* 3:1–4, 1990.

Peterson AH. *The American Focus on Satanic Crime,* Vols I and II. Millburn, N.J.: American Focus Publishing Co, 1989.

Peterson E, Gooch NL/Freeman L. *Nightmare: Uncovering the Strange 56 Personalities of Nancy Lynn Gooch.* New York, Richardson & Steirman, 1987.

Pfohl B, Coryell W, Zimmerman M, et al. DSM-III personality disorders: Diagnostic overlap and internal consistency of individual DSM-III criteria. *Compr Psychiatry* 27:21–34, 1986.

Philips DP. Natural experiments on the effects of mass media violence on fatal aggression: Strengths and weaknesses of a new approach. *Adv Exp Soc Psychol* 19:207–250, 1986.

Pitts WM, Gustin QL, Mitchell C, et al. MMPI critical item characteristics of the DSM-III borderline personality disorder. *J Nerv Ment Dis* 173:628–631, 1985.

Pope HG. Distinguishing bipolar disorder from schizophrenia in clinical practice: Guidelines and case reports. *Hosp Community Psychiatry* 34:322–328, 1983.

Pope HG, Jonas JM, Hudson JI, et al. The validity of DSM-III borderline personality disorder. *Arch Gen Psychiatry* 40:23–30, 1983.

Pope HG, Lipinski JF. Diagnosis in schizophrenia and manic-depressive illness: A reassessment of the specificity of "schizophrenic" symptoms in the light of current research. *Arch Gen Psychiatry* 35:811–828, 1978.

Prasad A. Multiple personality syndrome. *Br J Hosp Med* 34:301–303, 1985.

Pribor E, Dean JT, Yutzy SH. Personal communication, May 6, 1992.

Prince M. Some of the revelations of hypnotism. Post-hypnotic suggestion, automatic writing and double personality. *Bost Med Surg J* 122:463–467, 1890.

Prince M. Hysteria from the point of view of dissociated personality. *J Abnorm Soc Psychol* 1:170–187, 1906.

Prince M. Miss Beauchamp: The theory of the psychogenesis of multiple personality. II. "The Saint" (B-I) and "The Realist" (B-IV). *J Abnorm Psychol* 15:105–135, 1920.

Prince M. *The Dissociation of a Personality.* London, Longmans, Green, 1930.

Prince M, Peterson F. Experiments of psycho-galvanic reactions from co-conscious (sub-conscious) ideas in a case of multiple personality. *J Abnorm Psychol* 3:114–131, 1908.

Purtell JJ, Robins E, Cohen ME. Observations on clinical aspects of hysteria: A quantitative study of 50 hysteria patients and 156 controls. *JAMA* 146:902–909, 1951.

Putnam FW. The psychophysiologic investigation of multiple personality disorder. A review. *Psychiatr Clin North Am* 7:31–39, 1984.

Putnam FW. The scientific investigation of multiple personality disorder, in Quen JM (ed), *Split Minds/Split Brains: Historical and Current Perspectives.* New York, New York University Press, 1986, pp 109–125.

Putnam FW. *Diagnosis and Treatment of Multiple Personality Disorder.* New York, Guilford Press, 1989a.

Putnam FW. Pierre Janet and modern views of dissociation. *J Trauma Stress* 2:413–426, 1989b.

Putnam FW. Dissociative disorders in children and adolescents: A developmental perspective. *Psychiatr Clin North Am* 14:519–531, 1991a.

Putnam FW. Recent research on multiple personality disorder. *Psychiatr Clin North Am* 14:489–502, 1991b.

Putnam FW, Guroff JJ, Silberman EK, et al. The clinical phenomenology of multiple personality disorder: Review of 100 recent cases. *J Clin Psychiatry* 47:285–293, 1986.

Putnam FW, Loewenstein RJ, Silberman EK, et al. Multiple personality disorder in a hospital setting. *J Clin Psychiatry* 45:172–175, 1984.

Putnam FW, Post RM, Guroff JJ, et al. 100 cases of multiple personality disorder. Presented at the Annual Meeting of the American Psychiatric Association, New Research Abstract no. 77, New York, April 30–May 6, 1983.

Putnam FW, Zahn TP, Post RM. Differential autonomic nervous system activity in multiple personality disorder. *Psychol Res* 31:251–260, 1990.

Quill TE. Somatization disorder: One of medicine's blind spots. *JAMA* 254:3075–3079, 1985.

Reagor P, Ross CA, Anderson G, et al. Differentiating MPD and Dissociative Disorder Not Otherwise Specified, in Braun BG, Carlson EB (eds), *Dissociative Disorders: Proceedings of the 8th International Conference on Multiple Personality Disorder and Dissociation.* Chicago, Rush University, Dissociative Disorders Program, Department of Psychiatry, 1991, p 110.

Reich J. Multiple Personality Disorder: Diagnosis, Clinical Features, and Treatment (book review). *Am J Psychiatry* 148:1085, 1991.

Reich T, Rice J, Cloninger CR, et al. The use of multiple thresholds and segregation analysis in analyzing the phenotypic heterogeneity of multifactorial traits. *Ann Hum Genet* 42:371–390, 1979.

Resnick RJ, Goldberg SC, Schulz SC, et al. Borderline personality disorder: Replication of MMPI profiles. *J Clin Psychol* 44:354–360, 1988.

Resnick RJ, Schulz P, Schulz SC, et al. Borderline personality disorder: Symptomatology and MMPI characteristics. *J Clin Psychiatry* 44:289–292, 1983.

Rice J. Genetic epidemiology: Models of multifactorial inheritance and path analysis applied to qualitative traits, in Moolgavkar SH, Prentice PL (eds), *Modern Statistical Methods in Chronic Disease Epidemiology*. New York: John Wiley, 1986, pp 225–243.

Rice J, Reich T. Familial analysis of qualitative traits under multifactorial inheritance. *Genet Epidemiol* 2:301–315, 1985.

Rice JP, Reich T, Andreasen NC, et al. Sex related differences in depression: Familial evidence. *J Affective Disord* 7:199–210, 1984.

Richards DG. A study of the correlations between subjective psychic experiences and dissociative experiences. *Dissociation* 4:83–90, 1991.

Riley KC. Measures of dissociation. *J Nerv Ment Dis* 176:449–450, 1988.

Rivera M. Multiple personality disorder and the social systems: 185 cases. *Dissociation* 4:79–82, 1991.

Rix KJB, Pearson DJ, Bentley SJ. A psychiatric study of patients with supposed food allergy. *Br J Psychiatry* 145:121–126, 1984.

Robins E, Guze SB. Establishment of diagnostic validity in psychiatric illness: Its application to schizophrenia. *Am J Psychiatry* 126:983–987, 1970.

Robins LN. *Deviant Children Grown Up: A Sociological and Psychiatric Study of Sociopathic Personality*. Baltimore, Williams & Wilkins, 1966.

Robins LN, Helzer JE, Croughgan J, et al. National Institutes of Mental Health diagnostic interview schedule: Its history, characteristics, and validity. *Arch Gen Psychiatry* 38:381–389, 1981.

Robins LN, Helzer JE, Weissman MM, et al. Lifetime prevalence of specific psychiatric disorders in three sites. *Arch Gen Psychiatry* 41:949–958, 1984.

Robins LN, Schoenberg SP, Holmes SJ, et al. Early home environment and retrospective recall: A test of concordance between siblings with and without psychiatric disorders. *Am J Orthopsychiatry* 55:27–41, 1985.

Robins LN, Tipp J, Przybeck T. Antisocial personality, in Robins LN, Regier DA (eds), *Psychiatric Disorders in America: The Epidemiologic Catchment Area Study*. New York, Free Press, 1991, pp 258–290.

Rosenbaum M. The role of the term schizophrenia in the decline of diagnoses of multiple personality. *Arch Gen Psychiatry* 37:1383–1385, 1980.

Rosenbaum M, Weaver GM. Dissociated state. Status of a case after 38 years. *J Nerv Ment Dis* 168:597–603, 1980.

Rosenhan DL. On being sane in insane places. *Science* 179:250–258, 1973.

Ross CA. Diagnosis of multiple personality during hypnosis: A case report. *Int J Clin Exp Hypn* 32:222–235, 1984.

Ross CA. DSM-III: Problems in diagnosing partial forms of multiple personality disorder: Discussion paper. *J R Soc Med* 78:933–936, 1985.

Ross CA. Inpatient treatment of multiple personality disorder. *Can J Psychiatry* 32:779–781, 1987.

Ross CA. *Multiple Personality Disorder: Diagnosis, Clinical Features, and Treatment.* New York, Wiley, 1989.

Ross CA. Epidemiology of multiple personality disorder and dissociation. *Psychiatr Clin North Am* 14:503–517, 1991.

Ross CA, Anderson G. Phenomenological overlap of multiple personality disorder and obsessive-compulsive disorder. *J Nerv Ment Dis* 176:295–299, 1988.

Ross CA, Anderson G, Fleisher WP, et al. The frequency of multiple personality disorder among psychiatric inpatients. *Am J Psychiatry* 148:1717–1720, 1991a.

Ross CA, Anderson G, Heber S, et al. Dissociation and abuse among multiple personality patients, prostitutes, and exotic dancers. *Hosp Community Psychiatry* 41:328–330, 1990a.

Ross CA, Anderson G, Reagor P, et al. Differentiating MPD and schizophrenia, in Braun BG, Carlson EB (eds), *Dissociative Disorders: Proceedings of the 8th International Conference on Multiple Personality Disorder and Dissociation.* Chicago, Rush University, Dissociative Disorders Program, Department of Psychiatry, 1991b, p 158.

Ross CA, Heber S, Anderson G, Norton GR, Anderson BA, del Campo M, Pillay N. Differentiating multiple personality disorder and complex partial seizures. *Gen Hosp Psychiatry* 11:54–58, 1989a.

Ross CA, Heber S, Norton GR, et al. Somatic symptoms in multiple personality disorder. *Psychosomatics* 30:154–160, 1989b.

Ross CA, Heber S, Norton GR, et al. Differences between multiple personality disorder and other diagnostic groups on structured interview. *J Nerv Ment Dis* 177:487–491, 1989c.

Ross CA, Miller SD, Reagor P, et al. Schneiderian symptoms in multiple personality disorder and schizophrenia. *Comp Psychiatry* 31:111–118, 1990b.

Ross CA, Norton RG. Differences between men and women with multiple personality disorder. *Hosp Community Psychiatry* 40:186–188, 1989a.

Ross CA, Norton RG. Effects of hypnosis on the features of multiple personality disorder. *Am J Clin Hypn* 32:99–106, 1989b.

Ross CA, Miller SD, Reagor P, et al. Structured interview data on 102 cases of multiple personality from four centers. *Am J Psychiatry* 147:596–601, 1990c.

Ross CA, Norton GR, Fraser GA. Evidence against the iatrogenesis of multiple personality disorder. *Dissociation* 2:61–65, 1989d.

Ross CA, Norton GR, Wozney K. Multiple personality disorder: An analysis of 236 cases. *Can J Psychiatry* 34:413–418, 1989e.

Rush B. *Medical Inquiries and Observations Upon the Diseases of the Mind.* Philadelphia, Kimber and Richardson, 1812.

Salama AAA. Multiple personality. *Can J Psychiatry* 25:569–572, 1980.

Saltman V, Solomon RS. Incest and the multiple personality. *Psychol Rep* 50:1127–1141, 1982.

Savill TD. *Lectures on Hysteria and Allied Vasomotor Conditions.* New York, William Wood & Co, 1909.

Schreiber FR. *Sybil.* Chicago, Henry Regnery, 1973.

Schultz R, Braun BG, Kluft RP. Multiple personality disorder: Phenomenology of selected variables in comparison to major depression. *Dissociation* 2:45–51, 1989.

Schwarz DR, Frischholz EJ, Braun BG, et al. A confirmatory factor analysis of the dissociative experiences scale (DES). Paper presented to the 8th annual meeting of the International Society for the Study of Multiple Personality Disorder and Dissociation, Chicago, November 15–17, 1991.

Schwarz T. *The Hillside Strangler: A Murderer's Mind.* Garden City, N.Y., Doubleday, 1981.

Shea MT. Standardized approaches to individual psychotherapy of patients with borderline personality disorder. *Hosp Community Psychiatry* 42:1034–1038, 1991.

Silberman EK, Putnam FW, Weingartner H, et al. Dissociative states in multiple personality disorder: A quantitative study. *Psychiatr Res* 15:253–260, 1985.

Silver D. Psychodynamics and psychotherapeutic management of the self-destructive character-disordered patient. *Psychiatr Clin North Am* 8:357–377, 1985.

Silverstein ML, Harrow M. Schneiderian first-rank symptoms in schizophrenia. *Arch Gen Psychiatry* 38:288–293, 1981.

Simon GE, VonKorff M. Somatization and psychiatric disorder in the NIMH Epidemiologic Catchment Area study. *Am J Psychiatry* 188:1494–1500, 1991.

Simpson MA. Multiple personality disorder (letter). *J Nerv Ment Dis* 176:535, 1988.

Siomopoulos V. Hysterical psychosis: Psychopathological aspects. *Br J Med Psychol* 44:95–100, 1971.

Sizemore CC. *A Mind of My Own.* New York, 1989.

Sizemore CC, Pittillo ES. *I'm Eve.* Garden City, N.Y., Doubleday, 1977.

Skloot F. The night-side. *Runner's World,* December 1990, pp 70–74.

Skodol AE, Rosnick L, Kellman D, et al. Validating structured DSM-III-R personality disorder assessments with longitudinal data. *Am J Psychiatry* 145:1297–1299, 1988.

Slater E. Diagnosis of "hysteria." *Br Med J* 1:1395–1399, 1965.

Slater E, Roth M. *Mayer-Gross, Slater and Roth Clinical Psychiatry,* ed 3. London, Bailliere, Tindell & Cassell, 1969.

Slavney PR, McHugh R. The hysterical personality—an attempt at validation with the MMPI. *Arch Gen Psychiatry* 32:186–190, 1976.

Smith GR, Monson RA, Ray DC. Psychiatric consultation in somatization disorder: A randomized controlled study. *N Engl J Med* 314:1407–1413, 1986.

Smith JJ, Sager EG. Multiple personality. *J Med Soc NJ* 68:717–719, 1971.

Snyder S, Pitts WM, Goodpaster WA, et al. MMPI profile of DSM-III borderline personality disorder. *Am J Psychiatry* 139:1046–1048, 1982.

Solomon RS. Use of the MMPI with multiple personality patients. *Psychol Rep* 53:1004–1006, 1983.

Solomon RS, Solomon V. Differential diagnosis of the multiple personality. *Psychol Rep* 51:1187–1194, 1982.

Spanos NP. Hypnosis, nonvolitional responding, and multiple personality: A social psychological perspective. *Prog Exp Pers Res* 14:1–62, 1986.

Spanos NP, Weekes JR, Bertrand LD. Multiple personality: A social psychological perspective. *J Abnorm Psychol* 94:362–276, 1985.

Spanos NP, Weekes JR, Menary E, et al. Hypnotic interview and age regression procedures in the elicitation of multiple personality symptoms: A simulation study. *Psychiatry* 49:298–311, 1986.

Spencer J. *Suffer the Child.* New York: Pocket Books (a division of Simon & Schuster), 1989.

Spiegel D. Multiple personality as a post-traumatic stress disorder. *Psychiatr Clin North Am* 7:101–110, 1984.

Spiegel D. Dissociation, double binds, and posttraumatic stress in multiple personality disorder, in Braun BG (ed), *Treatment of Multiple Personality Disorder*. Washington, D.C., American Psychiatric Press, 1986, pp 61–77.

Spiegel D. The treatment accorded those who treat patients with multiple personality disorder (commentary). *J Nerve Ment Dis* 176:535–536, 1988.

Spiegel D, Cardena E. Disintegrated experience: The dissociative disorders revisited. *J Abnorm Psychol* 100:366–378, 1991.

Spiegel D, Fink R. Hysterical psychosis and hypnotizability. *Am J Psychiatry* 136:777–781, 1979.

Spitzer RL. More on pseudoscience in science and the case for psychiatric diagnosis. *Arch Gen Psychiatry* 33:459–470, 1976.

Steinberg M, Rounsaville B, Ciccheti DV. The structured clinical interview for DSM-III-R dissociative disorders: Preliminary report on a new diagnostic instrument. *Am J Psychiatry* 147:76–82, 1990.

Steinberg M, Rounsaville B, Ciccheti DV. Detection of dissociative disorders in psychiatric patients by a screening instrument and a structured diagnostic interview. *Am J Psychiatry* 148:1050–1054, 1991.

Stern CR. The etiology of multiple personalities. *Psychol Clin North Am* 7:149–159, 1984.

Stern TA. Malingering, factitious illness, and somatization, in Hyman SE (ed), *Manual of Psychiatric Emergencies*, ed 2. Toronto, Little, Brown, 1988, pp 217–225.

Stevenson RL. *Strange Case of Dr. Jekyll and Mr. Hyde*. London, Longmans, 1886.

Stoll AL, Tohen M, Baldessarini RJ. Increasing frequency of the diagnosis of obsessive-compulsive disorder. *Am J Psychiatry* 149:638–640, 1992.

Stoller RJ. *Splitting: A Case of Female Masculinity*. New York, Quadrangle, 1973.

Stone MH. The borderline syndrome: Evolution of the term, genetic aspects, and prognosis. *Am J Psychother* 31:345–365, 1977.

Sutcliffe JP, Jones J. Personal identity, multiple personality, and hypnosis. *Int J Clin Exp Hypn* 10:231–269, 1962.

Swartz M, Blazer D, George L, et al. Somatization disorder in a southern community. *Psychiatr Ann* 18:335–339, 1988.

Swartz M, Landerman R, Blazer D, et al. Somatization symptoms in the community: A rural/urban comparison. *Psychosom* 30:44–53, 1989.

Swartz M, Landerman R, George LK, et al. Somatization disorder, in Robins LN, Regier DA (eds), *Psychiatric Disorders in America: The Epidemiologic Catchment Area Study*. New York, Free Press, 1991, pp 220–257.

Taerk GS, Toner BB, Salit IE, et al. Depression in patients with neuromyasthenia (benign myalgic encephalitis). *Int J Psychiatr Med* 17:49–56, 1987.

Taylor WS, Martin MF. Multiple personality. *J Abnorm Soc Psychol* 39:281–300, 1944.

Thigpen CH, Cleckley H. A case of multiple personality. *J Abnorm Soc Psychol* 49:135–151, 1954.

Thigpen CH, Cleckley H. *The Three Faces of Eve*. New York, McGraw-Hill, 1957.

Thigpen CH, Cleckley HM. On the incidence of multiple personality disorder: A brief communication. *Int J Clin Exp Hypn* 32:63–66, 1984.

Time. Murderous personality: Was the Hillside Strangler a Jekyll and Hyde? May 7, 1979, p 26.

Tozman S, Pabis R. MPD: Further skepticism (without hostility . . . we think) (letter). *J Nerv Ment Dis* 177:708–709, 1989.

Trull TJ. Discriminant validity of the MMPI-borderline personality disorder scale. *Psychol Assess* 3:232–238, 1991.

Vaillant GE. The disadvantages of DSM-III outweigh its advantages. *Am J Psychiatry* 141:542–545, 1984.

Van der Hart O. News from the Netherlands. *ISSMPD&D News,* December 1991, p 9.

Van der Hart O, Boon S. Multiple personality disorder (letter). *Br J Psychiatry* 154:419, 1989.

Van der Hart O, Horst R. The dissociation theory of Pierre Janet. *J Trauma Stress* 2:397–412, 1989.

Van der Hart O, van der Kolk B. Hypnotizability and dissociation (letter). Am J Psychiatry 148:1105, 1991.

Varma VK, Bouri M, Wig NN. Multiple personality in India: Comparison with hysterical possession state. *Am J Psychother* 35:113–120, 1981.

Varma LP, Srivastava DK, Sahay RN. Possession syndrome. *Indian J Psychiatry* 12:58, 1970.

Veith I. *Hysteria: The History of a Disease.* Chicago, University of Chicago Press, 1965.

Velek M, Balon R. Multiple personality: Clinical syndrome of multiple etiology. *Res Staff Physician* 32:70–78, 1986.

Victor G. Sybil: Grande hysterie or folie a deux? (letter). *Am J Psychiatry* 132:202, 1975.

Völgyesi FA. *Hypnosis of Man and Animals: With Special Reference to the Development of the Brain in the Species and the Individual,* ed 2, revised in collaboration with the author by Gerhard Klumbies. MW Hamilton (trans). Baltimore: Williams & Wilkins, 1966.

Walshe F. *Diseases of the Nervous System,* ed 10. Edinburgh, Churchill Livingstone, 1963.

Ward WO, Farrelli L. *The Healing of Lia.* New York, McMillan, 1982.

Watkins JG. The Bianchi (L.A. Hillside Strangler) case: Sociopath or multiple personality? *Int J Clin Exp Hypn* 32:67–101, 1984.

Watkins JG, Johnson RJ. *We, the Divided Self.* New York, Macmillan, 1982.

Weissman MM, Bruce ML, Leaf PJ, et al. Affective disorders, in Robins LN, Regier DA (eds), *Psychiatric Disorders in America: The Epidemiologic Catchment Area Study.* New York, Free Press, 1991, pp 53–80.

Wessely S, Powell R. Fatigue syndromes: A comparison of chronic "postviral" fatigue with neuromuscular and affective disorders. *J Neurol Neurosurg Psychiatry* 52:940–948, 1989.

Westergaard C, Frischholz EJ, Braun BG, et al. The relation between the Dissociative Experiences Scale (DES) and hypnotizability. Paper presented to the 8th annual meeting of the Internation Society for the Study of Multiple Personality Disorder and Dissociation, Chicago, November 15–17, 1991.

Wetzel RD, Reich T, Murphy GE, et al. The changing relationship between age and suicide rates: Cohort effect, period effect or both? *Psychiatr Dev* 3:179–218, 1987.

Widiger TA, Frances A, Spitzer RL, et al. The DSM-III-R personality disorders: An overview. *Am J Psychiatry* 145:786–795, 1988.

Widiger TA, Rogers JH. Prevalence and comorbidity of personality disorders. *Psychiatr Ann* 19:132–136, 1989.

Widiger TA, Sanderson C, Warner L. The MMPI, prototypal typology, and borderline personality disorder. *J Pers Assess* 50:540–553, 1986.

Wilbur CB. Multiple personality and child abuse: An overview. *Psychiatr Clin North Am* 7:3–7, 1984a.

Wilbur CB. Treatment of multiple personality. *Psychiatr Ann* 14:27–31, 1984b.

Wilson A. A case of double consciousness. *J Ment Sci* 49:1640–1658, 1903).

Woerner PI, Guze SB. A family and marital study of hysteria. *Br J Psychiatry* 114:161–168, 1968.

Woodruff RA, Clayton PJ, Guze SB. Hysteria: An evaluation of specific diagnostic criteria by the study of randomly selected psychiatric clinic patients. *Br J Psychiatry* 115:1243–1248, 1969.

Woodruff RA, Clayton PJ, Guze SB. Suicide attempts and psychiatric diagnosis. *Dis Nerv Sys* 33:167–171, 1972.

Woodruff RA, Goodwin DW, Guze SB. Hysteria (Briquet's syndrome), in Roy A (ed), *Hysteria*. New York, Wiley, 1982, pp 117–129.

Yap PM. The possession syndrome: A comparison of Hong Kong and French findings. *J Ment Sci* 106:114–137, 1960.

Zahn TP. Psychophysiological approaches to psychopathology, in Coles MGH, Donchin E, Porges SW (eds), *Psychophysiology: Systems, Processes and Applications*. New York, Guilford Press, 1986, pp 508–610.

Zimmerman M, Coryell W. DSM-III personality disorder diagnoses in a nonpatient sample. *Arch Gen Psychiatry* 46:682–689, 1989.

Zoccolillo M, Cloninger CR. Excess medical care of women with somatization disorder. *South Med J* 79:532–535, 1986a.

Zoccolillo M, Cloninger CR. Somatization disorder: Psychological symptoms, social disability, and diagnosis. *Compr Psychiatry* 27:65–73, 1986b.

Author index

Adityanjee, 19, 21, 38
Aldridge-Morris, R., 11, 12, 15, 33, 37, 42, 63, 117, 122, 162, 170
Allison, R. B., 13, 18, 53, 122, 153, 177
Antens, E., 102
Armstrong, J. G., 74, 101
Armstrong, J. G., 55, 74, 106
Azam, E., 6

Bahnson, C. B., 61
Balon, R., 118, 150, 167, 189
Bechtel, S., 127, 218–21
Benner, D. G., 110
Ben-Porath, Y. S., 83, 100
Bernstein, E. M., 101
Black, D. W., 66, 169
Blatty, W. P., 117
Bleuler, E., 9, 10, 11, 119–20
Bliss, E. L., xii, 13, 16, 18, 27, 28, 29, 31, 32, 35, 44, 46–47, 48, 49, 52, 54, 65, 66, 78, 87, 95, 96, 109, 127, 165, 169, 206–08
Bliss, J., 127, 206–08
Boon, S., 108
Bowers, K. S., 6, 119, 159, 163, 171
Bowers, M. K., 65, 180
Bozzuto, J. C., 117, 122
Braun, B. G., 13, 18, 29, 44, 46–47, 49, 55, 58, 64, 65, 100, 154, 168, 176, 182, 216
Brende, J. O., 62
Breuer, J., 7, 52, 117
Briquet, P., 25, 52

Cardena, E., 100
Carlson, E. T., 102
Casey, J. F., 225–29
Castle, K., 126, 127, 218–21
Chase, T., ix, 127, 210–12
Chodoff, P., 17, 122
Clancy, T., 120
Clark, N. H., 127, 208–10
Cleckley, H. M., xi, 11, 15, 33, 60, 61, 118, 120, 127, 144, 168, 186–89, 200
Cloninger, C. R., 24, 54, 66, 164, 182

Cohen, M. E., 25
Coons, P. M., 3, 14, 15, 18, 20, 28, 32, 37, 38, 43, 44, 45, 46–47, 48, 49, 53, 55, 56, 59, 60, 62, 63, 73, 74, 78, 79, 81, 87, 88, 89, 90, 96, 98, 105, 109, 110, 134, 172, 180, 202
Coryell, W., 167
Cutler, B., 119, 158, 170, 177

Dahlstrom, W. G., 77
Dean, T., 104
Decker, H. S., 35, 116
Dell, P. F., 15, 23, 24, 57, 134
Dickes, R. A., 169
Drajier, N., 108
Dyce W., 4

Eisenhower, J. W., 15, 57
Eliot, T. S., 163
Evans, R. W., 90, 96

Fahy, T. A., 31, 117, 118, 119, 122, 167
Farber, I. E., 40
Farrelli, L., 127, 203–05
Feighner, J. P., 18, 25
Fine, R., 89, 90, 98, 172
Fleming, J. A. E., 12, 15
Fraser, G. A., 18
Fraser, S., 127, 216–18
Freeman, L., 127, 213–16
Freud, S., 5, 9, 21, 52, 116, 170

Ganaway, G. K., 21, 171, 180
Gartner, J., 79, 80, 91, 106–07
Gatfield, P. D., 176
Gilbertson, A., 103
Goettman, C., 14
Gooch, N. L., 127, 213–16
Greaves, G. B., 37
Greden, J. F., 63
Greene, R. L., 77
Griffin, R. B., 79, 88, 96, 106
Gruenewald, D., 9, 37, 159
Gunderson, J. G., 171
Gustin, Q. L., 96

Guze, S. B., 24, 25, 42, 52, 54, 59, 72, 82,
    125, 126, 132, 163, 169, 172, 176,
    177

Hacking, I., 11, 27, 35, 39, 115, 119, 121
Hawksworth, H., 127, 194–96, 200
Herzog, A., 37, 56, 62, 64
Horevitz, R. P., 46–47, 49, 55, 58, 64, 65,
    100, 168, 176, 182
Horton, P., 34
Heuman, B. A., 56

James, W., 59
Janet, P., 4, 6–11, 21, 25, 34–35, 52, 116
Jeppsen, E. A., 17, 18, 109
Johnson, R. J., 127, 205–06
Johnston, T., 20
Jones, J., 32, 34, 35, 162
Joscelyne, B., 110
Joyce, J., 116
Jung, C. G., 5

Keyes, D., 127, 198–200
King, S., 215
Kline, M. V., 20
Kline, N. A., 31
Kluft, R. P., xi, 15, 18, 20, 23, 27, 28, 30,
    31, 32, 33, 34, 38, 42, 44, 46–47, 48,
    49, 51, 55, 57, 65, 66, 67, 72, 109,
    110, 111, 115–16, 118, 122, 150,
    156, 164, 168, 173, 176, 177–79, 181
Kraepelin, E., 25
Kroll, J., 54, 96

LaCalle, T. M., 127, 212–13
Lachar, D., 77
Lancaster, E., 127, 186–89
Larmore, K, 38, 60, 61
Larson, B., 20
Larson, E. M., 54, 109
Lipton, S. D., 170
Liskow, B. I., 50, 80, 93, 97, 156, 171, 172,
    174
Loewenstein, R. R., 17, 55, 74, 101, 106,
    108
Ludolph, P. S., 32
Ludwig, A. M., 17, 38, 61, 62

Macnish, R., 117
Mai, F. M., 52
Martin, M. F., 4, 5, 11, 164
Mathew, R. J., 62

McCallum, K. E., 101, 104
McCurdy, H. A., 10
McDougall, W., 10
Merskey, D. M., 31, 52, 122
Miller, D., 34
Miller, S. D., 4, 63
Milstein, V., 45, 46–47, 49, 74
Mitchell, S. L., 4
Mitchell, S. W., 4
Moos, B., 111
Moos, R., 111
Morey, L. C., 56
Moricelli, G. E., 60
Mulhern, S., 20
Murphy, G. E., 183

Norton, G. R., 20

O'Brien, D., 135, 203
Orne, M. T., 13, 76, 134
Othmer, E., 12

Pabis, R., 32, 36, 118, 166, 167
Paracelsus, 4
Perley, M. J., 25, 52, 82, 126, 132
Peters, C. P., 127, 196–97
Peterson, A. H., 20, 60
Peterson, E., 127, 213–16
Pirandello, L., 116
Pittillo, E. S., 127, 186–89
Pitts, W. M., 79
Poling, J., 127, 186–89
Prasad, A., 31
Prevost, M., 116
Pribor, E., 101, 104
Prince, M., 6, 8, 9, 10, 52, 60, 127,
    185–86
Proust, M., 116
Purtell, J. J., 25
Putnam, F. W., 14, 15, 31, 41, 44, 46–47,
    48, 49, 56, 62, 63, 73, 115, 163, 166,
    170, 172, 178

Reagor, P., 101
Reed, J., 119, 158, 170, 177
Reich, T., 182
Resnick, R. J., 90, 96
Rice, J., 170, 172
Richards, D. G., 20
Richet, C., 116
Riley, K. C., 101, 102
Rivera, M., 2, 46–47, 49, 53

Robins, E., 24, 25, 42, 59, 125, 163, 172, 176, 177
Robins, L. N., 111
Rosenbaum, M., 170
Rosenhan, D. L., 40
Ross, C. A., xi, 7, 10, 12, 13, 17, 18, 19, 20, 21, 26, 29, 31, 37, 39, 44, 45, 46–47, 49, 50, 51, 52, 54, 55, 66, 101, 102, 107, 121, 132, 162, 164, 170, 171, 172, 181
Roth, K., 127, 208–10
Roth, M., 116
Rush, B., 4, 59

Saltman, V., 33, 59, 64, 65
Savill, T. D., 25
Schnitzler, A., 117
Schreiber, F. R., 127, 189–92
Schultz, R., 15
Schwarz, T., 102, 104, 127, 194–96, 196–97, 200–03
Shea, M. T., 182
Simpson, M. A., 33, 35, 36, 39, 45, 117, 118
Sizemore, C. C., 127, 186–89, 225
Slater, E., 116
Smith, J. J., 61
Snyder, S. 90, 96, 173
Stone, M. H., 175
Solomon, R. S., 28, 33, 59, 64, 65, 87, 178
Solomon, V., 178
Spanos, N. P., 34, 36, 37, 119, 121
Spencer, J., 127, 221–25
Spiegel, D., 37, 65, 100
Steinberg, M., 102, 107, 108

Stern, C. R., 20, 125, 180
Sterne, A. L., 73, 79, 88
Stoller, R. J., 127, 192–94
Sutcliffe, J. P., 32, 34, 35, 162
Sydenham, T., 24

Taylor, W. S., 4, 5, 11, 164
Thigpen, C. H., xii, 11, 15, 33, 60, 61, 118, 120, 127, 168, 186–89, 200
Tozman, S., 32, 36, 118, 166, 167
Trull, T. J., 96

Vaillant, G. E., 12
van der Hart, O., 178
Varma, V. K., 20
Veith, I., 5
Velek, M., 118, 150, 167, 189
Victor, G., 118

Ward, W. O., 127, 203–05
Watkins, J. G., 127, 140, 201, 205–06
Weaver, G. M., 170
Westergard, C., 104
Wetzel, R. D., 80, 82, 97
Widiger, T. A., 90, 96–97
Wilbur, C. B., 11, 27, 45, 64, 215
Wilde, O., 116
Woolf, V., 116
Wrobel,, T. A., 77

Yutzy, S., 104

Zahn, T. P., 63
Zola, E., 117

Subject index

Absorption Scale (Tellergen), 104
Adolescent and pediatric MPD, 15, 16, 56–57, 59
Allergies, 60
Alternate personalities, 144–46
  number per case, 15–16, 19, 44, 47, 144–45
American origins of MPD, 11–12
Amnesia, 28, 31, 35, 50, 52, 54
  in history of MPD, 7, 8, 14
Animal magnetism, 5
Anna O., 7
Antisocial personality disorder. *See* Personality disorder
Associationists, 3
Assortative mating, 141–42, 156–57
Autonomic nervous system activity, 60–61
Autohypnosis. *See* Self-hypnosis
Axis II diagnosis. *See* Personality disorder

Beauchamp, C., 10, 185–86
Beck Depression Inventory, 105
Behavior disorder. *See* Conduct disorder
Bianchi, K. (The Hillside Strangler), 35–36, 37, 115, 127
  summary of case vignette, 200–03
Biological psychiatry, 3, 23
Bipolar affective disorder, 18, 42
Borderline personality disorder. *See* Personality disorder
Briquet's syndrome. *See* Somatization disorder
British acceptance of MPD, 11–12

Cerebral blood flow, 61–62
Charcot, J. M., 5
Child abuse
  in association with hypnosis, 36
  in association with MPD, 31, 45, 59, 139–40, 156–57, 171–71
  in Briquet's syndrome (somatization disorder), 37, 104, 174
  in history of MPD, 9, 21
  prevalence in MPD, 47, 174

Chronic fatigue syndrome, 122–23
Clinical indicators of MPD, 28, 36
Clinical features of MPD, 44–47, 50–56
  antisocial features, 53–54
  other personality disorder features, 54–56
  post-traumatic features, 56
  psychotic features, 50–52
  somatoform features, 52–53
Cognitive testing, 73–74
Comorbidity, 48–50, 66–67, 110–12, 157–58
  in determination of disability, 45
  differentiation of MPD from comorbid disorders, 172–73
  model of conversion disorder, 169–72
  with personality disorders, 48–49, 66–67, 111
  in relation to nosology, 161, 164–66
  with somatization disorder, 48–50, 66, 111
  treatment of comorbid disorders, 178
Conduct disorder, 56–57, 138
Controversy over existence of MPD, 3, 23, 26
Conversion disorder, conversion symptoms, 52, 54
  association with MPD, 28, 31, 63
  in history of MPD, 7, 8
  prevalence in MPD, 49, 132–33
  relation to dissociation, 52, 169–70
Countertransference. *See also* Fascination, 64
Criminality. *See also* Personality disorder: antisocial; Homicide; Forensic cases

Definition of MPD, 14–15
Depression, major, 18, 59, 63, 83, 107, 171
Diagnosis of MPD, 28, 39
Diagnostic Interview Schedule (DIS), 12, 51
Diagnostic and Statistical Manual (DSM) of psychiatric disorders, 11, 14, 24–25, 131–32
Disability, 45, 66
Dissociation, dissociative disorders, 32, 37, 50, 104, 170, 177
  in history of MPD, 5–11, 14, 17, 21
  relationship to conversion, 52, 169–70

Dissociative Disorders Interview Schedule
    (DDIS), 12, 101, 107
Dissociative Experiences Scale (DES), 20,
    101–06
Duality of consciousness, 6

Eating disorders, 47, 104, 171
Electrodermal responses, 60
Electroencephalography (EEG), 60–63
Electromyography (EMG), 60–61
Epidemiologic Catchment Area study, 12, 51,
    52
Etiology, 177–78
    three-factor theory of Cutler and Reed, 177
Eve (of *The Three Faces of Eve*). *See*
    Sizemore, C.
Evoked potentials, 60–62
Exorcism, 5, 20, 181
Experiential time sampling, 108–09
Extrasensory perception. *See* parapsychology

Faking
    as etiology of MPD, 26, 39, 45, 61, 63,
        161
    in forensic cases, 36, 38,
False positive diagnosis, 12, 17, 121
Family histories, 58–59, 138–41, 156–57,
    170, 172, 175
Fascination, 33, 64, 118
Fictional accounts of MPD, 116–17
Folie a deux, 15, 35
Forensic cases, 37–38, 120–21
Freud, S., 52, 170
    in history of MPD, 5, 7, 9, 10, 21
    repression theory of, 9, 37, 170
    seduction theory of, 9, 37
Fugues, 6, 35, 52, 170
Fusion of personalities. *See* Integration of
    personalities

Galvanic skin response (GSR). *See also* Skin
    resistance, 60–62
Gender differences, 53–54
Global Assessment Scale (GAS), 100

Hallucinations, 8, 28, 31, 50–51, 132
    compared to pseudohallucinations, 51–52,
        111, 169
High functioning cases, 72, 156, 157
The Hillside Strangler. *See* Bianchi, K.
Histrionic personality disorder. *See*
    Personality disorder

Homicide, 115, 135
Hypnosis, 32
    as cause of MPD or additional
        personalities, 10, 28–29, 31, 40, 161,
        177, 179
    for diagnosis of MPD, 28, 36–37, 38
    in history of MPD, 5–6, 9–10, 20–21
    hypnotizability, 8, 28, 31, 54, 109, 170
    for treatment of MPD, 28, 32, 39, 65, 181
Hysteria. *See also* Somatization disorder
    in history of MPD, 5–8, 10–11, 19–21

Iatrogenesis. *See also* Suggestion
    as inadequate explanation for MPD, 28–29
    in etiology of MPD, 12, 17, 26, 31–37,
        39–40
    in history of MPD, 6, 9, 10
Imitation, 115–16, 118–19
Index Medicus, 11, 13
Integration of personalities, 88, 181
Intelligence tests, 73–74
    Shipley Hartford Intelligence Test, 74
    Weschler Adult Intelligence Scale (WAIS),
        73–74
    Weschler Intelligence Scale for Children,
        74
International Society for the Study of
    Multiple Personality and Dissociation
    (ISSMPD&D), 13
International trends in diagnosis of MPD, 19

Kluft, R. P.
    four-factor theory of etiology of MPD,
        111. 115–16, 177–78

Laboratory evidence; 29, 41, 59–64, 162.
    See also Physiologic differences
    between personalities

Malingering. *See* Faking
Mania. *See* Bipolar affective disorder
Mass media, 30
    as contributor to etiology of MPD, 36,
        115–24, 177
    in history of MPD, 8
    as source of public information on MPD,
        153–54, 158–59
Materialist approach, 3
Mesmerism, 5
Mind–brain controversy, 3
Minnesota Multiphasic Personality Inventory
    (MMPI), 28, 51, 56, 74–100, 174

in borderline personality disorder, 79–81, 86, 90, 93–94
in Briquet's syndrome (somatization disorder), 81, 86, 93–94
clinical scales, 81–98
  characterologic V, 88–89
  floating profiles, 86–87, 89
  Harris and Lingoes subscales, 81–84, 89
  high point codes, 86
  obvious-subtle scales, 77, 82
after fusion of personalities, 88
MMPI-2, 75
in MPD, 78–79, 81, 87–90, 93–94, 98–100
response set, 75–77, 95
schizophrenia scale, 83, 99–100
validity scales, 75–81
  CLS (carelessness) scale, 78
  critical items, 77, 89
  F scale, 76, 89
  F-K ratio, 76–77, 89
  inverted V pattern, 78
  K scale, 76
  L scale, 76
  Lachar-Wrobel critical item list, 79
  "neurotic" scales, 93
  "psychotic" scales, 93
  Q scale, 75
  TR (test-retest) scale, 78
Misdiagnosis, 17, 19, 27, 51, 142–44
Murder. *See* Homicide

Narcissistic personality disorder. *See* Personality disorder
Neurologic examination in MPD, 73
Neuropsychological functioning in MPD, 73
Nonfictional accounts of MPD, 117
Nonmaterialist approach, 3
Nosology of MPD, 161, 164–74, 178–182, 183
  "bigger syndrome" model, 168
  coordinate diagnosis, 112, 166–67
  severity marker, 168
  spectrum of disorders, 168–74, 170, 176
  subordinate diagnosis, 112
  superordinate diagnosis—symptom complex, 100, 112, 167–68, 170, 174–76, 178
  MMPI evidence, 87, 93
Not guilty by reason of insanity (MPD), 36, 120

Obsessive-compulsive disorder, 12, 17, 48, 55, 171
Occult experiences. *See* Satanic cults; Possession; Parapsychology
Organicists, 3

Paranatural experiences. *See* Parapsychology
Parapsychology, 5, 20, 21, 50, 151–52
Perceptual Alterations Scale (Sanders), 103–04
Perley-Guze criteria for Briquet's syndrome, 25, 128
Personality disorder
  antisocial, 66
    association with MPD, 134–35, 172
    overlap with MPD, 48–49, 53–54, 58, 156, 169, 172
    prevalence in MPD, 56
  borderline, 106, 107
    in nosology of MPD, 168, 170
    prevalence in MPD, 49, 54–55
    pseudopsychotic features in, 52
    overlap with MPD, 54–55, 57, 58, 66
    treatment, 181–82
  comorbidity with MPD, 49, 58, 164
  cluster B disorders, 92, 113
  histrionic, 55, 133–34
  MMPI, 79–81, 86, 90, 90–92, 93–94
  narcissistic, 55
  in nosology of MPD, 161, 171
  overlap with MPD, 54–56, 169
Personality fragment, 15
Physiologic differences between personalities, 26, 41–42, 59–64. *See also* Laboratory evidence
Politics of MPD movement, 13
Polysymptomatic, polysyndromic disorder, 48, 50, 54, 57, 98, 137
Possession by spirits or demons, 38
  in history of MPD, 3, 5, 6, 19–20, 21
Post-traumatic stress disorder (PTSD), 21, 48, 57
Prevalence of MPD
  among patients, 17
  in Briquet's syndrome, 53
  epidemic of MPD, 13–19, 36
  in general population, 12, 17, 44
  in publication rates, 13–14, 18
  in special populations, 17, 54
  with Westernization and industrialization, 19

Projective tests, 105–07, 109–13
  Rorschach, 106
Proponents of MPD, 23, 27–30, 39–42
Psychic experiences. *See* Parapsychology
Psychoanalysis, 21, 23, 39
Psychological testing. *See also* Minnesota
    Multiphasic Personality Inventory;
    Intelligence tests; Projective tests
Psychosis, psychotic symptoms, 28, 50–52
  compared to pseudopsychotic symptoms,
    51–52, 169
Putnam, F. W.
  theory of link of hypnosis to MPD, 31–32

Questionnaire of Experiences of Dissociation
    (QED), 101–04

Rape, sexual assault, 47, 137
Reinforcement of MPD symptoms, 34–37,
    65, 179
Role playing, 9, 19, 34, 36

Satanic cults, 20
  satanic ritual abuse, 20–21
Schizophrenia, 51, 58, 61, 83, 100
  confusion with MPD, 49, 119–20
  in history of MPD, 9, 11, 17
Schneiderian symptoms. *See* Psychosis
Secondary gain, 17, 33, 37–39, 118–19
Self mutilation, 54–55, 136–37
Self-hypnosis, 31–32, 54, 95, 161, 169, 177
Sexual history, 133
Simulation studies, 29, 36, 40, 62–63, 103–
    04
Sizemore, C. ("Eve", of *The Three Faces of
    Eve*), 36, 127, 150–51, 152, 153
  in history of MPD, 11
  as source of media information, 50, 115,
    117–18, 122, 150–51, 153–54
  summary of case vignette, 186–89
Skepticism, 15
  in Briquet's syndrome (somatization
    disorder), 12
  on existence of MPD, 18, 23, 26, 30–42,
    134
  extreme, 23–24
Skin resistance, skin conductance, 60–62
Social psychological theory of MPD of
    Spanos, 34
Sociopathy. *See* Antisocial personality
    disorder
Somatization disorder, 59, 63, 66, 104–05,
    113, 128

association with MPD, 16, 107, 130, 156,
    165
characteristics of, 12, 24–26, 32, 51–52
exclusion from MPD, 15, 112, 168, 172–
    76
in history of MPD, 7, 8
hypnotizability in, 54
nosologic relationship to MPD, 168
polysomatoform symptoms in, 28, 52, 58
pseudopsychotic features in, 52
similarities to MPD, 48–50, 52, 178
  in assortative mating, 142
  in comorbidity, 171–72
  in hypnotizability, 169
  in treatment, 149, 178
treatment of, 65–66, 179
Spiritualism, 5
Stanford Hypnotic Susceptibility Scale, 109
Structured Clinical Interview for DSM-III-R
    Dissociative Disorders (SCID-D),
    101–02, 107–08
Substance abuse, 18, 57, 65
  association with MPD, 16, 28, 38, 156,
    171
  family history of, 59, 173
  prevalence in MPD, 47–48, 130
Subtypes of MPD, 30
Suggestion. *See also* Iatrogenesis
  as inadequate explanation of MPD, 40, 45
  in etiology of MPD, 9–10, 26, 34, 159, 161
Suicide, 18, 115
  suicidal behavior, 28, 45, 47, 137, 169
Supernatural experiences. *See*
    Parapsychology
Sybil, 117–18, 127
  link with child abuse, 21
  as source of media information, 45, 50,
    122 150–51, 154
  summary of case vignette, 189–92

Transference, 10, 64, 148–49
Treatment, 45, 64–67, 146–48, 178–182
  excessive, 147–48
  outcome, 64–67, 100, 149–50, 174–76,
    178, 182

Validity of a diagnosis, 180
  Feighner criteria, 24
  five-phase procedure of Robins and Guze
    and colleagues, 24, 40–42, 59, 72,
    125
  of MPD, 21, 39, 162–63, 183
  of somatization disorder, 24–26